Caring for Older Adults Holistically

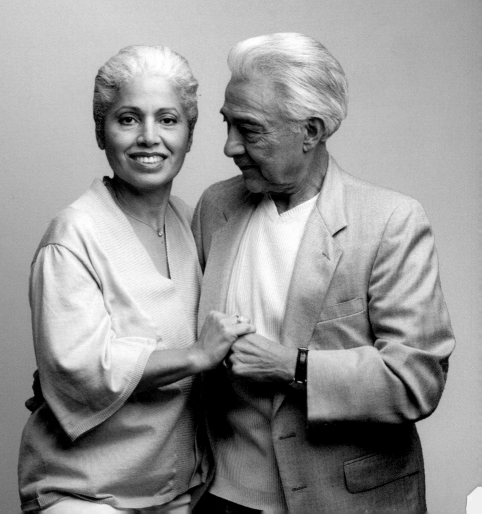

Davis*Plus*...

Online Resource Center

Davis*Plus* is your online source for a wealth of learning resources and teaching tools, as well as electronic and mobile versions of our products.

STUDENTS

Unlimited FREE access.
No password.
No registration.
No fee.

INSTRUCTORS

Upon Adoption.
Password-protected library of title-specific, online course content.

Visit http://davisplus.fadavis.com

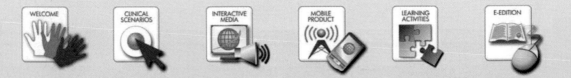

Explore more online resources from F.A. Davis...

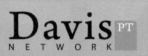
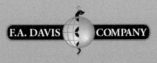
F.A. DAVIS COMPANY

www.fadavis.com

FIFTH EDITION

Caring for Older Adults Holistically

Mary Ann Anderson, PhD, APRN, BC
Fellow, National Gerontological Nursing Association
Retired
Sunset, Utah

F.A. Davis Company • Philadelphia

F. A. Davis Company
1915 Arch Street
Philadelphia, PA 19103
www.fadavis.com

Copyright © 2011 by F. A. Davis Company

Printed in the United States of America

Last digit indicates print number: 10 9 8 7 6 5 4 3 2 1

Acquisitions Editor: Lisa B. Deitch
Developmental Editor: Kimberly DePaul Mackey
Director of Content Development: Darlene Pedersen
Project Editor: Tyler Baber, Elizabeth Hart
Illustration and Design Manager: Carolyn O'Brien

As new scientific information becomes available through basic and clinical research, recommended treatments and drug therapies undergo changes. The author(s) and publisher have done everything possible to make this book accurate, up to date, and in accord with accepted standards at the time of publication. The author(s), editors, and publisher are not responsible for errors or omissions or for consequences from application of the book, and make no warranty, expressed or implied, in regard to the contents of the book. Any practice described in this book should be applied by the reader in accordance with professional standards of care used in regard to the unique circumstances that may apply in each situation. The reader is advised always to check product information (package inserts) for changes and new information regarding dose and contraindications before administering any drug. Caution is especially urged when using new or infrequently ordered drugs.

Library of Congress Cataloging-in-Publication Data

Caring for older adults holistically / [edited by] Mary Ann Anderson. — 5th ed.
       p. ; cm.
 Includes bibliographical references and index.
 ISBN-13: 978-0-8036-2500-6
 ISBN-10: 0-8036-2500-6
1. Geriatric nursing. 2. Holistic nursing. I. Anderson, Mary Ann, 1946-
 [DNLM: 1. Geriatric Nursing—methods. 2. Aging—physiology. 3. Geriatric Assessment—methods.
4. Holistic Nursing—methods. WY 152]
 RC954.A53 2011
 618.97'0231—dc22

                                                                                      2010047350

I have been very ill since the first of the year with cancer. I have had surgery, chemotherapy, and radiation, along with their accompanying side effects. I finished radiation therapy 3 weeks ago, and I am finally feeling better! It has been a long, but meaningful 8 months.

I have been delighted to be given care from many nurses who were formerly my students. What a pleasant experience to be greeted by someone who knows me and, in addition, is skilled and caring. There have been former students at every place I have gone for treatment. I am proud of them.

I am dedicating this book to my former students and, in a more personal way, dedicating it to those to whom I am closest. My dear friend, Karen Swank, who took me to up to five appointments a week. At each appointment, she has lifted my scooter chair out of the trunk of the car and then returned it when we were through. She brought her special brand of humor with her each day and has made me laugh! She has sat by my side for hours when I was so weak and unable to care for myself. She has been my beacon with her daily visits and caring personae.

My daughter Emily who has been my "True North." I have only one child and she is practically perfect! She travelled from Colorado to Utah, with her precious children, each time I was admitted to the hospital. At 8:00 every morning we were on the phone sharing the joys and sorrows of each day. Then she often called in the afternoon to see how I was doing. She taught her 5-year-old daughter, Kedzie, how to dial "* 3" so she could call grandma. We often are on the phone two to three times a day! What a joy. Kedzie's brothers, Ethan and Alex, also would talk to me on the phone, draw pictures and send them to me, and play with/for me on I-Cam visits.

I have five sisters and each one was both thoughtful and helpful. They are Lola, Linda, Merle, Vickie, and Iva. They took turns taking me to chemotherapy, called me, visited me, brought really good food, and one sister sent me a Get Well card every week.

My dear loved ones, this book is dedicated to you.
Thank you for being such caring people.

I want you, the reader, to know that I am in remission. I am slowly recovering from the treatments I have had, and life is good. In 3 weeks I am taking the grandchildren and their parents to Orlando for a week. In January, Karen and I are going on a Hawaiian cruise for my 65th birthday.

I am actually grateful for these past 8 months because I have learned and experienced many, many positive things. In addition, it has been wonderful to be supported by those I love.

All is well with me, and I wish each of you the very best life has to give.

Preface

I am amazed that this book has reached its fifth edition. The adventure has been tracking the progress of gerontological nursing throughout the years I have been writing and adding to it.

The book is a postmodern book, with content designed to assist students to enter the postmodern era of nursing. Students will study Dr. Jean Watson's Theory of Human Caring, Maslow's Hierarchy of Needs, and other current or well-established theories that will enhance their practice. Unique to this book are chapters on Gerotranscendence, transitions and caring theories designed for gerontological practice.

The foundation of this book is that of critical thinking. It is full of compelling questions that illustrate what it is to be a nurse. The critical thinking assignments draw the reader into the realm of wondering, "what if . . . ?" rather than thinking "this is . . ." It is designed to be reader friendly in that it conveys a feeling of conversation with a group of wise nurses who care deeply about nursing and its participants. This book also conveys a deep respect for every person who provides the most valuable kind of care, that art of caring for those who have gone before us and made the world a better place because of their effort; the elderly.

There is ample opportunity for students to use the computer with games, tests, and other interactive media to enhance their learning. For the faculty person there are tests and case studies at the end of each chapter and PowerPoint presentations, and a well-developed test bank. Each chapter has a presentation on what should be the priority focus of the chapter and assignments that can be done in or out of class, if the teacher chooses to use them. There also is a Focused Learning Chart in each chapter that brings the attention of the student to one critical aspect of the chapter.

Registered nurses, who maintain a clinical practice and value the role of the licensed practical nurse (LPN), wrote this book. The purpose of this book is to assist the future nurse to give informed and holistic care to the growing population of elderly persons who have the courage to live rather than die.

Contributors

Vickie Anderson, RN, CIC
Infection Control Coordinator
Intermountain Health Care
Salt Lake City, Utah

Tamara Chase, MSN, RN
Associate Professor
Weber State University
Ogden, Utah

Kathleen R. Culliton, APRN, MS, GNP
Associate Professor
Weber State University
Ogden, Utah

Judith Pratt, MSN, RN
Associate Professor
Weber State University
Ogden, Utah

Emily Ravsten, MSW
Thornton, Colorado

Alicebelle Maxson Rubotzky, RN, PhD
Associate Professor
Department of Nursing
Rhode Island College
Providence, Rhode Island

Reviewers

Holli Benge, MSN, RN
Coordinator
Professor
Tyler Junior College
Tyler, Texas

Belinda Douglas, GNP
Director of Nursing
Tennessee Technology Center
Ripley, Tennessee

Tammy Keith, RN, MS
Professor
Hocking College School of Nursing
Nelsonville, Ohio

Carmela Theresa de Leon, RN, BSN, MAN, PhD(c)
Collaborative Care RN
Didactic Faculty Member
Banner Gateway Medical Center
PIMA Medical Institute
Mesa, Arizona

Acknowledgments

As always, this book has been an adventure. Just when I think there is no more information to add to it, I find there is something new out there. That is an important truth regarding the aging process. There is always something new and dynamic to learn and add to one's practice.

I wish to acknowledge F. A. Davis editors Lisa Dietch, Tyler Baber, and Kim DePaul for their ever present and pleasant assistance. I also am giving recognition to the elderly persons who have had the courage to continue living, thereby, allowing us to assist and support them as professional nurses.

Most importantly, I want to recognize the gerontological nurses, in professional practice, who exhibit their caring skills to those who have grown older. The job you do is challenging and requires your very best. Thank you for being willing to do it!

Table of Contents

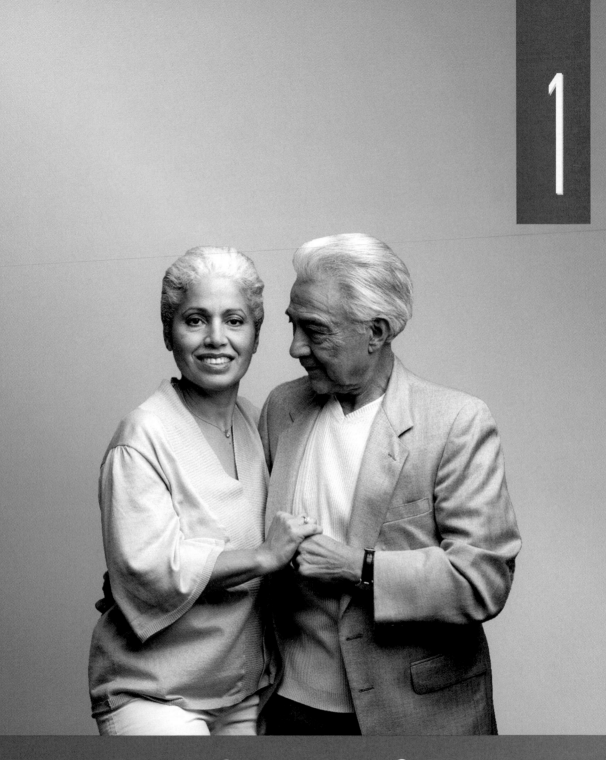

Foundations of Care
for the Older Adult

1

1 Holistic Caring

Mary Ann Anderson

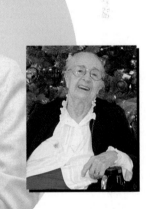

Learning Objectives

After completing this chapter, the student will be able to:

1. Define gerontological nursing.
2. Discuss the current demographics of people older than age 65 years.
3. Write a one-sentence nursing philosophy.
4. Define the word *holism* as it relates to gerontological nursing.
5. Discuss the theory "The Science of Human Caring" by Dr. Jean Watson as it relates to clinical practice.
6. Describe five examples of how you, as a novice nurse, can use Watson's theory as you give nursing care to older adults.
7. Define the concept of "gerotranscendence."

Welcome to gerontology! This is where you will learn information and skills that will assist you in being successful in all areas of nursing. "How can one class touch all segments of health care?" you may ask. "How" is by the simple growing number of persons older than age 65 who are living instead of dying. Caring for them is what gerontology is by definition. The growing number of older adults in the United States need, and will continue to need, health care because of the normal consequences of aging as well as the acute and chronic diseases that occur in all age groups. Older adults connect with all age groups, and because of their increasing numbers, we as nurses will be seeing them in more roles than ever before in our history.

GERONTOLOGICAL NURSING

It is important to understand the vocabulary that goes with the speciality of gerontological nursing. The word *gerontological* comes from the Greek words *gero,* meaning "related to old age," and *ology,* meaning "the study of." The word *gerontology* refers to the study of the complex world of human aging. It includes physical, emotional, social, spiritual, and economic considerations. It is an aspect of nursing that impacts all areas of society, including health care resources, politics, housing, education, business, and law making. Another commonly used word is *geriatrics.* The Greek word *geras* means "old age," and the word *iatro* means "relating to medical treatment." The word *geriatrics* refers to the medical speciality that deals with the diagnosis and treatment of elderly adults. The word *geriatrics* is very specific; it refers to medical treatment only. *Gerontology* covers several aspects of need for older adults. This definition is appropriate because of the holistic nature of nursing practice.

If you are a gerontological nurse, you are guaranteed a future in nursing because older adults are the fastest growing segment of the population in the United States. There are elderly people in home health settings, hospitals, homeless shelters, assisted living centers, and nursing homes. People older than age 65 occupy approximately 65% of the beds in acute hospital settings. They also are more frequently present in pediatric and neonatal intensive care units as the grandparents of crack-addicted or AIDS-infected babies whose parents are unable or

▲ PRIORITY SETTING 1.1

As you enter your new profession of licensed practical/vocational nursing, you will be expected to determine priorities that relate to the person receiving care, the environment, and the health-care team, among other things. In each chapter of this book, there will be a box titled "Priority Setting." It will focus on your development as a professional and the management of the priorities of care for the elderly people for whom you are responsible as a nurse. Setting priorities is a challenge. When you are licensed as a practical nurse, you will realize that others expect you to identify and meet the demands of patient-care priorities.

Thoughtfully read the Priority Setting boxes and work to incorporate the priorities identified into your nursing practice. Some may seem simple; others may seem a bit daunting. I want to assure you, though, that all of them are important in your role as an LPN.

Here is your first Priority Setting challenge.

The priority for this chapter is to incorporate within yourself holistic caring because this puts you on the cutting edge of health-care delivery and transforms you into a professional nurse.

As a nurse in the 21st century, you are expected to practice the skills of this profession on the cutting edge. Holistic approaches to care that are guided by what the literature refers to as a *caring ontology* (caring philosophy) are on that cutting edge. Historically, nurses have been very task-oriented. Such nurses carried the notorious list I referred to in the chapter. When everything was checked off the list, the nurse considered his or her work completed. There is more expected in this era of nursing. Everything on the list has to be done, as "the list" contains the critical interventions that will improve the health of the person receiving care—yet it needs to be done within the framework of holistic caring.

You will need to reread this chapter if you finish it and are unsure what the characteristics of holistic caring are.

◢ PRIORITY SETTING 1.1 — cont'd

Why? Because you need to start now and work to incorporate them into your philosophy of nursing and daily practice.

- You must learn to listen to people both verbally and nonverbally.
- You probably need to slow down. Don't rush people or even seem to be in a hurry when with a patient or family. This is especially true of older adults, who may need to do things more slowly because of the process of aging.
- Consider family members and significant others as critical to the care you administer. They need to be involved with every stage of treatment and are a valuable source of information.
- Give your *full* attention to the individual to whom you are giving care at the moment. Consider that person's feelings, personal needs, and strong individuality while you are with him or her. Learn from the individual as you teach him or her, and respect the person for the life that he or she has lived.

These are some of the components of transpersonal caring. Learn to live this concept as you practice your art of nursing.

unwilling to care for their ill children. You will be relating to and caring for older people throughout your career wherever you work.

Gerontology is a relatively new nursing specialty and has within it certified nurses, clinical specialists, and geriatric nurse practitioners who give care only to people older than age 65 years. There are nurses in the specialty who have a great deal of experience and novice (or new) nurses just like you. Together, all of us, experienced and novice nurses, make a valuable team for the frail and vulnerable older adults in need of nursing care and for the well elderly persons who are focused on health promotion. Gerontological nursing is exciting and varied, and I compliment you for being interested in this area of health care.

Early in my more than 40 years of experience as a registered nurse, I chose to be a gerontological nurse. I made this choice at a time when gerontological nurses were thought to be lesser skilled nurses. "If they were any good, they would be working in the intensive care units (ICUs), wouldn't they?" was a common comment. Fortunately, things have changed.

Gerontological nurses have a specific body of knowledge that they must master (similar to the ICU nurse) to be effective in their practice. For example, did you know that most elderly persons who have heart attacks do not have chest pain? In addition, medication doses for a middle-aged person may overwhelm the systems of an elderly person with devastating results. Aging brings with it stages of life development that are different from any previous stage; gerontological nurses need to know and understand these stages. The knowledge required to give gerontological care needs to be learned, understood, and implemented for the elders in this society to have the best quality of life possible.

In the current health-care environment, people respect gerontological nurses for their multiple skills and abilities. If they don't, those persons may be ageists, or prejudiced against older adults. Ageism has long been a social construct of the United States and is something every gerontological nurse should be willing to work toward eliminating. Who but a nursing-home nurse can pass medications to 42 residents twice in one shift without making a mistake?

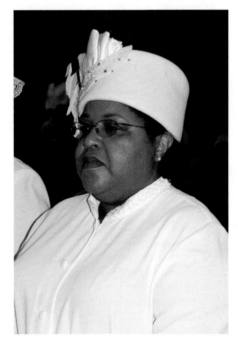

This elegant woman represents the growing number of older women in the United States who are living longer than older men.

Who has the skill and knowledge to calm a pacing, agitated older person with dementia by using validation therapy, a communication technique specifically for demented elderly persons? I am proud to be a gerontological nurse and willingly talk to others about how wonderful my career has been because of that choice made long ago to work with older adults.

⬤ DEMOGRAPHICS OF AGING

Old age is new. I find that simple statement to be true because of my age. I actually feel the consequences of aging. I am sure many of you reading this book do not notice from week to week or month to month that you are aging. I am 64 years old, have some chronic diseases, and feel them. Growing older is new for every person who experiences it, and it is new for our society as well. In the history of the United States, there never have been so many people older than age 65. The composition of the American population is different today from that of any previous generation.

The numbers of old people previously were small compared with the number of older adults who are age 65 and older today. In the 2002 U.S. census, there were 35.6 million older adults, and they constituted 12.3% of the population. It is predicted that 17% of the population will be age 65 and older by 2020. One in eight Americans was older than age 65 years in 2002. There were 20.8 million women older than age 65 but only 14.8 million men. The U.S. Census Bureau (2008) also projects that the number of people who are 85 years and older will increase from 4.6 million to 9.6 million by 2030.

What is the makeup of this growing number of older adults? The increase in number is attributed to the group referred to as the "baby boomers," who are people born between 1946 and 1965 after World War II. Baby boomers constitute 30% of the U.S. population. By 2011, they will begin to turn 65 and will qualify for Social Security and Medicare. This places federal financial concerns over paying for baby boomer retirement at the forefront.

⬤ POINT OF INTEREST

The increased numbers of elderly people in the United States have resulted in new definitions of aging. The term *young-old* is used for people 65 to 74 years old; *middle-old* is used for people 75 to 84 years old; *old-old* is used for people 85 to 100 years old; and *elite-old* is used for people older than 100 years. It is necessary to define the differences for each age group because of the health needs, medication dosages, and frailty that relate specifically to each age category.

Compare the previous numbers with the fact that, in 1776, when the Declaration of Independence was signed, a child born in the United States had a life expectancy of 35 years. In 1930, life expectancy was 59.7 years; in 1965, it was 70.2 years. Today, the average life expectancy is 79 years for women and 72.9 years for men (U.S. Census Bureau, 2008). When an older adult reaches age 65, that person can expect another 18.1 years, or to reach 82.9 years of age.

⬤ POINT OF INTEREST

The Bureau of National Health Statistics (2008) lists the following 10 diseases as the leading chronic diseases affecting people older than age 65 years:

1. Arthritis
2. Hypertension
3. Problems hearing
4. Heart conditions
5. Visual impairment
6. Deformities or orthopedic disability
7. Diabetes
8. Chronic sinusitis
9. Hay fever and allergic rhinitis
10. Varicose veins

Besides the sheer number of the aging baby boomers, other reasons for the increased number of older persons in our society include better nutrition, sanitation, and overall living conditions; lower infant mortality rates; and more effective medical management of acute and chronic diseases. There are specific trends, however, related to gender and race. Because more women reach 65 years of age than men, there are more older women than men in the older-than-85 category. This also means there are more single older women than single older men. The U.S. Department of Commerce (2010) states that there are fewer than 7 men to 10 women in the older-than-65 age group. The current trends show, however, that the ratio of men to women is slowly increasing. Unfortunately, even with the increase in life expectancy, it varies by race. Since the 1980s to the present, the gap in life expectancy between white and black elders has widened because the elderly black population has declined. This decline is attributed to death by homicide and AIDS (Eliopolous, 2010).

Older adults today have more education and financial resources than ever before in U.S. history. Because they initiated the fitness movement, they are more likely to have regular exercise programs. They also have fewer children to assist in their care.

Less than 5% of older adults live in nursing homes, assisted living centers, and other institutions. That leaves 95% living in homes either alone or with their aging spouses or family members.

NURSING PHILOSOPHY

I love working with older adults because doing so allows me to practice within the framework of my nursing philosophy. I was educated at a Catholic school of nursing and was taught to "Serve the Sick as Though They Were Christ in Person." I

CRITICALLY EXAMINE THE FOLLOWING

Think about the elderly people (older than age 65) in your family or among your other acquaintances. Identify three people and think about them. Use their name for the heading and list the characteristics of older people, just discussed, that apply to them. What are their race, gender, age, living conditions, general health, source of income, and other factors that contribute to their quality or lack of quality of life? The purpose of this exercise is to assist you in really seeing older adults. If you don't know the answers, go visit the people you chose and ask them just what it is like to be 65+ in the 21st century.

Geographically, older adults live in a variety of places. My home state of Utah, along with Alaska and Georgia, has the lowest percentage of older adults in the United States. The state with the highest percentage is Florida, followed by Pennsylvania, West Virginia, and North Dakota. In the past 10 years, Hawaii, Alaska, Nevada, and Arizona have had dramatic growth rates of older adults.

Understanding the diversity and uniqueness of older adults is important to giving them excellent health care. One professional aspect of yourself that will assist you in meeting the objective of excellence is a nursing philosophy.

embraced that philosophy and still practice it today. When I care for elderly persons in all settings, I am able to give them excellent physical and emotional care as well as to be caring. When I add holism to my caring approach, I have a successful format for delivering quality nursing care within the framework of my nursing philosophy. This book is based on the two concepts of holism and caring, and the purpose of this chapter is to share these critical concepts with you.

POINT OF INTEREST

Important definitions follow:

1. **Medicare:** Federal regulations that provide health care for individuals older than age 65 or who are permanently disabled.
2. **Medicaid:** State-supported health care for individuals who are financially disadvantaged.
3. **Social Security:** Federal benefit check paid to retired workers of a specific age, disabled workers of any age, and spouses and minor children of deceased workers.
4. **Supplemental Social Security (SSI):** Federal benefit check paid to persons older than age 65 or with disabilities that do not allow employment.

Have you considered what your nursing philosophy might be? As a beginning nurse, you may not know what a nursing philosophy is, let alone have defined one for yourself. This is a personal concept that has to come from within you. At this point in your career, you may find a philosophical statement that you like, and as you obtain more education and clinical experience, it is something you may change.

I have shared my philosophy with you. It is (1) simple and (2) specific and (3) has great meaning for me. These are three characteristics of a valuable nursing philosophy. Let me repeat it: "To serve the sick as though they were Christ in person." Obviously, I am a Christian; this philosophy would not work for someone of a different religion. I suggest you develop your own nursing philosophy to use as a guide and measurement for the work you do in nursing.

Holistic Nursing

The word *holism* or *wholism* is derived from the Anglo-Saxon root *hal,* which means "whole" or "to heal" (Random House College Dictionary, 2008). Its very definition makes the word and its concepts important to the profession of nursing. Holistic care refers to care of the body, mind, socialization, and spirit of the person for whom you are responsible. Holistic care occurs when you, the caregiver, make healing the whole person (all of the person's "parts") your priority. It goes beyond healing a surgical incision and includes all aspects of the individual that need attention so there is a wholeness of the person.

When you examine the career of Florence Nightingale in your nursing history class, it will be apparent to you that she was able to integrate holistic concepts into her personal nursing practice. She considered touch, light, empathetic listening, music, and quiet reflection essential components of good nursing care (Dossey et al, 2005). If she were not holistic, she would have considered just the soldier's wound and nothing else. You will learn that Nightingale is known as the "Lady with the Lamp." This is because when the other nurses had gone to bed, she would walk through the wards at Scutari with her lamp to check on the wounded; she wrote letters for them; and she spent her own money to buy them fruit and vegetables so they would have better nutrition. These are examples of holistic care.

Holistic nursing is something Florence Nightingale practiced without a textbook or a teacher to explain it to her. How did she, the Mother of Modern Nursing, capture the essence

CRITICALLY EXAMINE THE FOLLOWING

Ponder the idea of having a nursing philosophy to guide your clinical practice. Remember that it will change as you learn and grow in the profession. It could simply be:

1. Be kind and thorough in the care I give.
2. Always practice high-level physical and emotional care.

I am hopeful that by the end of this book or even this chapter, you will be able to say something like the following:

3. Practice holistic nursing based on the philosophy of caring.

Write a one- or two-sentence personal nursing philosophy and put it somewhere where you will find it again. It will be interesting to read it at the end of this class or at the end of your licensed practical nurse (LPN) education. Your instructor may want to have you share your philosophy in class.

of holism with her patients in Scutari? More importantly, how do we, as modern nurses, accomplish that vision today?

Basic Concepts of Holistic Care

According to modern writers (Savage & Money, 2005), understanding the concepts of holistic nursing is important for the practice of 21st-century nursing. It is a philosophy that weaves the demanding technical skills of nursing with the social science skills that enhance the humanity of the nurse and the person receiving care.

The philosophy of holism, which was first formulated in the 1930s, emphasizes the importance of understanding a person's whole being rather than treating only specific parts. When a patient is recovering from a total hip replacement, the patient definitely wants the hip fixed and fixed properly! There may be other needs, however, such as loneliness, fear about being able to live alone again, or a misunderstanding about medications. The person needs more than treatment for the hip.

The philosophy of holistic care should put an end to comments such as "the gallbladder down the hall," which ignores the person and focuses on the illness alone. A holistic identification of the "gallbladder down the hall" should be the person's name or something pleasantly descriptive, such as "the grandmother who knits all of the time."

Components of holistic nursing

Holistic nursing is based on the importance of understanding the whole person rather than treating parts of the person (IVs, wounds, oxygen).

Develop a Healing Relationship	Work with a Team	Excellent Clinical Skills
Unrushed time	Family, friends, and pets	Holistic communication
Truly listen	IDT	Medication administration
Determine what has worked in the past and discuss options	Other specialists	Assessment
		Bedside skills
		Management skills

If you are a holistic nurse, you will take an active role in developing a healing relationship with the patient. This relationship focuses on the multiple needs of persons who are ill and how they can best be resolved. The critical activity to promote holistic care is listening. This approach encourages people who are sick to be more involved in their care. The nurse should listen to what has worked in the past for patients and discuss their ideas as to what would be best for them in the current situation. The nurse needs to provide an environment in which the patient is able to make decisions that are honored by the health-care team.

Holistic nursing practice can be implemented in many ways. Following are four basic concepts:

Rule #1: Always follow the physician's orders. If the patient refuses the treatment or medication ordered, call the physician. That is an excellent way to validate that you are listening to the patient. Be sure to share the patient's concerns with the physician.

Rule #2: You will develop clinical expertise; use it.

Rule #3: Draw on the personal intuition and creativity patients have to resolve their own health problems. You will need to consider the patients' values and life experiences when devising treatments. Remember, all of the older adults you will be giving care to are the survivors; they are the people who did not die, and they are strong and smart and have lived with their body long enough to know what it needs. Can you imagine telling a man who endured imprisonment and torture as a prisoner of war how to manage his postoperative pain? I wouldn't do it. Instead, I would listen to what he had to say about it.

Rule #4: Take every opportunity to develop a closer relationship with family members or significant others. This is your true entry into getting support and assistance for the older person who is ill. You also will learn many things about the patient in your care.

Holistic Care Is Based on Teamwork

The holistic approach to nursing is effective when dealing with most populations, and it is an excellent way to deliver care to older adults. One of the principles of holistic care is that neither you nor the older person is alone. There always is a team of people working for the best outcome for the person needing care.

These teams look very different for each person. Most holistic teams have family members, although that is not always true. Some have a treasured family pet—a very valuable member. Others have an entire health-care team, such as an older adult in a nursing home who has the advantage of an interdisciplinary team. This is a team of professionals, such as a dietitian, physical therapist, nurse, pharmacist, social worker, and others, who work toward the best condition for the resident. They meet at least monthly to discuss each resident, and the resident and family members are invited to attend this meeting.

The premise is that you, the nurse, will work closely with the team members who are most important to the older adult. The focus of the teamwork should be to provide care, health promotion, and, if possible, cure. This means that you will advocate for the 15-year companion, Suzie the dog, to make regular visits to the nursing home. If you have a home health patient who needs assistance with getting into bed at night, you need to work to make arrangements with family, neighbors, or friends for the necessary assistance. If the person to whom you give care has six adult children and you get calls from each one each week, you need to be grateful that there are children who are willing to be involved.

A holistic nurse does not wait for the varied team members to come to the nurse. Instead, it is essential to be on the lookout for any sign or mention of the people who will make a difference in the life of the older person. I remember a blind woman who was brought to the hospital for terminal care. She was brought in an ambulance, and consequently none of her personal things accompanied her. She had no children, and her spouse was deceased, but she did have a dear older friend and neighbor. One morning I entered this woman's room and found her crying. With a bit of encouragement, she told me that she missed having her pictures with her. She had several treasured photos of herself and her husband, and she liked to hold them and think about the wonderful life she and her husband had shared. She was blind, right? But she still wanted those pictures! I located her neighbor, who brought her pictures to the hospital. I know that being able to hold her pictures assisted this woman in having a better quality of life before her death. It simply made her happier.

Some nurses would dismiss the need to be concerned about pictures for a blind woman, and others would not take the time to locate her friend. A holistic nurse would do both things because of the reality of caring about *every* aspect of *every* person in his or her care. Holistic care is a powerful concept and works best when complemented by the nursing theory of human caring.

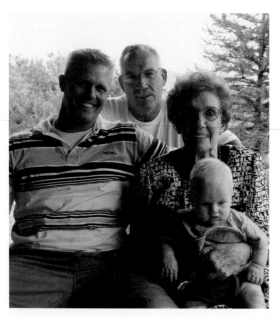

This elderly woman fell and broke her hip 10 days after this picture was taken. Her son and grandson were instrumental in her recovery. Her great-grandson brought her great joy when his parents brought him to see her at the hospital and nursing home.

⬤ HUMAN CARING

The Science of Human Caring is a nursing philosophy that was developed by Dr. Jean Watson, former Dean and Distinguished Professor at the School of Nursing, University of Colorado. Dr. Watson's theory is taught worldwide and serves as the basis of teaching and caregiving for many of the world's nurses. Watson (2000) proclaims that a theory assists us, as nurses, to "see" what it is we do more clearly. It is her hope that the individuals studying and using her theory of nursing will see the world of health care in a "new and different lens." She wants us to be open to new ideas that are based on caring, and she wants us to put them into our practice as nurses.

Watson (2000) focuses on looking at the person to whom a nurse gives care as a whole human being, with attention needed for the body, mind, and spirit. This theory calls on you, as a nurse-to-be, to use your imagination and creativity to solve problems in ways that are personal for the people to whom you give care.

When you base your nursing care on the foundation of caring, you will:

1. View all humans as valued persons to be cared for, understood, nurtured, and assisted.
   Scenario:
   You are working in a nursing home that takes care of a variety of older adults. After a thorough orientation to the facility, which includes their philosophy of human caring, you are assigned to work on the admissions unit. This is where all new admissions go for the first 3 days to evaluate where they should be placed to receive care specifically suited for their physical and emotional needs.

   The police bring in a 76-year-old intoxicated man to be admitted. The police tell you he is homeless and an alcoholic. He is dirty, smelly, and uncooperative. His hair is matted, and his beard is overgrown and crusted with food. He has been incontinent, his eyes are bloodshot, and he is drooling. The police remove his handcuffs and quickly leave the area.

   Your faculty person may want to discuss the following questions in class. I have listed some brief comments to start the group interaction. Please think about this situation and prepare more detailed answers to the questions.
   Questions:

1. "What is the reaction many people would have about being assigned to admit this man?"
   • Fear, disgust, negativism, anger.
2. "What is your reaction as an employee who is practicing 'The Science of Human Caring'?"
   • Look beyond the physical problems and into the mind and spirit of the man. This is done by understanding, by nurturing, and by assisting this human in need.
   • Place an emphasis on the human relationship and the relationship the person has with the environment.

3. "How can you put the relationship you have with this man as the highest priority?"
   Be gentle and quiet. Use his name (i.e., Mr. Lango, not Fred). Reach out and touch him if possible; make eye contact. There are many more things you can do. Think about the possibilities and be prepared to discuss them. Remember to use your imagination and creativity.
4. "What can you do to make the environment more conducive to the needs of this person?" Like you, the environment should be quiet, with minimal stimuli. Do not allow a group of people into the room. You may want one more person because Mr. Lango is drunk, but more than that will be upsetting and perhaps fearful for him. Do not rush him. Be prepared for him to be upset. Use patience.
5. "The Science of Human Caring" theory focuses on the human-to-human relationship. Dr. Watson refers to this as *transpersonal caring.* Put simply, it means that you focus on the other person while you are with him or her.

   You are not thinking about the medications you need to pass or what you will do for lunch. You are thinking about the patient or resident in your care totally and completely. The focus of transpersonal caring is to promote health and healing.

   Question:
   Treat the following as an essay question. List three to four examples of transpersonal caring that you could use with this resident. Do not use the behaviors listed in previous answers. Instead, think of *you* and how *you* could react to Mr. Lango. Some people would need to overcome a repulsion of his external appearance; some would need to overcome their fear of a person who is drunk. You need to control these thoughts so you can focus on him. Is he frightened? Hallucinating because of the alcohol? Hungry? In pain? Does he have any wounds? Why is he drooling and incontinent? There is much for you to do to promote his healing, and it will require your entire focus to be on him.

   There is much more to Dr. Watson's nursing theory, but for the moment, concentrate on the three concepts we just discussed. In summary, they are:

1. All human beings are valuable, and as a nurse, you have the responsibility to assist, nurture, and provide care for them.

Climate of caring: environmental management

Privacy	Personal Space	Safety	Stimulation/ Personalization
Knock on door before entering	Respect personal items	No clutter or throw rugs	Multiple opportunities for individual choice
Privacy with family members	Respect personal space	Proper shoes	Encourage independent function
Respect time to be alone	Use touch only if it is acceptable to the other person	Sometimes pets	Cherished furniture and decorations
Pull cubicle curtains		No frayed cords or broken furniture	Meaningful pictures

2. It is essential to focus on the human relationship you have with all persons in your care and their relationship with the environment.
3. Developing a human-to-human relationship is critical to being a caring nurse.

Why Study Caring?

Many nurses and other health-care providers tell me they are caring already and ask why they need to study it. I understand the question they are asking. Yet I often see acts of uncaring behavior, as demonstrated by the absence of the human-to-human connection. Here are just two examples.

Example 1:

One thing I often see are nurses with lists in their hands as they move quickly from room to room to reassure themselves of the safety of their patients or residents. Many times I have seen a nurse go into a room and say "good morning" without looking at the person and acknowledging him or her personally. Then, with list in hand, the rushed nurse checks the intravenous solution (IV), the bladder catheter, and any dressing or wound, says "good-bye,"

and leaves the room. Everything the nurse did should have been done, but something very serious was missing. There was no human connection, no transpersonal caring; the nurse was not at all holistic in his or her approach.

How could the same things (checking critical items) be done in a caring mode? First, on the same list with the IV and dressing information should be the person's name. Note it as you go into the room and use it. My personal rule of thumb is to use Mr. or Mrs. the first time I meet an older person. Then, if individuals ask me to use their first names, I do, but only if invited to do so. This is a respectful way to communicate. Look the person in the eye as you say "good morning." Really look at the person's face and see if it has good color, if there are grimaces from pain, or if the person seems sad or depressed. When you get close enough to the person, reach out to touch an arm or a hand if it seems appropriate. This action demonstrates an effort to use transpersonal caring, and it gives you the opportunity to feel if the skin is dry and hot or cold and clammy. Some of these things can be done while you are walking into the room, and none of them take any extra time. After you have connected with the person

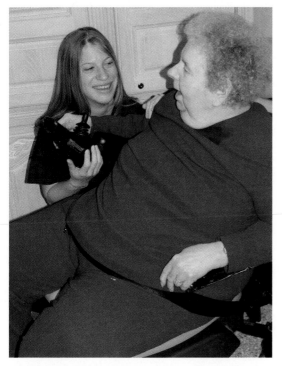

Notice how this LPN is touching the resident and looking directly into her eyes. She is down to the resident's level so the resident can see and hear as the LPN talks to her. What else does the LPN's nonverbal communication tell you?

Let the person know approximately when you will return.

Example 2:

Once when I had students at the local homeless center for clinical experience, an elderly man came into the center complaining of severe pain in his right shoulder. The other faculty person and I sat him down and removed his coat, which caused him a great deal of pain. We had a student take his vital signs and carefully role-modeled acceptance and concern for this dirty and disheveled person. The decision was made to call the paramedics because his pain was severe.

From the moment they came through the door, the two young male paramedics who came to the center could be heard complaining about being there. Their comments were something like, "This will just be some old bum who wants a hot meal and a bed for the night." I introduced them to the man with the shoulder pain, and the paramedics roughly took off his shirt so they could examine him. This action caused a great deal of pain for the older man. At this point, I intervened. I asked the paramedics to step around the corner with me. They knew I was a faculty person and willingly obliged me. I shared with them my point of view about valuing all people, respecting the elderly, and the standards of professional behavior (which they seemed to have forgotten). They were a bit shamefaced when they returned to the elderly man; they carefully assessed his shoulder and determined it was broken by the way it was hanging. That older man was genuinely in pain and deserved to be treated with the highest level of professional care. Truly caring behavior cannot allow prejudice, negative judgments, or disdain into the relationship.

(human-to-human connection), you can check the IV, the wound, and the catheter. Then lean close so that the older person can see you and hear you, and tell him or her "everything is all right," or "I need to check with the registered nurse (RN)," or whatever is appropriate. Be honest and pleasant in all of your communications.

 POINT OF INTEREST

Remember the list of 10 chronic illnesses most common for people older than 65? Visual and hearing problems were on that list. With that information, can you understand why it is so important to move in close so that an older adult can see you and hear you?

 POINT OF INTEREST

When speaking to older adults, some people address them as "honey," "dearie," or "sweetie." This is an example of the caregiver treating the patient or resident as a child. It is called *paternalism*. Think for whom those comments are generally reserved; it is children. You may hear others use such terms, but you should talk to gerontological patients as the older adults they are rather than as children. It is a matter of respect.

Expanding the Concept of the Science of Human Caring

To truly be a caring person, as defined by Watson, you need to use her principles in all aspects of your life. I do not know your personal or family environment, but I do know that you can choose to behave in any way you wish. I have been screamed at by family members of older adults, but I never scream back. I simply let them "get it out." While they are screaming, I observe them and really listen to their words so I can understand the problem. When the screaming is done, the person generally is crying with sorrow or fear. I keep in mind that there is a reason for every behavior, and I consider it my responsibility to learn the reason for the behavior before I react.

This one application of caring theory in your personal life will improve your ability to relate well to the people you care for the most. Other examples are to listen to people when they are talking and respond thoughtfully. Caring people "get into it" and help others when they need it. This could mean cooking a meal for a sick neighbor, working with the community to make a vacant lot a safe play area, or telling your mom that you love her. (Being a mom, I really like that idea!) I am simply saying that to be a caring nurse, you need to be a caring person, too.

GEROTRANSCENDENCE

Eric Erickson spent his life studying the psychological developmental tasks of people. His concept was that people would have good psychological health if they fulfilled the developmental tasks associated with each age group. Developmental tasks are the skills and knowledge learned through life experiences that allow us to meet the challenges that occur as we age. Erickson identified eight life stages with specific tasks that need to be accomplished. They are the following:

- Infancy: Trust vs. Mistrust
- Toddler: Autonomy vs. Shame
- Early childhood: Initiative vs. Guilt
- Middle childhood: Industry vs. Inferiority
- Adolescence: Identity vs. Identity diffusion
- Adulthood: Intimacy vs. Isolation
- Middle age: Generativity vs. Self-absorption
- Old age: Integrity vs. Despair

If older adults have accomplished integrity, they have likely experienced *gerotranscedence,* which is one of the critical tasks of old age.

Tornstam (2005) identified the concept of gerotranscendence. He states that older adults desire a life with more connections to other people, a life that is significant to self and others. This concept indicates that aging involves a transition to a lesser concern with material possessions, meaningless relationships, and self-interest. With gerotranscendence, older people are satisfied with the lives they have led and look forward to living a full life for the rest of their days; without gerotranscendence, older people are more likely to feel despair with their lives—past, present, and future. These ideas and other insights into gerotranscendence will be integrated throughout this book in an effort to provide you with information that will assist you to help older adults achieve satisfaction with the lives they have lived.

CONCLUSION

I am confident that you can see how holism and caring complement each other. If you are caring, you look at the body, mind, and spirit of the person. If you are holistic, you also look at the entire person. Both approaches look at how the environment affects the person, and they work with the individual to make the environment more healing. Family members and other loved ones also are essential to delivering both types of nursing care, and understanding gerotranscendence is key to helping older adults feel more satisfied with the lives they have lived so far. There is much more to these concepts. My goal is for you to have an understanding of the basic principles of each approach to nursing care. Then it makes sense for you to discuss, think about, and put into practice the things you have learned. If you can gradually incorporate the material in this chapter into your daily caregiving, you will be the type of nurse you would want to take care of the people you love most. Best wishes for the journey!

You have been out of school for 1 year, and although you have learned a great deal as you have been working, you are aware there still is much to learn. You enjoy your job at the Country Meadows Nursing facility, where you work full-time on the day shift. It is a bright, open place that actually is surrounded by country meadows.

You work on the locked Alzheimer's disease (AD) Unit and have learned to love the residents there. Even though there is a great deal of agitated behavior, you understand the phrase, "There is a reason for every behavior." This is because you take the time to observe and listen to residents carefully to understand what is going on inside their minds. Then you act on what you have seen and understood. You seem to do this naturally, based on your knowledge of holistic and caring nursing care, and have received compliments from your nurse manager on your skills.

The nurse manager has hired a new certified nursing assistant (CNA), and she has asked you to orient him to your philosophy of care for persons with AD. You have worked with him for two shifts and are concerned about some of his behaviors. You have noticed the following:

1. He consistently calls the residents "honey," "dearie," and "sweetie."
2. He is impatient when the residents are slow in walking, eating, or asking for things.
3. He refuses to learn their names.
4. You noticed one resident who did not have her glasses on or teeth in, and it was 10:00 a.m.
5. He got into an argument with an older man who was confused and wanted to leave the building.
6. He does not listen to you or treat you with respect.

Make a narrative summary of your thinking regarding the following questions. Be prepared to submit your answers to your faculty person. Add more ideas and comments to your paper than what is listed in the solution. Apply the principles you read in this chapter. Expound on the list noted in the solution. Use it as a foundation of thinking only.

• How does the CNA's behavior conflict with your holistic and caring philosophy?
• What are you going to do about the problem?

Solution

• How does the CNA's behavior conflict with your holistic and caring philosophy?

It seems that he has not embraced either concept into his caregiving, even after you have role-modeled and discussed appropriate behaviors for him.

1. He is not respectful. Examples are the "cutsie" names he uses rather than learning the residents' names and his disrespect toward you.
2. He does not listen. An example is the argument he got into with a demented resident. If he would have listened to the resident, he would have understood the "reason behind the man's behavior."
3. He is not caring. An example is his impatience with the slowness of older persons.
4. He does not give good technical care. This CNA not only is *not* caring or at all holistic, but he doesn't give good physical care. We know this because of the glasses and teeth that were not in place by mid-morning.

• What are you going to do?

It is only day 2 and there already are many problems with this employee. You are a relatively new LPN, but you know how nursing care should be delivered. His care is dangerous. What if he got into another argument with a resident and hit the person? It is a serious point of concern.

You have role-modeled for him and tried to explain things to him, yet he hasn't changed. This indicates that he doesn't want to change and probably won't. His lack of respect for you also is a point of concern in terms of how decisions are made on the unit. There will be many times when he will need to do what you tell him to do. You must question if he actually will do what you ask. This puts residents at risk.

You should carefully document his actual behaviors, both positive and negative. Then make an appointment with the nurse manager *before* he comes to another day of work. Carefully and objectively explain everything to her and leave the decision as to what to do with her. If she asks you to assist in continuing to evaluate or teach him, do as you are asked in a caring manner. If the CNA is terminated, that is the responsibility of the nurse manager and not your responsibility.

Select the best answer to each question.

1. Gerontological nursing refers to the nursing care of:

   a. the "old-old" population.

   b. people who are older and in need of assistance.

   c. people age 65 and older.

   d. a specialized body of knowledge regarding holistic and caring principles of nursing.

2. Older adults constitute:

   a. 12.3% of the U.S. population.

   b. 8.4% of the U.S. population.

   c. 25% of the U.S. population.

   d. 10% of the U.S. population.

3. The underlying concept of holism is:

   a. to include family and pets in the care plan.

   b. to recognize persons as individuals and to see them as an entire or whole person

   c. to identify team members who will make the nursing care easier.

   d. to look at the patient's face and note how he or she looks.

4. The purpose of a nursing philosophy is to be able to:

   a. think like a philosopher.

   b. have something positive to write on a job application.

   c. talk to other nurses about philosophy.

   d. have a personal conviction of the type of nursing care you will give to others.

5. "The Science of Human Caring" is:

   a. a nationally accepted philosophy of nursing.

   b. authored by Dr. John Wadsworth, former Dean and Distinguished Professor at the University of Colorado.

   c. a philosophy that addresses the body, mind, and physicality of all human beings.

   d. a philosophy of nursing that calls for the practice of individual caring.

6. Gerotranscendence is:

   a. one of the critical tasks of old age.

   b. based on Dr. Watson's developmental task of integrity vs. despair.

   c. a concept that refers to an elderly person's transition to a more materialistic mindset.

   d. a task that, when accomplished, makes older people despair the lives they have led.

2 The Aging Experience

Mary Ann Anderson

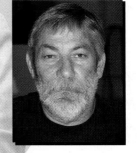

Learning Objectives

After completing this chapter, the student will be able to:

1. Define the term *ageism*.
2. Discuss six common theories of aging.
3. Identify age-related changes in the following body systems:
   Cardiovascular
   Respiratory
   Musculoskeletal
   Integumentary
   Gastrointestinal
   Genitourinary
   Neurological
   Special senses

INTRODUCTION

The aging experience is a significant part of personal and societal living. Throughout most of human history, only 1 in 10 people could expect to live to the age of 65 years. Today, 80% of Americans can anticipate reaching that age or older (Eliopolous, 2010). Two-thirds of all men and women who have lived beyond the age of 65 in the entire history of the world are alive today. Sometimes called "the graying of America," this dramatic change in our population has many ramifications in politics, economics, health care, recreation, and entertainment. All facets of life, not just health care, are affected by the fact that many more older adults are living today than lived in the past.

People 65 years old and older constitute 12.7% of the population in the United States—that is more than one in every eight Americans. There are many numbers I could share with you in this section, but I find most students do not want to read demographic data unless they have to in order to pass a test. I would prefer you learn the importance of the numbers rather than just memorize them.

Here are two important pieces of demographic information that will impact your practice as a licensed practical nurse (LPN):

1. The older white population will grow more slowly than before, and in the next 40 years, it will begin to decline compared with African American and other ethnic minority groups. Current minority populations are projected to represent 25% of the elderly population in 2030.
2. The fastest-growing segment of the population in the United States is people who are older than 85 years of age. Projections indicate that the size of this age group will double between 2000 and 2040. At present, there are more people having their 85th birthday every day in the United States than babies being born.

IMPACT OF AGING ON NURSING

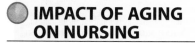

The great increase in the number of older people means that nursing practice must be different from what it has been in the past. Dr. Robert Butler (1969), a geriatric specialist, said that all graduates going into health-care work today will spend 75% of their working lives caring for older people. Current national statistics state that 65% of all patients in acute-care hospitals are age 65 or older, as are 83% of people in home care and 92% of residents in nursing homes. In 2000, Tim Porter O'Grady, a nursing futurist, said that if a nurse was not preparing for a job in gerontology, that nurse was not preparing for the nursing jobs of the future. The graying of America calls for gerontologically qualified nurses who can work in diverse health-care settings. The purpose of this book is to assist you to meet that objective.

CRITICALLY EXAMINE THE FOLLOWING

Before reading the next section, take the time necessary to complete this critical thinking exercise. Critical thinking is an essential component of nursing. These exercises are a positive way to begin to develop that all-important skill.

How Will It Impact Your Nursing Practice to Have:

1. Increasing numbers of old-old people as your clients?
2. Increasing numbers of nonwhite older adults as your clients?

I am going to answer the questions as though I were a student. It is hoped that this will assist you in considering how you will answer the questions. Your faculty person may request this assignment to be turned in at the next class session, or it may be used as a point for class discussion. However it is used, it is an opportunity for you to think critically and compare your thinking with your classmates. Here are my responses:

1. When I planned on going to nursing school, I wanted to be an obstetrical nurse. I was excited to think about working in labor and delivery, and I cannot imagine anything nicer than working in the newborn nursery. However, if the population of older people, especially the very old, is growing, I need to consider working in gerontology. If that is where I am going to be because of the need for nurses, I am going to become very good at taking care of fragile old-old or elite-old people. They sound like my type of challenge!
2. I live in Utah, where 95% of the population is white. I will have an adjustment to make when my patients are not mostly white and of the same working-class, emigrant society. I need to learn about the cultures of other ethnic groups so that I can be an effective nurse and meet their needs on a high level.

Health care has changed in various ways because of the number of people who are aging. As a group, older citizens are a very powerful political force; they have influenced the actions of Congress and the President on health-related issues and will continue to do so. Congress passed legislation providing insurance coverage for catastrophic medical events for individuals under Medicare, which added a relatively small amount to the cost of Medicare insurance paid by recipients. The new plan was unacceptable to older adults, however, and as a result of numerous calls and letters, Congress was persuaded to rescind its legislation.

Older adults want and expect to have a say in the kind of health care they receive, where they receive it, and from whom. They are better educated than any other generation of older adults and have the knowledge to make more sophisticated demands on the health-care system. For instance, demand is growing for home-care services from older people who need assistance and nursing care but prefer to be cared for at home.

This population of new clients in the health-care system requires you, the nurse, to consider them in a new way. Never before have nurses had to care for such a large number of older adults who have survived the Great Depression, two world wars, the Holocaust, the Korean and Vietnam Wars, and rock and roll! Because the survival experiences and life skills of these elderly people are new to health care, they require society to address them in a new way.

⬤ ATTITUDES TOWARD AGING

The study of aging is a very important part of nursing. Many myths, stereotypes, and prejudices about old age exist in our culture, and nurses need to be able to separate myths and prejudices from fact. Modern researchers are

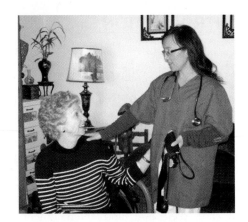

Home health care is one of the health-care changes that elderly people have demanded as part of their health-care options. People want to stay at home and be near family, friends, and the things that are familiar to them.

intently studying the aging experience (another indication of the importance of this topic in today's world). This chapter draws from their findings to represent a realistic picture of the processes and effects of aging.

Myths and prejudices about old age are pervasive in our society. Browsing through a greeting card display reveals some very good examples of the stereotypes and fables of aging:

"I won't say you're old," reads one greeting card, "but in horse years, you'd be glue on this envelope."

"Happy birthday, Hot Stuff! Who says people our age can't still live in the fast lane?" reads another. The inside message: "Voila! Adult diapers with racing stripes."

As the contents of many of the cards imply, old age conjures up images of rocking chairs, dentures, memory loss, and incontinence. People laugh at the humor in the birthday cards, but a serious societal danger lurks in such negative and prejudicial images. Stereotypes, myths, and

---

➡ POINT OF INTEREST

Dr. Robert Butler, mentioned earlier, coined and defined the words *geriatrics*—the medical study of older adults—and *gerontology*—the nursing study of older adults. You need to know the definitions of both words to discuss gerontological issues knowledgeably.

A former colleague of mine joined a tour group led by a sincere, well-intentioned young man. He tried to exchange a friendly word with every person in the group. He spoke to a healthy-looking man, who may have been in his late 70s, in a raised voice as though he assumed that the man was hard of hearing. "What did you used to be?" he asked. After a pause, the older man replied, "I still am." The behavior exhibited by the young tour guide is an example of ageism.

distortions concerning aging and old people lead to actions that discriminate against the aged. American culture glorifies youth. Print and television advertising, clothing fashions, and other expressions of the desirable norm all push the image of zestful youth. Because today's adults have grown up in this culture, they pick up its values and prejudices without realizing it.

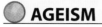 AGEISM

The term *ageism* was coined in 1968 by Robert Butler (1969) to describe negative attitudes and practices that were directed toward old people. He defined ageism as a systematic stereotyping of and discrimination against people simply because they are old. Ageism is very similar to racism and sexism, which discriminate against people because of skin color and gender. We as a society are outraged by acts of racism and sexism, but we seem to accept ageism as a norm for behavior. Old people are categorized as confused, rigid in thought and manner, and old-fashioned in morality and skills. Yet older adults are as individual and unique as people of all other age groups. It simply seems easier to place them in a negative category and ignore them. Ageism allows the younger generation to see older people as different; they subtly cease to identify with their elders as human beings.

In the decades since Dr. Butler first wrote about ageism, a steady improvement in attitudes toward the aged has been seen. This change partly resulted from general public education, increased attention in the media, and broadening of education about gerontology in colleges and universities. Seriously negative attitudes toward the aged still exist. They appear subtly, covertly, and even unconsciously. Similar to racism and sexism, ageism is still persistent.

An example is the cosmetic industry, which thrives on the sale of products that eliminate age spots, smooth away wrinkles, conceal gray hairs, and make one look younger than one's actual age. Growing old is represented as a calamity, and being old as having a dreaded disease. The last years of life are pictured as time spent in death's waiting room.

In reality, elderly people do not offer a panorama of doom and death. Many senior citizens live well into their 80s and 90s with "youthful vigor," in relative physical comfort and safety, and in good health. Many others do have chronic health problems, but because the problems are well managed and well controlled, such

▲ PRIORITY SETTING 2.1

As Robert Butler has said, you will spend 75% of your career taking care of older adults. The priority you need to take from this chapter is that of recognizing and combating ageism. Why is that the priority I chose? Ageism is a powerful, negative form of discrimination.

Because you are going to be giving care to older adults, you need to be their champion and assist them in combating this negative influence in their lives.

When you read Chapter 7 on culturally specific care, you will realize that many cultures revere and value their elderly citizens. In China, when an older member of the family can no longer be left alone during the day, the extended family organizes a way for one member of the family to stay home and give the necessary care to the older person. The remaining members of the family support the caregiver. That is not the societal attitude of the United States.

How can you meet this priority of recognizing and fighting ageism?

- Start with becoming acutely aware of what ageist behavior is. It could be something as simple as not laughing at the discriminatory cards that mock older people and the aging process. They simply are not funny. Look for age-based discrimination. Once you can recognize it, you can begin to change within yourself if that is needed.
- Look at older adults as "wise and wonderful." They really do have the wisdom of the ages. Just think of all the problems they have solved by living in a war-torn and tumultuous world (world wars, the Great Depression). They deserve to be heard, so listen!
- Be patient with older people. Their bodies are wearing out because of the *normal* process of aging. Don't hold that against them.
- Along with patience, speak up, move in close so you can be seen, touch if it seems appropriate, smile, and learn to enjoy your time with someone older. You may need to start with enjoying your grandparents or older aunts and uncles. Both generations have so much

Continued

to offer each other. Don't be too busy to take advantage of this opportunity.

- Be brave! Speak up when someone says or suggests doing something that is ageist. You don't need to be aggressive, but you should state your opinion. You don't need to defend what you say because the statement should speak for itself.
- Read about ageism, ponder what you read, talk to others about it, consider how you would like to be thought about and treated when you are older. If you don't like what you foresee, how can you change it?

people consider themselves healthy and lead active, fulfilling lives. Still others have significant limitations that affect their independence and activity, but they are able to enjoy a rich and varied existence because they live with family members or in other protected environments.

Negative images of nursing homes envisioned by some people are in part an expression of ageism. Most nursing homes give excellent care to a frail and vulnerable population that cannot be cared for elsewhere. Another point of information, unknown by many people, is that only 5% of people older than 65 years are in nursing homes at any one time (Eliopolous, 2010). Today's nursing home is characterized by a concept of *rehabilitative,* not *custodial,* care, a perspective that calls for nursing interventions intended to support the highest possible level of independence despite physical and cognitive limitations.

It is easy for society to judge, criticize, and ignore an older person. Do an internal examination to determine if you are ageist. Do you get impatient when an older person is in front of you driving on the freeway? I tell my gerontology students that they will not pass the class until they have conquered that type of impatience. I give them assignments to sit down and unhurriedly talk to a well elderly person. I suggest they go to lunch or shopping, even to the grocery store. The students are encouraged to ask the person about living with ration cards, going to war, or being left a widow or widower after 50 to 60 years of marriage. The ageism in our society has kept most of us from knowing about the aging process and respecting those who survive it. It is time for this situation to change.

An important concept to remember is the uniqueness of the individual. Just as every child and every middle-aged adult is unique in some way, so is every older adult. The mistaken belief that one old person is just like another is an expression of ageism, and this perception can lead to potentially harmful treatment. Physicians and nurses sometimes treat older patients as they might treat a child, calling them by their first names without asking how they wish to be addressed or, worse yet, calling them "honey" or "dearie." Caregivers often are guilty of "infantilizing" the elderly. It is easy to see how such treatment increases dependence and frailty, rather than fostering independence, even for a person with limitations. Not all old people are cranky and gloomy, although a man or woman who was cranky and gloomy at age 40 is probably more so at age 80. People tend to become more and more like themselves as they age. All individuals who work in the health-care field need to examine their own attitudes and biases about older adults in general and about frail or ill older adults in particular to battle ageism successfully.

THEORIES OF AGING

Theories of aging are a scientific effort to assist people to understand what contributes to aging in a positive or negative manner. As a nurse, you need to understand the basic theories to assist and support your older adult patients and residents to live healthier lives. There are physiological and psychological theories to assist you in understanding aging. There are many theories available for study; the following are three from each category that will assist you in giving effective nursing care.

Physiological Theories of Aging

Genetic Factors

The theory of genetic factors is easy to understand if you critically examine yourself and your family members. You already know that you may have inherited your hair and eye color, height, and body size from your ancestors. There are many other things you also may have inherited, such as musical or athletic ability. Have you considered that the aging of your body also is inherited? This theory says that it is. Interview your grandparents or older aunts and uncles. Are their siblings still alive? How long did their parents and grandparents live? I know of a family in which all of the men died before

CRITICALLY EXAMINE THE FOLLOWING

What are three things you can do to overcome your personal ageism?

1.
2.
3.

What are three things you can do to assist others in overcoming their ageism?

1.
2.
3.

I will not answer these questions because I do not think you need an example. It is more important for you to share your thinking. Spend time pondering the issue of ageism. Really grasp what it means for you on a personal level. This can be done by talking to your colleagues and peers and, more importantly, by talking to older people.

CRITICALLY EXAMINE THE FOLLOWING

Spend time with your parents or older relatives and discuss the genetic factor theory with them. Ask questions about your ancestors, and identify traits that you may have inherited from them. Inquire about the longevity of your ancestors as well as their major diseases. When you have enough information, predict how long you will live and the predominate diseases you will have. Justify what you predict from your family history. Prepare the information into one paragraph that could be read in class.

the age of 50 with heart disease, but the women lived to be in their 70s. I know a family of six sisters who all went through menopause at age 52. I have a friend whose mother had 11 brothers and sisters; they all lived to be in their 80s.

This theory claims that animals and humans are born with a genetic program that predetermines their life span. This may seem discouraging to people who are working hard to obtain or maintain optimum health. A healthy diet, exercise, and stress control, among other things, will certainly support a higher quality of life, however, if not add to one's longevity.

Just as nurses interview people about their family history regarding diseases, it would be appropriate use of this theory to ask about their parents and siblings and their aging process. This information may assist you in working with the patient or resident. The most important aspect of this theory is for you to recognize that it is one way to accept aging as the inevitable process it is. With that acceptance, you should develop an additional acceptance of the normal and abnormal aspects of aging and the eventual death of each of us. According to this theory, it is predetermined and inevitable.

Wear and Tear

If you were to go to a senior citizen center or a nursing home dayroom, you would easily identify the basis for the wear and tear theory. As people age, their body parts show the effects of the complex and sophisticated work the body

does through the years. People will be walking with canes or walkers; some will be on oxygen; others will simply moan when they get up from a chair. Similar to all fine-tuned machinery, body parts wear out or become less effective. Knees need to be replaced because of the lack of cartilage that comes with aging, joints develop arthritis, and hips break because of decreased bone mass or lack of balance leading to a fall.

Think of all the running and jumping you did as a child. Perhaps you were an athlete during high school. Think of how you use your body now that you are in school. The body is well used and sometimes abused, and its parts simply wear out.

Understanding this theory should assist you in accepting that older adults walk slower, hear less effectively, and need to stop and rest and overall do things at a slower and safer pace. If you understand and accept this theory, you will accept the changes that require your attention in giving care to specialized, older people.

Nutrients

Chapter 6 in this book is devoted to nutrition. The focus is on nutrition for older persons. When considering the nutrient theory, however, you should focus on your own nutritional intake. This theory states that aging and the quality of aging depend on a person's nutrition intake over the span of his or her life. This is easy to understand because, as a health-care worker, you recognize the negative effects of obesity, lack of exercise, and high cholesterol, all of which are attributed to food consumption. The quart of chocolate ice cream, mountain of french fries, and large steak are not ways to promote a successful aging process. The nutrient theory states that good nutritional intake at any age assists in improved health as one ages.

The longer you eat healthy foods, the longer you will live with a better quality of life. Now is a good time to start.

Whenever you are giving care to an older person, you should examine the individual's eating habits and determine if you can teach him or her something new that will improve health. Ask the nurse manager about having a dietitian visit the person or arrange for fresh fruits to be available for snacks if that would help. You need to take care of yourself and share your knowledge with those you love. Teach them the things you will learn in the nutrition chapter and apply the principles to yourself as well. There is little in life that is better than a healthy old age!

Psychological Theories

Developmental Tasks

Eric Erikson (1963) is famous for his eight stages of personal development of individuals. He begins with infancy and progresses through old age. His focus is on ego development, which gives people the strength to manage their lives. The task for old age, according to Erikson, is Integrity vs. Despair. If older people can find meaning in the life lived, then they will have the ego integrity to adjust and manage the process of aging. If they do not have integrity, they will be angry, depressed, and feel inadequate; in other words, they will feel despair.

You may encounter older persons who are feeling despair. They complain constantly and keep saying they wish "this" or "that" had happened in their life. Also frequently heard is the phrase "if only . . . ." Such people need your time and acceptance of them and their lives. Ask them to talk about their life experiences and reinforce the valuable things they have done. Help them to see what they have contributed to the world. Your efforts should focus on identifying the actions in their life that will assist in building the feeling of ego integrity.

Subculture Theory

This theory defines older people as a subculture. In anthropological terms, this theory indicates that older people have their own cultural norms and standards. This includes attitudes that cross over to multiple members of the group and beliefs, expectations, and behaviors that make them different from others.

You will study the cultural and ethnic differences in people throughout your education. It is important to understand people, their differences, and their needs. This theory indicates that elderly people are another group worthy of your study. You need to observe older people and note their similarities. They will not be the same because, similar to all people, they are strongly individualized, but they will exhibit similarities. In reference to this theory, you need to note their similarities. An interesting political group is the Gray Panthers. This group of older adults has the power to influence votes on the national level as well as locally. They are a power that you should examine to help understand this theory.

Continuity Theory

In simple terms, the continuity theory states that as people change, their basic personality and behavioral patterns do not change. If you are an angry person at age 20, then you will be even better at being angry at age 70. The same is true of a teacher, who will find a way to keep teaching as he or she ages. A loving mother will find a way to continue to mother people (perhaps her grandchildren or children in the neighborhood), musicians will keep playing, and athletes will still keep trying to win.

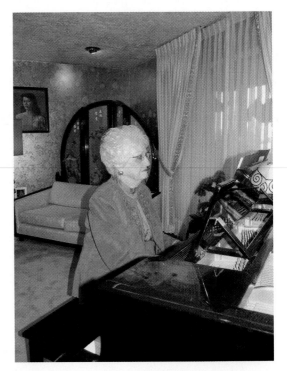

This 82-year-old woman has always played the piano and organ, and currently she plays every Sunday at her church. Now that she is older, she is better at it than ever before in her life. Which psychological theory does this demonstrate?

The continuity theory recognizes the unique and individualized characteristics of people and their ways of adapting to aging. This theory is easy to apply to your practice. You simply need to talk to the older person and the family members about what type of person your patient was in his or her youth or adulthood. Then you will know what type of behavior to expect now that he or she is an older adult. Don't try to change older people; rather, respect them for who they are.

NORMAL AGING PROCESS

Since the early 1950s, much research has been done in Europe and the United States on identifying and classifying common physiological and psychosocial changes that occur as people grow older. These changes have been termed *normal* because they represent alterations in body structure and function that occur gradually throughout life. In this context, aging is seen as a natural process, and the changes associated with it are considered to be expected and continuous. If you are curious about your potential normal aging changes, you need to look at your grandparents. What acute and chronic diseases do they have? At what age do people in your family die? Do the men go bald; do the women develop osteoporosis? We all will age until we die. To me, that comment makes aging the desirable choice between the two. I would sooner grow old than die young.

To understand the normal aging process fully, nurses must realize that aging is a normal developmental event and that patterns of aging vary dramatically among older adults. Although the profession studies normal age changes that are universal, every person ages in a particular, individualized way. No two individuals are alike; the number of ways in which people age may be seen as equal to the number of people who have lived into old age. As individuals age, they

FOCUSED LEARNING CHART

Theories of aging

Physiological Theories	Psychological Theories
Genetic Factors *Born with a genetic program that predetermines life span.*	**Developmental Tasks** *Eric Erickson defined eight developmental tasks from infancy to old age. The task for old age is integrity versus despair.*
Wear and Tear *All life is a fine-tuned machine. Body parts wear out as they age.*	**Subculture Theory** *Defines old people as their own subculture with cultural norms and standards.*
Nutrients *Aging and the quality of life depend on the person's nutritional intake over his or her life span.*	**Continuity Theory** *People change physiologically as they age, but their basic personality and behavioral patterns do not change.*

become more diverse, not more alike. The range of "normal" aging characteristics is wide, and each individual exhibits a unique interplay of physical, social, and environmental influences that define the personal aging experience.

Older adults often have a chronic or acute illness superimposed on age-related changes, but development of disease is not a normal part of aging. It is essential for you, the LPN, to understand this perspective and develop a positive approach to normal aging. It also is important to remember that most older adults live actively and independently in the community and cope successfully with age-related changes and chronic illnesses (remember that only 5% of them are in nursing homes). Health for older adults might be defined as the ability to function at an individual's highest potential despite the presence of age-related changes and risk factors.

Essential facts about the normal aging process can be summarized as follows:

- As individuals age, they become more diverse, not more alike.
- Age-related changes develop in each individual in a unique way.
- Normal aging and disease are separate entities.
- Normal aging includes gains and losses and does not indicate decline.
- Successful adaptation to the aging process is accomplished by most older adults.

NORMAL PHYSIOLOGICAL CHANGES ACCORDING TO BODY SYSTEMS

Specific age-related changes are described in terms of the body systems with which they are associated. Common functional changes experienced by older adults as a result of physiological alterations also are discussed. The term *function* refers to an older adult's ability to perform activities of daily living (ADLs) and independent activities of daily living (IADLs) and takes into consideration the quality of life of the individual. As the older adult experiences an increase in the number and intensity of age-related changes, functional independence is often jeopardized. Nursing approaches to prevent losses and promote self-care in light of age-related changes also are considered in this section.

Cardiovascular System

The cardiovascular system loses its efficiency with age, but because older adults require less oxygen at rest and during exercise, many people effectively compensate for changes in circulatory function. The high incidence of cardiovascular disease in the older population often makes it difficult, however, to distinguish normal age-related changes from changes related to sickness. One of the "good news" facts about cardiovascular disease and elderly people is that it is no longer the number one cause of death as it has been for decades. Older adults now know more about taking care of themselves, which improves their cardiovascular system. Cancer is now the leading cause of death in older adults.

Age-Related Changes

Heart
- Cardiac muscle strength is diminished.
- Heart valves become thickened and more rigid.
- The sinoatrial node, which is responsible for conduction, is less efficient, and impulses are slowed.

Blood Vessels
- Arteries become less elastic.
- Capillary walls thicken and slow the exchange of nutrients and waste products between blood and tissues.
- The greater rigidity of the vascular walls increases systolic and diastolic pressures.

Blood
- Blood volume is reduced owing to an age-related decline in total body water.

POINT OF INTEREST

Function is the ability to take care of one's ADLs—basic personal needs, such as eating, dressing, washing, toileting, and moving. Function also refers to the ability to live independently in one's community, performing IADLs including cooking, shopping, taking medications properly, cleaning, traveling locally, and managing finances.

- Bone marrow activity is reduced, which leads to a slight decrease in levels of red blood cells, hematocrit, and hemoglobin.
- Heart contractions may be weaker, blood volume decreases, and cardiac output declines at a rate of about 1% per year below the value of 5 L normally found in a younger person.

In summary, with normal aging, some atherosclerosis is expected as well as decreased cardiac output, but cardiovascular response remains adequate if cardiac disease is not present.

Respiratory System

Respiratory functioning shows minimal age-related decline in healthy older adults. The age-related changes that affect the respiratory system are so gradual that most older adults compensate well for these changes.

Age-Related Changes

Skeletal Changes
- The rib cage becomes rigid as cartilage calcifies.
- The thoracic spine may shorten, and osteoporosis may cause a stooped posture, decreasing active lung space and limiting thoracic movement.

Accessory Muscles
- Abdominal muscles weaken, decreasing inspiratory and expiratory effort.
- The diaphragm does not seem to lose mass.

Intrapulmonary Changes

- Lung elastic recoil is progressively lost with advancing age.
- Alveoli enlarge and become thin, and although their number remains constant, the number of functioning alveoli decreases overall.
- The alveolus-capillary membrane thickens, reducing the surface area for gas exchange.

Functional Changes

Structural changes in the respiratory system affect the rate of airflow into and out of the lungs as well as the rate of gas exchange at the alveolar level. Because of limited elastic recoil, residual volume increases; less ventilation occurs at the bases of the lungs, and more air and secretions remain in the lungs. In addition, the shallow breathing patterns of older adults—secondary to postural changes—contribute to this reduced airflow. Decreased chest muscle strength contributes to a less effective cough response and places an older adult at greater risk of pulmonary infection. The shallow breathing pattern also affects gas exchange. Oxygen saturation is diminished. For example, the partial pressure of oxygen in alveoli (P_{AO_2}) is about 90 mm Hg for a healthy young adult, whereas a value of 75 mm Hg at age 70 years would be acceptable. This decline may result in a decreased tolerance for exercise and the need for short rest periods during activity.

Musculoskeletal System

Most older adults experience alterations in posture, changes in range of motion, and slowed movement. These changes account for many of the characteristics normally associated with old age.

Bone Structure

- Loss of bone mass results in brittle, weak bones.
- The vertebral column may compress, leading to reduction in height.

Muscle Strength
- Muscle wasting occurs, and regeneration of muscle tissue slows.
- Muscles of the arms and legs become thin and flabby.
- Muscles lose flexibility and endurance with inactivity.

Joints
- Range of motion may be limited.
- Cartilage thins, so that joints may be painful, inflamed, or stiff.

Functional Changes

Loss of muscle mass is a gradual process, and most older adults compensate for it well. Regular exercise has been shown to reduce bone loss, promote increased muscle strength, and improve flexibility and muscle coordination. Conversely, immobility and sedentary lifestyles lead to loss of muscle size and strength.

Loss of bone mass and bone density results in osteoporosis and porous, brittle bones that are at greater risk of fracture. This problem can be due to estrogen deficiencies and low serum

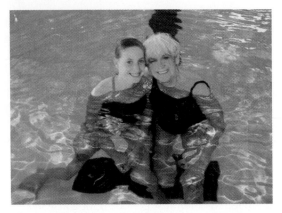

This grandmother and granddaughter team go swimming together twice a week. It provides a special time for them to be together and a great opportunity for meaningful exercise.

calcium levels; calcium supplements and estrogens are often prescribed. More recent research has raised some questions, however, about the use of estrogen therapy. This should be discussed with the older person's physician.

In summary, changes caused by osteoporosis, lack of joint motion, and decreased muscle strength and endurance may affect the functional ability of the older adult. An effective exercise program, together with adequate diet and a healthy outlook that includes independence and an active lifestyle, can reverse or slow down musculoskeletal changes. The phrase "Use it or lose it!" directly applies to an older adult's musculoskeletal functional ability.

Integumentary System

Changes involving the skin and hair probably are symbolic of the aging process more than those of any other system. The formation of wrinkles, the development of "age spots," graying of the hair, and baldness are constant reminders of growing old. In addition, no other system is so highly influenced by previous life patterns and environmental conditions, particularly exposure to the sun.

Age-Related Changes

Skin
- The skin loses elasticity, leading to wrinkles, folds, and dryness.
- The skin thins, giving less protection to underlying blood vessels.
- Subcutaneous fat diminishes.
- Melanocytes cluster, producing the skin pigmentation known as age spots.

Hair
- Decreased activity of hair follicles results in thinning of the hair.
- Decreased rate of melanin production results in loss of original color and graying.
- Women may develop hair on the chin and upper lip.

Nails
- Decreased blood flow to the nailbed may cause nails to become thick, dull, hard, and brittle, with longitudinal lines.

Sweat Glands
- Decreases in size and number occur.

Functional Changes

Intact skin is the first line of defense against bacterial invasion and minor physical trauma. Age-related skin dryness and decreased elasticity increase the risk of skin breakdown and skin tears, leading to increased potential for injury and infection. Body temperature regulation is impaired by decreased sweat production. Because of this, older adults may not exhibit diaphoresis with elevated body temperatures.

Conversely, the loss of insulation in the form of a fat layer may make older adults feel cold. They often ask for extra sweaters when younger adults are comfortable with the ambient temperature. Nurses need to be aware of temperature discomforts when bathing, dressing, or examining an older adult and respond appropriately to the older adult's concern.

Age-related changes in the integumentary system affect the essential mechanisms of body protection and temperature regulation and greatly influence one's perception of aging. Earlier health practices related to nutrition, grooming, bathing, and physical activity as well as genetic, biochemical, and environmental factors are powerful determinants of integumentary status. An older adult who has followed a healthy lifestyle often takes pride in the moistness and softness of aging skin and reveals newfound beauty in gray hair and wise wrinkles.

Gastrointestinal System

Changes in the gastrointestinal (GI) system, although not life-threatening, often cause the greatest concern to the older adult. Indigestion, constipation, and anorexia are common GI problems that greatly affect functional status.

Age-Related Changes

Oral Cavity
- Reabsorption of bone in the jaw may loosen teeth and reduce the ability to chew.
- People with dentures must have them checked regularly to maintain a proper fit.

Esophagus
- The gag reflex weakens, causing an increased risk of food aspiration.
- Smooth muscle weakness delays emptying time.

Stomach
- Decreased gastric acid secretions may impair absorption of iron, vitamin B_{12}, and protein.

Intestines
- Peristalsis decreases.
- Weakening of the sphincter muscles leads to incompetent emptying of the bowel.

Functional Changes

The slowing of peristalsis and the loss of smooth muscle tone delay gastric emptying so that a feeling of "fullness" is present after eating only small amounts of food. In addition, delayed gastric emptying time and reduced gastric acid secretions may lead to indigestion, discomfort, and reduced appetite. Frequent small meals, rather than three large ones, may be better tolerated. Decreased peristalsis also contributes to slower transit time in the large intestine and allows more time for water reabsorption and hardening of the stool. Because of this factor, the nurse must recommend a diet adequate in fiber and fluids.

Fatigue, discomfort, activity intolerance, and sensory losses may make food preparation difficult for an older adult living at home. This problem could result in a nutritionally inadequate diet. In summary, effective GI functioning creates peace of mind for the older adult and greatly influences well-being.

Genitourinary System

Changes in the genitourinary system affect the basic bodily functions of voiding and sexual performance. These issues are often difficult for an older adult to discuss. A commonly held belief is that genitourinary problems, such as incontinence and decreased sexual response, are normal results of aging. They are not, but the belief that they are often causes an older adult to delay seeking treatment. Helping the older adult to maintain optimal genitourinary function is often a challenge for the nurse.

Age-Related Functions

Renal Function
- Renal blood flow decreases because of decreased cardiac output and reduced glomerular filtration rate.
- Ability to concentrate urine may be impaired.

Bladder
- Loss of muscle tone and incomplete emptying may occur.
- Capacity decreases.

Micturition
- In men, increased frequency owing to enlargement of the prostate is possible.
- In women, increased frequency may be caused by relaxation of the perineal muscle.

Female Reproduction
- The vulva may atrophy.
- Pubic hair may fall out.
- Vaginal secretions diminish, and vaginal walls thin and become less elastic.

Male Reproduction
- Testes decrease in size.
- The prostate may enlarge.

Functional Changes

Despite decreased renal blood flow and the loss of kidney mass, the genitourinary system continues to function normally in the absence of disease. Functional impairments result from decreased bladder capacity and include urinary frequency, nocturia, and retention of urine. These changes may eventually cause dysfunction, leading to infection, urgency, and incontinence. Although urinary incontinence is not a normal outcome of the aging process, loss of perineal muscle mass may contribute to one of the most common forms of incontinence in women—stress incontinence. This condition involves leakage of urine that occurs with coughing, sneezing, laughing, or lifting. Pelvic floor exercises are an effective strategy to strengthen muscle tone and prevent involuntary leakage. Vaginal changes may lead to painful intercourse, vaginal infections, and intense itching.

Enlargement of the prostate, which occurs in most elderly men, is most often benign. It can cause, however, urinary retention, frequency, overflow incontinence, and, eventually, renal damage. Older men should have regular examinations of the prostate.

Changes in voiding, particularly incontinence, and changes in sexual response may dramatically alter genitourinary function and contribute to embarrassment and general discomfort for an older adult. By showing sensitivity and acceptance, the nurse can intervene effectively to improve genitourinary functional response.

Nervous System

Age-related changes in the nervous system affect all body systems and involve vascular response, mobility, coordination, visual activity, and cognitive ability. Most misconceptions about normal age-related changes involve the nervous system. For example, there is a misconception that mental decline or "senility" is inevitable with aging or that intellectual capacity diminishes with age. The nurse needs to teach older adults that general decline of neurological function is not an automatic response to aging and that, in the absence of disease, the older adult's neurological system functions adequately.

Age-Related Changes

Neurons
- Neurons are steadily lost in the brain and spinal cord.
- Synthesis and metabolism of neurotransmitters are diminished.
- Brain mass is lost progressively.

Movement
- The kinesthetic sense is less efficient.
- Balance may be impaired.
- Reaction time decreases.

Sleep
- Insomnia and increased night wakening may occur.
- Deep sleep (stage IV) and rapid eye movement sleep decrease.

Functional Changes

As motor neurons work less efficiently, reaction time slows, and the ability to respond quickly to stimuli decreases. Research studies indicate that although response time may be prolonged, older adults are willing to give up speed for accuracy and tend to respond more slowly but with greater precision. There seems to be little correlation between brain atrophy and cognitive loss. Older adults are generally well oriented to time, place, and person, with minimal changes in memory performance despite decreased synthesis of neurotransmitters and diminished brain size.

Older people are particularly at risk for falls, owing to a slower reaction time in maintaining balance and the potential for hypotensive reactions secondary to decreased blood volume. Resulting symptoms of dizziness, lightheadedness, and vertigo contribute to impaired balance. Nurses should allow older adults adequate time for position change; dangling at the bedside and standing briefly before ambulation may be indicated.

Older adults generally sleep less at night but take naps during the day, so that cumulative sleep time is usually adequate. The frequent awakenings may cause restless sleep and abrupt wakefulness that are often troubling to an older adult. Thorough sleep assessment is necessary to determine actual sleep time. Additionally, the nurse may suggest afternoon exercise and a decrease in stimulants at bedtime. Environmental changes, such as noise control and regulation of room temperature, may be helpful.

Common age-related changes of the nervous system, particularly slowed reaction time, affect movement, sleep, and cognition, the functions of which are vital to optimal performance of ADLs.

Special Sense Organs

The sensory organs of sight, hearing, taste, touch, and smell facilitate communication with the environment. Loss of sensory function, particularly vision and hearing, severely alters an older adult's self-care abilities and quality of life. Age-related changes that result in loss of sensory function may be the most difficult for a person of any age to accept and cope with effectively. The nurse must be extremely sensitive to sensory changes and their impact on each person.

Age-Related Changes

Vision
- Ability to focus on close objects is diminished.
- Increased density of the lens occurs, and lipid accumulates around the iris, causing a grayish yellow ring.

- The production of tears decreases.
- The pupils decrease in size and become less responsive to light.
- Night vision decreases, and the iris loses pigment so that eye color usually becomes light blue or gray.

Hearing

- The ability to hear high-frequency tones decreases.
- The cerumen contains a greater amount of keratin so that it hardens and becomes more likely to become impacted.

Taste

- Ability to perceive bitter, salt, and sour tastes diminishes.

Touch

- Ability to feel light touch, pain, or different temperatures may decrease.

Functional Changes

Despite normal age-related changes in vision, most older adults have adequate visual function using corrective lenses for self-care activities. Because dark and light adaptation takes longer, simple activities, such as entering or leaving a theater or going to the bathroom at night, put older people at risk for falls and injury. Yellowing of the lens makes vision for low-tone colors (violet, blue, green) difficult; use of yellow, orange, or red colors on signs or on bedroom walls increases the older adult's ability to read. Decreased production of tears by the eye may contribute to irritation and infection; artificial tears are often prescribed.

Functional hearing changes result initially in an inability to hear high-pitched tones. The nurse should speak in a normal tone of voice without shouting and without increasing pitch.

Because it takes more sensory stimulation to trigger the taste experience, older adults may use more salt to produce a salt taste on their food effectively. Sensory changes have a profound impact on the functional ability of older adults. The nurse must always determine whether the patient uses corrective lenses or a hearing aid and ensure that the older person has these assistive devices available at all times.

Later in this book, the reader will be able to compare abnormal physiological changes of older adults with the normal changes explained here. As a future gerontological nurse, you should have a thorough understanding of both aspects of physiological aging.

CONCLUSION

This chapter has pointed out the importance of understanding the older adult in today's society. As the number of aged individuals increases, and as more and more older adults require nursing care, you need to develop a strong knowledge base in gerontological nursing content. It is equally important to explore the myths, stereotypes, and prejudices about old age to begin the process of seeing older adults as unique individuals who have special histories and life experiences. Understanding the various theories of aging can promote a more positive attitude toward the process. Normal aging changes each person in a unique way. As you acquire the specific knowledge and skills to be an effective caregiver of older adults, it is hoped that you will embrace the attitude that all older adults are unique and should be encouraged to function at their full potential. With this critical understanding, you are the generation of nurses who will define the application of gerontological nursing. Best wishes with the task!

Ms. B. is 76 years old and lives in a duplex with her 83-year-old sister. Last year, the sister had a mild stroke, leaving her with left-sided weakness. Ms. B. manages the household and coordinates her sister's care, including home health aides, physical and occupational therapy, and visits to the doctor's office.

Ms. B. describes herself as healthy. She also comments, "Okay, I had cancer of the colon 2 years ago, but I had surgery and some chemotherapy too, and now I'm okay. Oh, I sometimes get constipated, but that has nothing to do with the cancer."

She states that she tires more easily these days and tries to rest every afternoon. Still, she maintains a full schedule of grocery shopping, visiting friends, cooking and cleaning, and caring for her sister's needs. She has no breathing problems, and her appetite is excellent. "I can't eat as much as I used to at each meal, but my sister and I have a snack in the afternoon and at bedtime."

She does complain about nocturnal voiding two or three times a night and has had two urinary infections this year. "Sometimes I dribble urine, and I use those pads."

Both sisters are always cold; their home is kept very warm, and they always seem to be wearing sweaters and heavy stockings. Every Sunday is beauty day at the B.'s residence, when they apply face and hand cream to dry skin, style their thinning hair, and care for their nails, which are getting thick and brittle. Both claim that they have become shorter in the past few years; Ms. B. often feels weary at night because of joint pain. She has learned to adjust her daily schedule to changes in endurance. She says, "No matter where I go, I take my time, sit down, and pace myself. I know where every bench and restaurant is in south Philadelphia."

Ms. B. has noticed that she needs to wear her glasses all the time when reading or paying bills; she invested in 100-watt light bulbs for every lamp "because we both need stronger light to read by these days." She is never without her sunglasses to avoid glare; every shade is always lowered at their house during the day. Ms. B. claims, "I don't think as clearly lately as I used to; it takes me longer to figure things out and make decisions." But she continues to manage the household and lead an active life.

"I have my friends, my neighborhood, my home, and, of course, my sister. We have been together all of our lives. We care about each other, and we do pretty well, taking each day as it comes, each day expecting another good day."

Discussion

1. What age-related changes has Ms. B. experienced?

2. Would you consider Ms. B. to be a healthy older adult? Explain.

Solution

1. Ms. B. has experienced age-related changes in all the following areas:

Cardiovascular
Decreased activity tolerance
Fatigue with increased activity

Musculoskeletal
Loss of muscle strength
Height loss
Joint pain

Integumentary
Dry skin
Brittle, thickened nails
Thinning hair

Gastrointestinal
Delayed gastric emptying leading to fullness
Reduced GI motility

Genitourinary
Urinary retention, which may contribute to infection
Urgency and stress incontinence

Nervous
Delayed reaction time

Special Senses
Diminished ability to focus on close objects
Inability to tolerate glare
Poor vision in reduced light

2. Ms. B. is a healthy older adult because she functions at an optimal level despite the presence of age-related changes. She feels good about her life and about her coping skills. She expects continued "good days."

Select the best answer to each question.

1. Your client is 84 years old. What normal change in vital signs would you expect to assess?

   a. A higher than normal temperature

   b. A slower pulse

   c. A shallower breathing pattern

   d. A lower blood pressure

2. Immobility or sedentary lifestyles have what effect on the older adult?

   a. Loss of muscle size and strength

   b. Decreased serum sodium levels

   c. Loss of skin elasticity

   d. Thinning of cartilage in joints

3. Mrs. Jones, aged 86 years, complains of fullness after eating only small amounts of food. This is primarily due to which GI change?

   a. Delayed gastric emptying time

   b. Increased gastric acid secretions

   c. Hypertonicity of gastric muscles

   d. Loss of ability to chew

4. Mrs. Smith, aged 79 years, is admitted to the hospital. Based on your understanding of normal age changes in the nervous system, what behavior might you expect Mrs. Smith to exhibit?

   a. Decreased intellectual function

   b. Forgetfulness and confusion

   c. Lack of orientation to time and place

   d. Longer response time to questions

5. Which of the following statements most accurately describes normal aging changes in an older adult?

   a. As individuals age, they become more diverse.

   b. Most older adults experience chronic illness and functional impairment.

   c. Age-related changes are similar in each older adult.

   d. Normal age changes most commonly describe decline and loss of function.

3 Supporting Life Transitions and Spirituality in the Elderly

Mary Ann Anderson

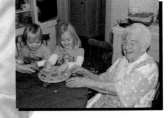

Learning Objectives

After completing this chapter, the student will be able to:

1. Identify the significance of transitions and spirituality in the lives of elderly people.
2. Describe what a transition is and the impact it has on people.
3. List four to six activities the nurse can perform that will facilitate a successful transitional outcome.
4. Define how the "progressively lowered stress threshold" concept can assist in the management of negative behaviors in older adults.
5. Discuss three transitions common to older adults.
6. Compare and contrast spirituality and religion.

INTRODUCTION

With today's harried workloads in health-care environments, you, the licensed practical nurse (LPN), may think that there is not time to deal with the issues of transition and spirituality. There are too many medications, too many treatments, and definitely too much paperwork! In addition, there are not enough licensed nurses and too many budget cuts. It is challenging and difficult for this generation of nurses to be able to deliver humanistic (vs. mechanistic) care. Transitions are a consistent part of life, however. Even the choice to be a more humanistic, holistic nurse requires a transitional period, during which time the nurse needs to work out the details of how to treat elderly people in a more caring and holistic manner, while still fulfilling all of his or her responsibilities on time. This chapter will assist you in understanding transitions and spirituality so that you can learn to incorporate holistic care into your daily practice.

SIGNIFICANCE OF TRANSITIONS AND SPIRITUALITY

Whatever your age, you have experienced a lifetime of *transitions,* which are the moments between what was old and what is new. One author describes transition as the moment when you let go of a trapeze bar (the old life) and are soaring through the unknown until you reach the second trapeze bar (the new life). That time between the bars, when you are hurtling through space, is frightening, unpredictable, and lacks familiar reference points. The time of the unknown, which is usually marked by the stress provoked by the change, is the *transitional* moment.

You experienced transitions after you chose to attend school. The need to pay for school, arrange child care, complete house work and school work, and maintain a part-time job are some possible challenges that you faced during the transition. Do you remember the stressful feelings you had until you worked out the details successfully? That period of stress and the unknown was the transitional period. You eventually resolved the stress of the changes and are now a successful student.

Youth is a period of constant growth and learning. A child learns to ambulate by first crawling, then standing up, and then walking; the child may then learn to ride a tricycle and then a bicycle. All of these instances involve periods of uncertainty as the child learns the new skill. Adults, too, experience transitions as they commit to an education and career, a spouse, and possibly children.

As people reach older adulthood, there is still much to learn and many new skills to master; however, it is also a time when more of life's changes include loss. I am referring to children leaving their parents' home for work, school, or adventure, among other choices. One's parents may die and siblings or friends may move or succumb to accident or disease. Retirement is a big change for most people, resulting in a loss of work friends, income, and often social position. As people age, some develop the chronic diseases of normal aging and other diseases such as heart disease, diabetes mellitus, or a debilitating stroke that results in physical and emotional losses.

Many of the life occurrences that accompany aging are challenging experiences, and all of them require older adults to make a life transition. No one experiences only one transition in a lifetime, and sometimes there is more than one transition at a time. Each loss or change requires transitional effort from the person experiencing it.

For example, I have a young-old friend who lives out of state, and she called me recently. She had fallen while attempting to do yard work; although she lives alone, a neighbor noticed that she was lying in her front yard crying with pain. She was found to have a broken wrist and a wrenched rotator cuff (shoulder). Her wrist was put into a brace, her arm was placed in a sling, and she was instructed to see an orthopedic surgeon that upcoming Monday. Yet on Sunday, she had so much pain in one of her teeth that she had an emergency root canal (I am not making this up!). She is a strong woman who has lived her life well. When I talked to her this morning, however, she was feeling despair. The changes she was dealing with were major and painful, and she was managing them alone. She needed assistance to move through the changes: someone kind who would keep her informed, provide honest hope regarding her situation, and care for her as the total person she is rather than the crying older woman she appeared to be. Humanistic health-care providers can assist her and people like her through this transition.

Now let us consider how spirituality fits into the concept of transition. *Spirituality* is often part of the process of transition for older people. Most people have a belief in God, the Divine, or a greater power. With this belief, there is a connection with something more powerful than oneself. When individuals have this connection, it links them to others with a similar belief. It also can be a link to nature or to familiar rituals and behaviors. Spirituality is comforting and can provide for many people a method for understanding the losses that are being experienced.

Spirituality can also provide the purpose for moving forward, for accepting and adapting to the losses that are occurring, and for finding the strength to deal with one's life changes. This ability to "move on" results in an improved quality of life and death. Let us return to my friend. She is a very religious person, and I know that she would want to see a clergyman and would appreciate someone to pray with her. I realize that you may not believe in God and may not pray. If that is the case, as her nurse you could offer to sit with her while she prays, and you could offer to call the clergyman. Because her religious beliefs have helped her through previous transitions in her life, she will benefit from

them again. Accepting and accommodating a person's spirituality to the best of one's ability is one of the many ways a holistic nurse can help a person through a transition.

UNDERSTANDING TRANSITIONS

Ralph Waldo Emerson, a poet, essayist, and philosopher who is described as belonging to the tradition of "wisdom literature," commented, "Not in all his goals, but in his transitions a man is great." Emerson understood change and its powerful impact on the life quest for individuals. Transitions are significant, universal human experiences. Because transitions are interconnected with the growth of the person and, consequently, the world, understanding transitions has rich significance for your personal and professional life and for your practice of human caring.

As a holistic nurse, your objective is to assist the older person in your care to be successful in making the transition and managing the stress. Doing so alleviates despair and promotes integrity for the individual, and it achieves your objective of excellent caregiving. Most people have experienced a critical transition; if you assist people in remembering the behaviors that were helpful to them in the past, they can use those behaviors again to help them through the transition that they are currently facing.

Common Transitions

High school graduation, sudden loss of a job, marriage, significant illness, death of a loved one, pregnancy, divorce, and relocation to a new home are some of the life events you may have experienced. These events are marked by beginnings and endings and a new phase of life change (the time between the trapeze bars). Joy and celebration at a transition are common, although some transitional events result in a deep sense of loss and sadness. Whether pleasant, painful, anticipated, unexpected, temporary, or permanent, all transitions, by their nature, evoke some degree of stress.

Patients often face health-illness transitions, which occur when changes in health status result in a change in role relations, expectations, and abilities. Multiple transitions occurring simultaneously are common and particularly challenging. For example, a health-illness transition precipitated by a severe stroke can require a person to relocate to a hospital, which could be followed by a second or even third relocation to a nursing home or rehabilitation center. In addition, there are the physical losses from the stroke: perhaps the loss of one's job and social role as the breadwinner. Dependence on others often is a difficult transition for most people to make.

The time span of a complex transition, such as having a stroke, extends from the first anticipation of transition until a sense of stability in the new situation has been achieved. A transitional period can last weeks or months, which indicates the critical need for nursing staff to know and understand the concept of transition. Only by understanding can the nurse be therapeutic.

Four Common Features of Transitions

Transitions are serious, life-altering experiences. They are processes of change that are lasting in their effects; they force one to give up how they view the world, and they necessitate the development of new thinking and skills. Transitions generally cause great emotion and require the

person experiencing the transition to work hard to survive the change. Transitions warrant the attention of health-care professionals.

According to researchers, there are four common features to transition:

1. A phase of turmoil
2. Disturbances in bodily function
3. Mood and cognition changes
4. An altered time perspective

These four characteristics are commonly seen in older adults in health-care facilities. Have you had experience with an older person who was in a state of turmoil, was unable to control bowel or bladder, seemed confused, and did not know the time or date? I realize that this could be a person with mental illness or any form of dementia, that a loss in bodily function is expected when someone has a stroke, and that time confusion is something that happens to people who are no longer tied to work schedules or routines.

So are these characteristics being exhibited because of illness or because of transition? All of these behaviors demonstrate a change for the person experiencing them, and so they are due to transitions. As a nurse, you can play a strong role in assisting a person to make sense of the change and to manage it with minimal symptoms. The objective is integrity vs. despair. With your thoughtful application of transition theory, you can assist the older people in your care to achieve integrity and improve their quality of life and death.

⬤ HOW TO INFLUENCE A TRANSITIONAL OUTCOME

You can influence the outcome of transitions for elderly people. The following factors have been identified as having a strong influence on transitional outcomes:

1. Degree of choice in the transitional process
2. Extent or degree of change
3. Preparation for the change

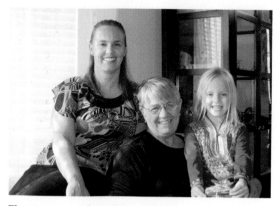

The moments of our lives combine to make a lifetime of transitions. This picture of a grandmother, mother, and daughter is symbolic of that concept.

4. Characteristics of the individual experiencing the transition
5. The individual's perception of the change
6. The characteristics of the prechange and postchange environment, including support systems

Let's examine these influences and see how nurses can use these influences to help ease older people into necessary transitions.

Give People a Degree of Choice and Respect Their Decisions

People who think they have freely chosen the transition are more likely to embrace it or own it. Think of the differences between your decision to come to LPN school and the fact that you "had" to go to high school. Choice is an essential part of being human, and it should be honored and respected.

I spent some time as a consultant at a large (700-bed) nursing home on the East Coast. While I was there, I learned some valuable lessons. The most profound lesson that I learned occurred on the very large Alzheimer's Unit. Everyone, and I mean *everyone*, included the residents in the decision making. For example, a resident refused his medication, and the polite and caring nurse agreed with the decision and came back within 10 minutes and tried again (successfully). She understood that the resident had the right to refuse any treatment, had the need to have some control over his life, and that—within just a few minutes—would forget that he refused the medication and might be amenable to taking it later. When the housekeeper asked to clean a resident's room and was told no, the decision-making authority to the resident was respected and the housekeeper did not go in, but returned when the resident was not in the room. The housekeeper accepted the negative answer, but did not neglect professional responsibility. Everything was done, just at a slightly later time.

Make the Extent or Degree of Change More Manageable

Transitions can be made smoother if the apparent obstacles are removed and the changes are manageable. A family asking their aging mother to relocate from a rural farmhouse to a city apartment to be closer to health-care services would require their mother to make a huge change, which would be very disruptive for the older woman. To ease their mother into the transition, a family member who lives in the city could invite her to stay for either a long weekend or a 2-week period so that she could get a feel for city life. Additionally, when the family members find an apartment that meets the physical requirements necessary for their mother, they could verify that there are people near their mother's age who live in or around the complex. Is there a senior citizen's center nearby where she can crochet with newly made friends? Is there a grocery store that is within walking distance? All of these are thoughtful considerations of a loving family that would make their mother's transition easier. They represent humanistic caring rather than mechanistic caring. The mechanistic solution would be to find an apartment that meets the location and safety needs of the mother, while doing nothing to make the transition less stressful. Which approach would you like someone to use with you?

Help Prepare People for the Transition

Although preparation for a transition is something logical to do, reflect how often people fail to prepare for a transition even though it is expected. Retirement is an excellent example. Death is something we all will experience, and yet it seems difficult for people in our society to discuss it and plan for it. Psychologists often say that the closer a family is, the easier it is to discuss the topic. When transitions are identified as part of one's future, preparation is a key factor in being able to manage them.

Talk to your patients and residents about changes that are anticipated. Give them all appropriate information and be willing to repeat it as often as necessary. You should involve the family members as well. Use your creative thinking and do all you can for each individual to prepare him or her for changes that are coming.

Consider the Characteristics of the Individual

Transitions can be very threatening to persons who are cognitively impaired or who require a high degree of structure and predictability in their environments. Research has shown that relocating people who are mentally ill or confused is associated with higher death rates compared with people with similar impairments who are not moved. Some people who are cognitively intact don't deal well with change either. It is common for people to fear or avoid change.

A person's personality, past experiences, and coping skills are important factors to consider when helping that person through a transition. Generally, being in good health increases resiliency during stressful times. Adequate sleep, nutrition, exercise, and satisfying social relationships are also important to transitional outcomes.

Learn How the Person Perceives the Transition

All of us create meaning and give our experiences labels. Different individuals can view the same transition as an opportunity, blessing, crisis, challenge, or disaster. Use your communication skills to listen to how a person perceives a transition and gain insight into the unique meanings that are attached to it for the person.

CRITICALLY EXAMINE THE FOLLOWING

Think back to your decision to go to school. What fears did you experience? Were there changes that you tried to avoid? Now think of an older adult in your life, either someone to whom you have given care or someone who is a friend or family member who has recently experienced a transition. Did you recognize their fears or resistance at the time? Do you see them now? They are there even if you did not recognize them.

It is dangerous to assume that you know what someone is thinking. It is better to invite their reflection on the transition and accept that there are differences in the way people think.

Remember the example of the woman who needed to move to the city from her farm? It is possible that she would love to be closer to her grandchildren, that she is excited about being near a wider variety of stores for shopping, and that she recognizes that she needs to be closer to health-care services.

Help Improve Environmental Characteristics

We all live in an environment with its variable aspects. When you walk onto a unit in a hospital or nursing home, can you sense what the environment really is like? I am not talking about cleanliness or colorful or drab decoration schemes, although they are important for a healing environment. I am referring to aspects of the environment such as cheerfulness, relaxation, nurturance, and respectfulness. These environmental components are the opposite of harsh, demanding, restrictive, and joyless environments. In caregiving situations, nurses have the power to cocreate with the older adults there healing environments that are loving, empowering, and respectful.

● PROGRESSIVELY LOWERED STRESS THRESHOLD

The "progressively lowered stress threshold" (PLST) is a care concept (Hall & Buckwalter, 1987) designed to be used when planning personalized, holistic care for elderly individuals. The concept of PLST originates from the importance of personal freedom and control. According to the PLST theory, dysfunctional or negative behaviors of humans often occur because of increased anxiety. If people perceive that they have lost their personal freedom or their control over a situation because of an increasing amount of outside stressors, they can become anxious and stressed, which leads to frustration and anger.

A classic example with which most people are familiar is getting children to eat their vegetables. Imagine a scene at the family dinner table when parents tell their children to eat their vegetables. By telling the children to do something, the children's personal freedom and control are taken away. Generally, this situation results in a power struggle (*note: no one* wins in a power struggle) and in the children not eating their vegetables.

An elderly person's freedom is restricted during the time he or she resides in a health-care facility. In hospitals and nursing homes, meals are generally served at set times, and baths are given at the convenience of the staff rather than of the patient or resident. No one is encouraged to stay up late and watch or read a good mystery! There are rules in health-care facilities, and they usually are enforced.

When people have limited control over their life, there is a higher likelihood that stress will occur. With unresolved stress comes frustration, and unresolved frustration leads to anger. That is a normal human reaction. What does anger look like? It is different for every person because of individual personality traits, but it can include raising one's voice, screaming, hitting, or a high level of criticism of the environment and the people in it. If you perceive that the reason behind the anger is stress because of lack of control, you can apply your understanding of PLST to your practice and work at giving the people in your care as much personal control over their lives as is safe for them.

CRITICALLY EXAMINE THE FOLLOWING

Take some time and think back to any recent experience when you were told what to do. How did you feel? Did it make you feel like a child? That is the feeling that comes to me. I like suggestions, interesting information, even metaphors, but I do not like being told what to do. I have learned over the years how to handle this feeling so that a situation does not degenerate into a power struggle, but I still have to take time to consider my reaction.

Write a brief paragraph regarding how you feel when someone imposes on your personal freedom. Note how you handle being told what to do and what your thought processes are regarding it. Then consider how your feelings compare with those of any elderly person with whom you have had experience. Does the older adult like being told what to do? How does he or she handle the situation? Be prepared to share your ideas in class either verbally or by handing in the paragraph.

Common Stressors

Five common stressors that tend to result in the highest levels of stress for older persons are:

1. Fatigue.
2. Change in environment, routine, or caregiver.
3. Misleading or inappropriate stimuli (sounds or noise are examples).
4. Internal or external demands to achieve that exceed one's functional ability.
5. Physical stressors such as pain, discomfort, infection, acute illness, or depression (Hall & Buckwalter, 1987).

I am sure that you can immediately see the relationship between transition and these five stressors. It is like "the perfect storm." Changing living environments is tiring (stressor 1), and it is a dramatic change in environment, routine, and caregiver (stressor 2). The person going through the transition may have great expectations from self to "do well" so as not to worry "my daughter" or to assure a return to one's home (stressor 4). Deteriorating health or a new illness (stressor 5) may be the very reason the elderly person was moved.

With this basic information on PLST, do you see how transitions and most other stressors will, in all likelihood, result in the older person showing signs of stress? It is a given for most of us and is something that needs to be recognized as a reality in giving care to susceptible older people.

Application of Progressively Lowered Stress Threshold

Your objective, each day you go to work, needs to be to decrease the stress of the persons in your care. This often includes the certified nursing assistants (CNAs) and other people in your work environment. Settle disputes among the staff, keep noise levels low, provide places of rest for elderly people in the facility to avoid fatigue, and expect stress-related behavior to occur.

When such behavior does occur, don't be upset and get involved in the problem. Instead, use your knowledge, and work to eliminate the stress. Perhaps taking an elderly man who is angry and combative off the unit for a "special walk" with you will remove him from what is upsetting him. Try to find out what is the stressor for any person who is acting stressed, and involve the other members of the health-care team in correcting the problem.

I remember a cold and snowy winter afternoon in Utah. My daughter, one of her friends, and I were traveling in the car. The girls were laughing and playing noisy games in the backseat, the radio was blaring something I didn't recognize, and, unknown to me, the temperature was falling. I recognized the fall in temperature the moment my tires started to slide on the newly formed ice into a monstrous snowdrift on the side of the road. If I corrected the slide, I would head into the oncoming traffic. I was stressed!

Within a brief second my entire personality changed. I turned off both the heater and the radio, I literally yelled at the girls to be quiet, and then miraculously (or so it seemed to me) I was able to stop the car with minor damage caused by the snowdrift. When the initial stress was over, I spoke with great concern and tenderness to the girls, turned the heater back on, and got out my cell phone to get the help I needed.

Why did my behavior change so abruptly? It was because of the stress. Without thinking, I turned off the radio and heater because they were stressors to me. Much to my chagrin, I yelled at the girls because their noise was a stressor as well. Then, with less external stress, I could handle the immediate situation.

Have you seen exasperated mothers of young children raise their voice at them in a store? A man swearing out loud because of a flat tire? Two children or two adults hitting each other? I observe that they usually are exhibiting such behavior because they are stressed. Relate the concept of stress and the resulting behavior to yourself. Once you understand how it affects you, you will have a better understanding of how and why it makes a big impact on elderly people, who often have fewer physiological resources.

Remember the initial premise of the PLST model. It is to give as much control as possible to the individuals in your care. After all, they are adults who are accustomed to making their own decisions, and, in most situations, they should be allowed to continue. This premise requires the entire health-care team to understand and agree to provide such an environment.

Transition is challenging, and being older can be difficult. The role of the LPN is to do everything possible to make these realities less stressful and enhance the quality of daily life for older adults.

Read the following poem. It is charming and meaningful. Read the poem to enjoy it, and then read it again to look for the impact of transition and PLST on human life.

Sunshine Acres Living Center
Marilyn Krysl, RN

The first thing you see up ahead is

Mr. Polanski,

wedged in the arched doorway,

like he means absolutely

to stay there; he shouldn't

be there in the first place, put here

by mistake, courtesy of that grandson

who thinks he's a hotshot, and too busy

raking in the dough to take time

for an old man.

If he had anyplace to go, you know he'd

be out instantly, if he had any money.

So he intends to stay in that doorway,

not missing a thing, and waiting for
trouble.

Which of course will come.

And that could be you—you're handy,
you look

likely, you have the authority. And you're

new here, another young
whippersnapper,

doesn't know ankle from elbow, but has

been given the keys.

Well, he's ready, Mr. Polanski. So you go
right

to him. "Mr.Polanski, good morning." You

say it in Polish, which you learned a
little of

when you were little, and your grandmother

taught you a little song about lambs,
frisking

in a pen, and you danced a silly dance
with

your grandmother while the two of you
sang.

So you sing it for him in the dim,
institutional

light of the hallway, light which even you
find

insupportable, because at that moment

it reminds you of the light in the hallway

in the rest home where, when your

Grandmother died, you weren't there.

So you're also singing to console yourself.

And at the moment you pay her this silly

little tribute.

Mr. Polanski steps out of the doorway. He

who had set himself to resist you, he who

made himself a first, Mr. Polanski,

> contentious

> often combative

> and always inconsolable

hears that you know the song. And he
steps out

from the fortress of the doorway, begins to
shuffle

and sing along.

This poem captures many aspects of human relationships and struggles. You may want to discuss your insights about the poem's message with fellow students or family members. As an LPN, you will have many opportunities to meet people like Mr. Polanski.

Understanding the mediating factors of control and decision making, preparation, support, meaning and perception, and maintaining optimal health will assist you in your own transitions as well as in supporting and caring for older people.

● COMMON TRANSITIONS FOR OLDER ADULTS

As I have stated, transitions occur at every stage of life. It is important to examine the transitions that commonly occur in the lives of older adults to anticipate them and develop the knowledge base to be supportive when they occur. As you know, not all transitions happen for everyone, but some can be anticipated because of their frequency in the aging process. Job changes and retirement, family role changes, and health changes are common impetuses for transitions that occur with older people.

Job Changes and Retirement

Job changes and retirement can have a dramatic impact on the aging population. Common changes include the following:

1. *Role change.* When an older person retires, the role change can be a very difficult transition. The person retiring has to adjust to the loss of what was their purpose and position for 8 or more hours a day.
2. *Lower income.* A retiree's income often is decreased. This can be the cause of several other changes. Health care can be reduced because of the financial need to maintain the house or replace a furnace. Good nutrition may be impacted because of the expense of essential medication. Plans of traveling or other leisure activities may have to be cancelled.
3. *Dissatisfaction with employment status.* Older adults generally were raised with a strong work ethic and believe that unemployment is an unacceptable situation whatever the cause.
4. *Unpreparedness for the future.* Many people do not prepare for their eventual retirement. They have not developed interests outside of work, prepared financially for a decreased income, or nurtured their dreams. Without preparation, retirement can be fraught with profound losses for the individual.

5. *Loss of identity.* For some people, the loss of their job, with retirement or other factors, threatens their identity. Most people derive their identity from the work they have done throughout their lifetime. Be it mother, physician, teacher, or nurse, part of who we are rests solidly on what we do. When that crucial role is gone, it is a struggle to redefine one's personal identity, and that struggle is not always successful.

6. *Lack of social interaction.* Someone who has been focused on their work setting often has many friends there. With retirement comes a separation from those people. This can be a serious transition unless the retiree has been wise enough to maintain relationships outside of work. Without friends to join in social activities, life can be very lonely.

Family Role Changes

Family roles and relationships change as each of us age. Common changes in old age are the following:

1. *Grandparenting.* Because of the aging of America, more people experience grandparenting, and many are able to enjoy this phase of life longer than ever before in U.S. history. There can be serious transitional concerns, however, with the various roles grandparenting can take.

2. *Distant family members.* Adult children move out of the house, and many are scattered throughout the United States. Older people of today frequently were raised with the responsibility to build their adult lives in a location near their parents to promote family closeness and to care for their aging parents. Today's grandparents often have to adjust to not seeing children and grandchildren as frequently as they would like, and they cannot count on adult children to assist them to remain in their homes as they age.

3. *Parenting for parents.* Some grandparents are assisting single parents by providing child care or are tending children while both parents work. For many older adults, this can be too much responsibility in the day-to-day activities of their children and grandchildren.

4. *Role crisis.* Parents eventually die. In some situations, the illness and death are lingering, which requires the caregiver to be part of what is known as the "sandwich generation." This role often goes to the woman. The sandwich generation caregiver is a person who is raising children while caring for aging parents. As this person ages, the children leave the home, and the parents die. This can cause a role crisis because there is no one left who needs the "sandwiched" person.

5. *Death of spouse.* The death of a spouse is more common as people age. It is an event that has a dramatic impact on all aspects of life for the surviving partner. Although divorce did happen in the "olden days," it did not happen as often as it does currently. When an older spouse dies, the survivor has lost the person with whom they have spent most of their life. The intimacy that was shared is gone as is the help, understanding, and often part of the income. Their experiences together can be the most significant happenings that have occurred during their lifetime. With the deceased person go dreams, plans for the future, and a lifelong companion. The loss can be intolerable.

6. *Insufficient income.* More women than men experience the death of a spouse. Because of their age, many older women have not worked outside of the home and are poorly prepared to supplement their income. Their life role generally has been focused on their spouse and children. These women end up alone, without the income they need, and with fewer friends because most of their

CRITICALLY EXAMINE THE FOLLOWING

What can you do now to prepare for your retirement? Think in terms of financial, physical, and emotional health. Seriously ponder what it is you want to be able to do when you retire and what it would take to fulfill those plans.

POINT OF INTEREST

According to Charlotte Eliopolous (2010), more than one in six older adults live in poverty. She also states that of the people who are currently in the work force, only half of them will retire with a pension plan.

previous friends were couples. If their children and grandchildren are living in other states, the situation is even more difficult because they are truly alone.

Health Changes

Health changes are complex concerns for older adults. They can affect every system in the body and cause a change in one's health that has a life-altering impact. Some common health changes are as follows:

1. *Illness and disability,* which are major reasons that older adults need assistance and support. Older people generally have one to three chronic diseases that, it is hoped, can be managed, but are never cured. More than one-third of the elderly people in the United States have a disability that limits doing yard work or housework. This may extend to cooking as well. Along with the disappointment over what they are unable to do, older adults with disabilities often worry about being placed in an institution such as a nursing home or assisted living facility. The overall fear is the loss of independence.

2. *Acute diseases.* It could be the flu or pneumonia, a heart attack, or some type of infection. Regardless, older adults often do not have the strength to fight such acute illnesses as they did when they were younger. The immune system commonly is weaker because of aging. Every winter, numerous older people die of pneumonia because their bodies are no longer strong enough to ward off the disease.

3. *Body image.* Adjusting to a new body image is another challenge of growing older. There may be crippling from arthritis that interferes with routine activities such as cooking or walking. The older body gains weight and becomes shorter, hair color changes, and vision and hearing diminish. There are also changes related to acute and chronic diseases. All of these conditions can cause an altered body image or lower one's self-esteem.

4. *Longer physiologic response time.* The aging body does not work as efficiently as it once did. Fatigue is often a daily occurrence along with decreased memory function and slower response time.

It is important for you to keep these transitional situations in mind as you care for older people. For example, even if you have seen numerous people put into wheelchairs because of the pain and danger of arthritis, remember that it is each person's first time doing so. During the transition, there is fear and concern on the part of the older adult and the need for support and understanding from you. Preparing yourself to assist people through the transition is a critical aspect of giving holistic nursing care.

⬤ SIGNIFICANCE OF SPIRITUALITY

In the lifelong search for integrity vs. despair, spirituality has a significant role. Most people feel they are part of something very important when a spiritual bond connects them to others. There is a commonality in belief and understanding of the universe. The belief system often provides a social system as well. These aspects of spirituality are supportive to someone going through one or several transitions.

Religion and Spirituality

There is a difference between religion and spirituality. *Religion* is the organized practice of one's belief regarding God or a higher power. Most religions have a formal building for worship and prescribed actions (prayer) or practices (partaking of the sacrament). Some religions worship personages other than a God or simply believe in a Divine power. Religion is an organized practice, whereas *spirituality* is the feeling within that communicates to individuals there is a higher power at work in the universe. Many spiritual people do not belong to a religion but practice beliefs they feel strongly about regarding a higher power.

Humans, by their nature, are spiritual. This makes awareness of and concern for another's spiritual and religious needs a significant aspect of nursing care. Being supportive while sharing and participating in a person's spiritual beliefs is an important aspect of holistic care.

Realizing their connection to something greater than themselves assists all people to rise above their challenges. For older adults, this sense of connection to a greater being is very important because of the numerous losses and transitions they make as they age. Spirituality and the practice of formal religion can assist people to overcome their problems, manage their despair, and find the peace that will help them to accept the change that is occurring. Spirituality and religion help provide the essential step toward integrity and gerotranscendence.

Assessing Spiritual Needs

Assessing people for their spiritual needs and identifying how you can assist in meeting them may be a new skill for you. Most health-care facilities list the religious preference of the person on the chart. That is the place to start. Use your observation skills to identify religious jewelry or other artifacts in the person's personal belongings. Are there religious books in the room such as the Koran, Book of Mormon, or Bible?

The facility where you work may have a spiritual assessment. If not, think about what it is you need to know to be helpful. The information you need should include the following:

1. Does the person belong to a formal religious group? If so, does he or she want the leader of the group or other members to visit? Are there special rituals the person would like to have performed, such as a blessing for health, a prayer circle, or something else?
2. You need to know the person's specific spiritual beliefs, so ask. Then inquire if there are any specific practices the person would like to see performed. This may include a Shaman from the Navajo Indian culture, being allowed out of bed to pray on the floor facing East for a Muslim, incense burning, or specific foods. You cannot meet an individual's spiritual needs unless you know what they believe.
3. When a person in your care is found crying, exhibits depression, or simply does not seem interested in what is going on in the environment, these could be symptoms of spiritual distress. A person may continuously question, "Why is God doing this to me?" or, "What have I done to deserve all of these problems?" Comments of this type often are expressions of an unmet spiritual need.
4. Some people exhibit anger at God or the Divine power because of the severity of the transition that must be made. Loss of basic physical ability because of a severe stroke or unmanageable pain from cancer could be examples. An older adult may feel betrayed by God and express unusual anger. This symptom of unmet spiritual needs should be addressed with understanding and empathy.

Resolving Spiritual Needs

Research indicates that a meaningful spiritual or religious practice promotes health and healing in many people. Because of this fact alone, you need to strive to identify unmet spiritual needs.

When you have identified such needs, determine interventions that will help the older adult in your care. You should do all you can to assist the person to meet the unmet needs. This may require quiet listening, meaningful discussions, and the involvement of outside people from the religious or spiritual groups of the person.

To learn what you need to be helpful, you need to *listen attentively*. Ask questions if you do not understand what has been said. Plan time so that you can stay with the person until he or she is through with what they what to say. Then take this new understanding to your nurse manager and, together, identify a way to resolve the spiritual need.

It is essential that you *accept the beliefs* of the person in your care, even if you do not agree with them. Your support of another's belief system is as important as your support when you assist someone to walk. Work with the family and spiritual leaders to provide the spirituality that will assist with comfort and healing.

Provide the people in your care with time alone so that they can participate in religious activities. This time could be spent praying, reading scriptures or other meaningful books, or meditating in solitude. Solitude is a valuable asset for most spiritual people. Do all you can to provide it for your patients while still caring for their physical needs.

Remember the spiritual need that is expressed with anger toward God or a Divine power? It generally is based on the need to make sense of the transition that has occurred. *Do **not** be judgmental* when you hear this anger. Be empathetic, and do all you can to understand the person's point of view. Look at the situation as if you were the person so that you can more readily understand the frustration being expressed. Let's be honest: Some things are not fair, but nevertheless they do happen. Do not join in the anger and do not criticize the anger; rather, listen and make nonjudgmental comments designed to be comforting.

Prayer is a common tool for spiritual people. I realize you may or may not pray; however, if a person in your care requests someone to pray with, please do what you can to assist the person. You might hold a hand or sit near and be reverent during the prayer. If you are uncomfortable with prayer, find a coworker who can assist the person. The objective is to support the person with unmet spiritual needs so that he or she can achieve management of the illness or problems being faced. You play a crucial role in that goal achievement.

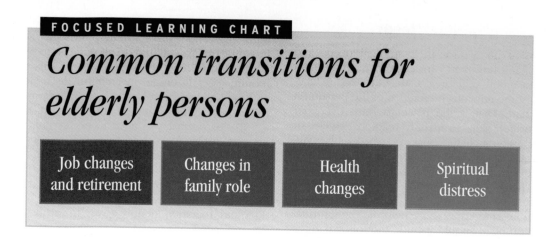

Common transitions for elderly persons

| Job changes and retirement | Changes in family role | Health changes | Spiritual distress |

⬤ RESOLVING TRANSITIONAL PROBLEMS

At this point, you understand the basics of transitional and spiritual care. I hope that you also understand the importance of meeting the needs that arise based on those concepts. Meeting such needs contributes greatly to improved health, the ability to manage distress, and the all-important objective of achieving integrity and eventually gerotranscendence. Gerotranscendence allows an older person to live life without regret and to die well, which is something we all would like to achieve. That makes finding a way to implement the resolutions to transitional situations a quality-of-life as well as a quality-of-health issue.

I realize that your workloads are heavy and that fulfilling the medical orders and personal care needs of the individuals to whom you give care is essential for you to do. If you believe in holistic care, however, assisting an older adult who is under the stress of seemingly insurmountable transitions is also essential and needs to be addressed. You may need to talk to your nurse manager and determine if family members or volunteers could be thoroughly oriented to the skills needed to take over that responsibility. If volunteers are used, ensure that there is an effective way for them to communicate with you regarding what they learned. Perhaps the patient or resident mentioned a spiritual person or ritual he or she would like to be with or experience, or perhaps there is a person the patient or resident wronged and wish to apologize to before death. It is important you learn of the unmet needs so that these can be resolved, if possible.

One way to help older people resolve transitional problems and move toward integrity and gerotranscendence is life review. Staff members who value the lives of older people are also key to providing holistic care and guidance to aging residents and patients.

Life Review

The objective of this activity and the activities described subsequently is to assist older people to review their lives and appreciate them. If there are items the older adults feel need to be resolved, life review also gives them that opportunity.

I often hear families complain about having to listen to the same stories over and over again from their elderly parent or grandparent. This storytelling is not unhealthy behavior. Instead, it is exactly what the older adult should be doing to achieve integrity. When health declines and the older person's social system gets smaller, it is healthy to reflect on the accomplishments of one's life. In that reflection, the older person can identify strengths that will assist with current transitions as well as feel the satisfaction of good deeds and good times.

This crucial behavior requires time from you or others assigned to do life reviews. Volunteers with maturity and a deep sense of responsibility can be taught to do effective reviews.

Sometimes there is an event in life about which the person feels shame and remorse. It may be difficult for you or the volunteer to listen to older persons reveal their mistakes and talk about the people they have hurt. Yet, this information should be shared. Talking about life errors to a kind and attentive listener is therapeutic

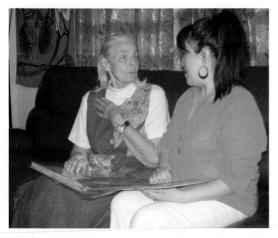

This home health nurse is assisting her patient with reminiscence therapy. Notice how involved the older woman is in telling her story or memory after seeing pictures in her scrapbook.

and should be encouraged. Sometimes referrals to a counselor or therapist should be made. This is a strong reason for you to keep in close contact with volunteers who may do life reviews on the unit. In addition to verbal life reviews, written and visual life reviews can be created by the older adult and their caregivers and loved ones.

Writing One's Life Story

When writing a life story, many adults do not feel as if it is something they can do. It is especially difficult if they hand-write rather than use a word processor. This is where a volunteer would be very effective. Initially, the volunteer needs to develop a relationship with the older person. It can be determined if a tape recorder or simply talking would be the best way to share the person's life story. The volunteer would need to be able to write on a word processor while the older person is talking or interview the older person while using a tape recorder. Then the information on the recorder would need to be typed. There is a great satisfaction in recording one's life events. It is even better when there is a willing listener and facilitator for the project.

Imagine the satisfaction of having your life recorded, even if it is just you who reads it. That is seldom the case, however. This type of life review meets the same needs as previously discussed. Perhaps the family could be involved and copies made for the children and grandchildren. A copy of a life story could be put on each chart or in a specific file so that staff members could read it and know the person better. Keep in mind that you would need permission from the person, whose story it is, to share it with the staff.

Collecting and Organizing Photos

Many people I know have boxes of photos that are unlabeled and disorganized. When those boxes exist for an older adult, it could represent the disorganization they are feeling in their life. Suggesting to a family member or recruiting an effective volunteer to assist in the organization and labeling of, quite literally, one's life is a significant thing to do. This is another way to do a life review. It provides the opportunity for the older person to relive precious moments, note the voids in pictures because of a family argument, or simply enjoy the grandchildren's pictures when they were babies.

The final product, the photo album, often becomes a treasured item to be shared with others. The significance of one's life is then visually apparent. The scrapbook provides the opportunity to reassess one's life and experience a sense of accomplishment.

Staff Who Value the Lives of Older People

If you are working on a unit that has a large percentage of older adults, or if you work in a nursing home, I hope that people who value the lives of older people surround you. As you go through your daily workload, take the time to ask older adults about the Great Depression, World War II, or what it was like to grow a Victory Garden. Hopefully you know about the person and his or her culture and can ask questions that have significance for the person. When you ask a question, take the time to listen. Be especially alert for coping mechanisms that worked in the past for that individual. Listen for accomplishments and success stories that can be shared with the staff, and hopefully someone will ask to have the story told again.

Think of your own transitional stress and what helped you, then provide the same support for your patient. Consciously strive to be a truly holistic nurse by embracing the body, mind, and spirit of the person to whom you give care. You do this by following the medical plan of care (body), addressing transitional stress needs and all that accompanies those needs (mind), and meeting spiritual needs (spirit).

CONCLUSION

Transitions are an undeniable part of life. It is important to provide elderly patients and residents with holistic and humanistic care, assist them as they develop or hone the skills they need to manage their transitions, and support them in their religious beliefs and their spirituality. My hat (oops! My nursing cap) is off to you as you work at adapting to the transitions that come to you as a nurse. Accept the challenges, resolve the problems, and move the profession forward.

Mrs. Goldstein, age 82, was living at the local Hebrew Nursing Home after the death of her husband 8 months ago. She was admitted because she confused her heart medication with her arthritis medication and became dehydrated and fell. The fall resulted in a broken left humerus. She adjusted well to the nursing home and was allowed to bring in two of her favorite pieces of furniture, pictures of her husband and son, and artwork for the walls. Mrs. Goldstein is an Orthodox Jew who continued to practice her religion while in the home.

Mrs. Goldstein became confused during the night and fell while trying to get out of bed. She fractured her femur and bumped her forehead. After assessing her, the nursing home sent her by ambulance to St. Mary's hospital. You are Mrs. Goldstein's nurse postoperatively.

As Mrs. Goldstein is being wheeled down the hall to her room, from surgery, you hear her crying out and repeatedly saying, "My head, what have you done to my head?" She is grabbing at her head while she repeats her question.

Discussion

1. You immediately go to her and attempt to determine what is wrong.
When she is recovered enough to eat something other than clear liquids, you bring her a light supper. On the tray are cheese, crackers, Jell-O, and a small slice of turkey. She immediately demands to know who fixed the food and where it was prepared. She pushes the tray away, and by doing so, knocks it onto the floor.

2. Determine what has caused this behavior and how you can assist her with what seems to be a problem.
The next day is Saturday, and Mrs. Goldstein refuses to go to physical therapy. This is very serious because the therapy department is closed on Sunday.
3. How will you resolve this problem?
Consider all three problems and determine what you can do to help Mrs. Goldstein.

Solution

1. Quietly approach Mrs. Goldstein after she has been transferred to her bed. Be calm and do not react to her crying out. Instead, calmly ask her "what is wrong?" Gently touch her arm, if she is receptive. Maintain eye contact; do not move quickly.

The problem is that this patient is an Orthodox Jew. It is part of her religion to keep her head covered as a statement of humility. When she awoke to find her head uncovered she was very upset. She explained to you that she would not have to worry about such things at the Hebrew Home. She requests to go back there immediately.

You cannot return her to the nursing home as quickly as she wishes, but you can find her scarf or locate something suitable so that she can cover her head. She calms down and then you feel you can do her postoperative assessment.

As you leave her room, you recognize that it may be a transitional stress for her to be at a Catholic hospital rather than a Hebrew nursing home. You plan to ask her about her spiritual needs as well.

2. You were thinking about Mrs. Goldstein and how to help her transition to an acute hospital when the certified nursing assistant (CNA) comes out into the hallway looking frantic. She announces that Mrs. Goldstein threw her dinner on the floor. You rush to the room, and once again ask, "what is wrong?" "This is not kosher food," she screams. "You are trying to kill me!"

The CNA timidly followed you into the room, and you send her for a kosher tray for Mrs. Goldstein. Apologize to her for not recognizing that her diet should be kosher. Ensure that the hospital prepares kosher meals all of the time and that the mistake will not happen again. Stay with the patient because she is very upset. Sit and look relaxed; listen to what she has to say about her husband's death. Listen for clues to what helped her with that major transition, and determine if it would be helpful in the current situation. If it is possible, stay

Continued on page 50

with her until her tray comes, and make sure it is satisfactory.

3. You are back on duty Saturday morning and Mrs. Goldstein refuses to go to physical therapy (PT). By this time, you had anticipated the problem. This woman is very serious about her religious rituals, and you and the staff were unaware of their importance to her. You go in and talk to her about PT. You discuss the significance of having PT the day after surgery, and you ask her if there is any type of compromise she can make. With some effort, the two of you work out a partial PT schedule for the day. Then you talk to the staff for Sunday, when PT is closed, and see if they will assist her with some basic exercises.

When you come back on Monday, you bring the picture of her husband and son from the nursing home. She cries when she sees it and states that she can do anything if Fred (her husband) is with her. She is wearing her headscarf, cheerfully eating a kosher breakfast, and is excited about working with the physical therapist. Her recovery will be challenging simply because of the seriousness of the fracture and her age, but you can see that you have made it easier for her.

1. The overall objective of recognizing and assisting clients with transitions is to:

   a. Resolve shame vs. doubt

   b. Lessen the complaints filed on your unit.

   c. Achieve gerotranscendence.

   d. Arrive at the top of Maslow's hierarchy of needs and be fulfilled.

2. The importance of understanding PLST is to:

   a. Give firm directions to older adults so they won't feel insecure.

   b. Provide health-care environments where older people have complete freedom to make decisions.

   c. Lower the stress threshold of the environment where older adults are given care.

   d. Assist older adults in making the decision to make a transition or to perform PLST.

3. The difference between spirituality and religion is:

   a. One is done in a formal building; the other can't be.

   b. One is a feeling that comes from within.

   c. The age of the person determines the difference.

   d. Spirituality is a category of highly functioning religious people.

4. Research with spirituality and religion indicates that:

   a. It does not impact people who believe in a Divine power only.

   b. It does promote health and healing.

   c. It should not be considered when planning nursing care.

   d. It is too personal to discuss with patients and residents.

5. The value of life review is to:

   a. Find something useful for the volunteers to do.

   b. To keep older people busy while they are hospitalized.

   c. To publish a book of older adults' lives and sell it as a fundraiser project.

   d. To gain understanding into one's successes and mistakes.

6. The importance of working with staff members who value older adults is:

   a. Everyone is the same and it makes the workload easier.

   b. It supports the philosophy of caring and holistic nursing care.

   c. You can share your transitions with each other.

   d. You know each other well enough to cover each other's shifts.

4

The Use of the Nursing Process and Nursing Diagnosis in the Care of Older Adults

Kathleen R. Culliton

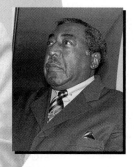

Learning Objectives

After completing this chapter, the student will be able to:

1. Describe the nursing process as a problem-solving technique in the context of assessment of the older adult, plan of care, nursing interventions, and nursing documentation.
2. Identify the use of the nursing process minimum data set (MDS) and resident assessment protocols (RAPs) in developing nursing care plans for residents in nursing facilities.
3. Use the nursing process to develop a care plan for the presented case study.

INTRODUCTION

Licensed practical nurses (LPNs) work in a variety of care settings. Each setting may require the LPN to function in a different capacity, yet each practice area expects the practical nurse to be involved with the assessment, planning, implementation, and evaluation of older adults and the care they receive.

▲ PRIORITY SETTING 4.1

There is a great deal of information in this chapter, and all of it points you toward the behaviors and thought processes of a licensed nurse. One of the unwritten objectives for you in attending school is to learn to think like an LPN, and this chapter provides the foundation for that type of thinking. Your priority for this chapter is to learn and put into practice the nursing process.

Using the nursing process in your everyday life will assist you in learning to think like a nurse. Remember the five stages of the process:

- Assessment
- Nursing Diagnosis
- Planning
- Implementation
- Evaluation

I suggest that you purposefully think in those five stages. It would work in most everyday situations. For example, when fixing dinner, you need to assess the number of people who will be eating and their likes and dislikes as well as the food you have on hand. Your nursing diagnosis would be the selection of food you choose to serve to a specific number of people. Then you plan the actual meal, implement the plan by serving the meal, and then evaluate the meal by obtaining feedback from those who ate it.

I know this seems simplistic, but it is critical to learn to think like a nurse. By going through the steps several times a day, you soon will think that way automatically.

ENVIRONMENTS OF CARE

Home Care

A relatively new practice area for LPNs is working in home care. LPNs in home care work under the direction of a registered nurse. They provide nursing care such as changing dressings, monitoring blood glucose levels, administering medications, and assessing the status of chronic disease processes in the older adult's home.

Hospital Care

LPNs work in various capacities with acutely ill older patients in the hospital. Often, the LPN is paired with a registered nurse to form a care team in providing nursing care. Other care delivery models may require the LPN to have specific tasks on the unit, such as treatments or passing medications for all of the patients on the unit.

Long-Term Care Facilities

The LPN may be employed in many types of long-term care facilities. *Skilled nursing facilities* and nursing facilities were previously thought of as nursing homes. These facilities generally provide a high level of nursing intervention. *Assisted-living facilities* provide care to older persons who may need assistance with activities of daily living (ADLs) but who do not require complex, skilled intervention (Eliopolous, 2010). *Continuing care retirement communities* have several levels of care, including skilled nursing, assisted living, and independent living apartments. Wellness clinics are frequently provided for residents living in independent apartments. LPNs could be employed in any one of these long-term care settings.

In the long-term care environment, the practical nurse collects admission data, provides input to the plan of care, carries out the nursing interventions that are outlined in the plan of care, and evaluates the effectiveness of these interventions in meeting the goals of the care plan for the older adult. Often, the LPN confers with the interdisciplinary health-care team (IDT) to share observations and clarify the plan of care. The LPN in these settings very often is responsible for working with nursing assistants to ensure the plan of care is carried out. Practical nurses often call physicians to clarify orders and to report changes in the

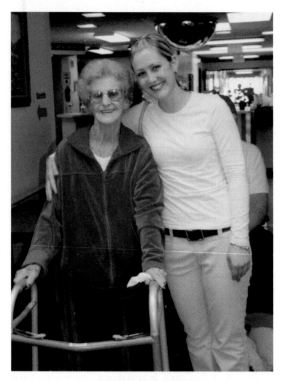

This woman soon will be discharged from the nursing home where she has been for the past 8 weeks because of a fractured hip. While at home, she will receive nursing and physical therapy as home care. Because of the multiplicity of services available to her, she spent only 5 days in the hospital and will be home much quicker than she would have been a decade ago.

airway. After the nurse does the abdominal thrusts, the resident is assessed for respiratory movements. If the person is breathing again, the nurse takes a deep breath, cuts the resident's meat into smaller pieces, and observes the resident eating the rest of the meal. If the resident is not breathing, the nurse may attempt another abdominal thrust or reposition the resident so that another abdominal thrust can be done from behind.

This short scenario is an example of the nursing process (Fig. 4.1). When the LPN entered the room and saw the older person with hands clenched on the throat and turning blue, the nurse was collecting data. In a split second, the nurse identified the resident's problem as choking. The nurse's next thought was to set a goal for this resident's care: the resident will expel the food that is causing the choking. With the goal of expelling the lodged food, the nurse designs the plan from nursing knowledge and immediately implements abdominal thrusts. After the nursing intervention, the nurse evaluates the situation to determine whether the resident has expelled the food. If the resident has not, the nurse must rethink and redesign the plan and immediately implement the revised nursing actions.

Nurses are faced with many patient-care or resident-care problems every day (note that residents are people who have been admitted to long-term care facilities). The nursing process provides a structure for nurses to plan and give high-quality, individualized care.

resident's health status. The practice of LPNs in nursing facilities is the practice model referred to in this chapter.

NURSING PROCESS

The nursing process is a problem-solving model that describes what nurses do. It identifies the way nurses approach patient care, and it recognizes the ongoing and changeable nature of the care that nurses provide, care that is based on the individual needs of the patient. Consider the following example.

An LPN in a long-term care facility walks into a resident's room and finds the resident with a supper tray in place. The resident is unable to talk and is turning blue. The nurse thinks that the resident is choking. Quickly, the nurse moves the meal tray out of the way and uses a two-handed thrust under the resident's diaphragm to attempt to dislodge the food that is obstructing the

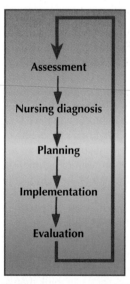

FIGURE 4.1. Nursing process model. The circular nature of this model demonstrates that the process is ongoing.

Assessment

The first step in the nursing process is to collect all of the information the nurse will need to identify clearly the older person's strengths and current and potential problems. Usually, the assessment starts with the call or written summary from the agency or department that is transferring the older adult to your nursing care area. Before the actual transfer takes place, your nursing care area should have the following information regarding the incoming patient or resident:

- Name, age, and insurance identification numbers
- Medical diagnoses, advanced directives, and disease prognosis
- Family support
- Need for equipment (Does the person need special equipment, such as a special bed, oxygen, intravenous [IV] setup, or feeding pump?)
- Functional ability (How does the person transfer, ambulate, move in bed, bathe, toilet, and eat?)
- Medications (Which prescription and over-the-counter medication does the person take?)
- Cognitive ability (Is the person oriented? How is the person's memory?)
- Special needs (Is the person depressed or at risk for skin breakdown or other health risks?)

This information is very important for the preparation of the older person's bed and room and makes the transfer to your care as smooth as possible.

After the older person is transferred, the nurse makes a focused assessment that culminates in a comprehensive assessment. The admission assessment includes a nursing history, observations, physical examination, review of laboratory values, and an interview with the older adult and his or her family.

In 1987, the federal government enacted legislation that set minimum standards for the assessment and care-planning processes in nursing facilities certified for Medicare reimbursement. This legislation is known as the Omnibus Budget Reconciliation Act of 1987 (OBRA 1987). This legislation was followed by OBRA 1990, which clarified some of the questioned areas of OBRA 1987. The minimum data set (MDS) and resident assessment protocols (RAPs) were a part of the legislation that had been implemented across the United States in nursing facilities that

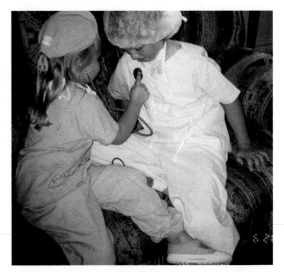

Although these children are only "playing nurse," they are illustrating what each reader of this book needs to do—practice, practice, and practice physical assessment skills until you have confidence in them.

accept Medicare and Medicaid funding as reimbursement for the care they provide. The MDS and the RAPs are two components of the mandated assessment process entitled the Resident Assessment Instrument (RAI). I realize that I just threw three abbreviations at you, so I want to go over them again. It is important that they become automatic language for you when you work in a long-term care facility.

Resident Assessment Instrument (RAI)

Every person admitted to a long-term care facility *has to have* a Resident Assessment Instrument (RAI) form completed, and the form must be updated every 3 months. If a long-term care facility is reimbursed by federal monies, that is the law. There is a sample RAI for you to work with when you complete the case study at the end of the chapter and in the Appendix at the end of the book. It is an important form and one you will need to understand and be able to contribute to as you assess the residents. Simply repeat it several times and it will begin to grow on you! Just think RAI, RAI, RAI!

Minimum Data Set (MDS)

The minimum data set (MDS) is just that—the absolute smallest amount of information that must be collected on every resident. It is the minimum. Nurses in long-term care facilities walk around asking each other "… have you done the MDS on Mrs. Hashamoto?" "… on Mr. Nay?" and others. The MDS contains information from all disciplines that work with the resident (i.e., nursing, social work, physical therapy, and dietary). When you work in long-term care, you will, I hope, become obsessed with completing the MDS.

Resident Assessment Protocols (RAPs)

When the MDS is completed, it provides a comprehensive assessment as well as indicators of risk for the resident. These are known as the "resident assessment protocols (RAPs)." The RAPs are the reason the RAI is done because they guide all caregivers as to how to give individualized care to the resident. In addition, the RAPs and RAI are caring and holistic.

What does a nurse do with all of the information that has been collected during assessment? The MDS refers care providers to a list of problem areas that must be addressed in the plan of care. Each of these problem areas

also has a RAP that lists areas that require further assessment and consideration before designing the plan of care (Box 4.1).

Frequently, RAPs are not actually incorporated into the assessment process. These protocols extend the assessment, however, from the minimum information of the MDS and offer a more thorough review of the identified problem areas.

Nursing Diagnosis

Developing the nursing diagnosis is a primary responsibility of the registered nurse. It involves the use of diagnostic reasoning to reflect the older person's strengths, problems, and potential problems. The registered nurse considers the assessment data and organizes them to decide whether they meet criteria for a specific nursing diagnosis. The North American Nursing Diagnosis Association (NANDA) has identified diagnoses that are widely accepted and understood by multiple disciplines and are viewed as

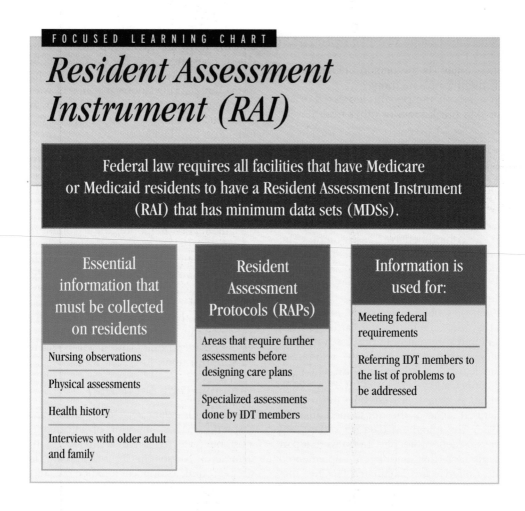

FOCUSED LEARNING CHART

Resident Assessment Instrument (RAI)

Federal law requires all facilities that have Medicare or Medicaid residents to have a Resident Assessment Instrument (RAI) that has minimum data sets (MDSs).

Essential information that must be collected on residents

Nursing observations

Physical assessments

Health history

Interviews with older adult and family

Resident Assessment Protocols (RAPs)

Areas that require further assessments before designing care plans

Specialized assessments done by IDT members

Information is used for:

Meeting federal requirements

Referring IDT members to the list of problems to be addressed the national standards for nursing diagnoses. The NANDA diagnoses are not specific to older people, but they are useful in providing consistent expression of nursing diagnoses for all disciplines and in all settings. An example of a NANDA diagnosis is the following: *Comfort altered, Pain, related to: degenerative joint disease.*

In the long-term care setting, nurses often prefer to use nursing diagnoses that incorporate the MDS language and format. An example of an MDS-related nursing diagnosis is the following: *Potential for joint pain due to degenerative joint disease.* Common nursing diagnoses for older adults include the following:

- Self-Care Deficit
- Physical Mobility, impaired
- Nutrition, altered: less than body requirements
- Injury, high risk for
- Urinary Elimination, altered
- Constipation
- Thought Process, altered
- Skin Integrity, impaired: high risk for

The registered nurse is responsible for ensuring that nursing diagnoses address the comprehensive assessment. The nursing diagnosis is an important part of the nursing process and addresses the potential and actual problems of the older adult.

Nursing Diagnosis and Medical Diagnosis

There are two basic ways to communicate the nature of an older adult's health problems. One way is by medical diagnoses, and the other is by nursing diagnoses. Medical diagnoses are made by a physician and describe a disease or a disease process. Diseases are diagnosed by identifying a specific group of signs and symptoms. For example, diabetes mellitus is diagnosed when a person has elevated fasting blood glucose levels, weight loss, thirst, and a large urine output. A person who has an area of dead brain tissue on magnetic resonance imaging (MRI) and computed tomography (CT) scans, along with speech and swallowing difficulty and left-sided paralysis, would be diagnosed with a cerebrovascular accident. Both of these medical diagnoses are common for older adults and communicate information to the nurse about what physical or psychological processes are happening to the person.

The major problem with planning care based only on medical diagnoses is that they do not describe the individual problems of the older adult or the impact the disease has on the person's day-to-day life. Nursing diagnoses are specific to the individual older person's nursing care needs and frequently relate to the areas in which the older person has difficulty functioning. For example, an obese person who is newly diagnosed with diabetes mellitus may have the following nursing diagnoses:

- *Nutrition, altered: more than body requirements and knowledge deficit related to poor dietary practices.*

A patient with long-term diabetes may be experiencing problems with a heel ulcer that will not heal. In this case, the nursing diagnosis would be as follows:

- *Skin Integrity, altered.*

Both of these people have the same medical diagnoses but different health-care needs, as shown in their nursing diagnoses.

Planning

After organizing the assessment data and noting the nursing diagnoses identified by the registered nurse, you, the LPN working with the older adult, the family, and the health-care team, begin the planning part of the nursing process. The planning portion of the nursing process includes setting priorities, identifying goals and outcomes of care, and designing and documenting interventions.

Setting Priorities

The nurse reviews the nursing diagnoses and places them in priority order. Remember the example at the beginning of this section? Removing the lodged food so that the resident could breathe would be a higher priority than putting on the resident's shoes!

One of the most popular models used to assist the nurse in setting priorities is Abraham Maslow's hierarchy of needs. This framework gives life-sustaining needs the highest priority. These needs are followed by safety and security needs, love and belonging needs, self-esteem needs, and self-actualization needs.

Because the nursing process is focused on the older person as an individual, it also is necessary to consider the priorities of the resident. Often, a resident will state that the highest priority is to go home. The resident may refuse treatments, medications, and activities that would maintain personal health because no one is assisting in the patient's discharge. Although discharge may not be realistic (at this time), you, as the nurse, will probably be more successful in providing nursing care if the plan of care addresses discharge to home as a high priority.

Following is an example of how the nutrition nursing diagnosis can be considered:

- *Nutrition, altered: less than body requirements*
  - Resident refuses to eat and drink.
  - Discuss with the resident what is usually eaten at home and how it is prepared.
  - Review how the resident's current health status would affect the ability to buy food, prepare it, and eat at home.
  - Discuss strategies and plans for ensuring that the resident is able to eat after returning home.
  - Include the resident's food preferences in meals.

Goal Setting or Identifying Outcomes

After identifying the priorities for the resident's care, the nurse identifies goals or outcomes for each of the nursing diagnoses. Setting goals is something that most of us do all of the time. Sometimes our personal goal may be to clock out on time or to survive a busy day. The goals that are part of the planning process describe the specific resident outcomes and identify the goals that direct nursing care. To direct care and describe outcomes, goals must be:

- *Measurable*—measurable outcomes need to be identified. "Eating 100% of a meal" can be measured, whereas it is difficult to measure "appetite will improve."
- *Realistic*—the goal must fit in with the resident's abilities. "The resident will recall the correct date and time" is probably an unrealistic goal for a person with Alzheimer's disease.
- *Specific*—the goal should identify certain behaviors or conditions to aid in their attainment and evaluation. "The resident will feel better" is not specific. It could be better worded as, "The resident will state that he has less nausea."
- *Timely*—a time frame needs to be established for the attainment of each goal. "The resident will walk 100 feet" does not specify a time frame for achievement of this goal. Adding "by the end of December" provides a time frame.
- *Attainable*—the goal should be written in such a way as to communicate a motivating factor to the resident and the nursing care staff. For an older adult with left hemiplegia, a goal such as "The resident will be independent in self-care by the end of the year" may be a strong motivator to work harder at the occupational and physical therapy sessions.

In nursing facilities, the documentation regulations under OBRA 1987 and OBRA 1990 require that the status of goal attainment be systematically addressed. These documentation requirements are

---

> **POINT OF INTEREST**
>
> Did you notice how many times the term *resident* was used in the previous explanation on outcomes? In the 1987 OBRA Act, the federal government determined that persons living in a long-term care facility are to be referred to as residents. The reason is because they live there; they are residents of the facility.

the monthly summaries (a comprehensive review of outcomes every 30 days) and the quarterly reviews (comprehensive interdisciplinary review of the resident's plan of care every 90 days) (Box 4.2). With new admissions or specific insurance carriers, the nurse may be required to conduct monthly comprehensive assessments of the outcome of care. This provides a 30- or 90-day time frame in which goals can be designed. It also helps the nurse think about what is realistic in that specific time frame. For a resident who is rehabilitating after having a hip replacement, "Ambulate independently" may be a realistic goal in 6 months. "Stand and walk 10 steps with a walker" may be a more realistic goal for 30 days. Following are examples of goals:

- The resident will eat more than 75% of each meal for the next 30 days.
- The resident will toilet independently when reminded to go to the bathroom for the next 90 days.
- The resident will attend one activity daily for the next 90 days.
- The resident will have no signs and symptoms of a urinary tract infection for the next 90 days.
- The resident's supplemental oxygen needs will be decreased to 1 L in the next 30 days.

Look back at these goals. What do you notice about them? Each goal identifies something that the resident will or will not do or will or will not experience. The resident's behavior is the major focus of goals as outcomes. Nursing care is not part of the goal. "Bathe the resident" is a nursing intervention, not an outcome or a goal. Nursing standards also are not part of the goal statements. "Administer all medications within 30 minutes of their ordered time" is a nursing standard, not a resident goal.

BOX 4.2 Assessments Needed for Each Nursing Home Resident

Comprehensive admission assessment including Resident Assessment Instrument (RAI)
1. Minimum data set (MDS)
2. Resident assessment protocols (RAPs)
3. Ongoing nursing assessment
Annual reassessment including RAI
Significant change in status assessment including RAI
Quarterly assessment including part of MDS

Designing and Documenting the Plan of Care

After the goals or outcomes of care are identified, the LPN, along with the other members of the IDT, begins to plan the activities that will help the older person reach the goals. The planning phase involves discussion and pen-and-paper activity. Discussing and documenting the plan of care allows input from all members of the team to be communicated to all staff members who are providing care for that resident. Standards of nursing practice and federal regulations require that each resident have a written, comprehensive, and interdisciplinary plan of care. The plan of care includes the problem or potential problem to be identified, the actions or interventions to be taken to address the problem, the person or discipline responsible for each action, and the goals to be achieved. An example of interventions in an interdisciplinary plan of care follows:

- Document percentage of food eaten at each meal—*nursing*
- Feed resident and assess swallowing ability—*speech therapy*
- Review dietary preferences—*dietary services*
- Promote feeding of self—*restorative nursing*

The focus of this chapter is on developing interdisciplinary plans of care using the nursing process. All disciplines caring for the resident need to be represented in an actual plan of care. This is an important criterion for planning interventions: planned interventions must complement the interventions of other therapies. For example, it would be confusing for the resident to be ambulated with a walker by physical therapy and encouraged to walk with two canes by the nursing staff.

It is crucial that members of all disciplines discuss and develop the components of the interdisciplinary plan of care so that confusion among the staff does not occur. Residents who are asked to perform one way in physical therapy and another way on the nursing unit can become confused as to how they should perform. A coordinated approach between physical therapy and nursing helps residents improve quickly and maintain function longer. A coordinated approach among all disciplines enhances the effectiveness of the care given to the resident and minimizes duplication of efforts.

Nursing interventions also must consider the safety of the resident. "Administering a diuretic and a sleeping pill at bedtime" is an unsafe nursing action. The resident may fall while going to

To be successful and effective, nursing interventions must be developed with input from certified nursing assistants (CNAs). CNAs are important members of the interdisciplinary team. Nursing assistants spend more time with residents in nursing facilities, assisted living facilities, and retirement communities and sometimes in the older adult's home than any other member of the IDT. They can offer important specific information for the assessment of the older adult. Because CNAs are so familiar with the daily routine and functioning of the residents, they can offer pertinent, realistic suggestions for individualized interventions to deal with specific problems. They also are frequently the first people to notice subtle changes in clients' conditions that may indicate onset of a new problem or success or failure of an intervention. A care plan meeting, including representatives of all disciplines, is generally held to discuss assessment information and develop the interdisciplinary plan of care. The CNA who works with the resident to be discussed should be invited to this meeting, and arrangements should be made to facilitate the CNA's attendance. The time away from the unit for the CNA is minimal compared with the value of the CNA's input into the care-planning process.

Successful nursing interventions require the resident's input and should be important to the resident. A resident may not want to "lift weights to strengthen and increase flexibility of his arms" but may be very willing to "comb his hair and wash his face." "Encourage the resident to drink 1000 mL of water" may not work as well as "encourage the resident to drink 1000 mL of fruit juice and water."

Nursing interventions also must include continuing assessment and monitoring of disease processes and effects of medications and treatments. If a resident has an IV, the IV site must be "assessed every shift for signs of infiltration, irritation, and infection." If a resident is receiving therapy with digoxin (Lanoxin), the "apical pulse must be taken and recorded before each dose." Residents with congestive heart failure (CHF) should be "assessed for edema and dyspnea."

The plan of care is part of the resident's permanent record. It needs to be routinely reviewed and updated as the resident's health status improves or declines. The monthly and quarterly review times provide excellent opportunities to revise the care plan to ensure that the resident is receiving appropriate nursing care.

the bathroom at night if still groggy from the sleeping pill. Transferring a resident who is able to stand only with the assistance of one staff member may place that resident at risk of falling.

Selected nursing interventions should help to attain the identified goal. If a resident's goal is to "lose 1 lb a week," then giving "dietary supplements between meals and at bedtime" would not assist in achieving this weight loss. When the resident's goal is "will ambulate 100 ft by the end of the month," a nursing intervention must state that the nursing staff will assist the resident to ambulate.

Nursing interventions also must be realistic for the resident, staff, resources, and equipment. A reality in the workplace is that there often is not extra time for staff to talk to the residents. Providing 30 minutes of one-on-one time every shift to discuss pain with the resident is an unrealistic intervention. Stating that each staff member "will ask the resident about hip pain whenever he or she interacts with the resident" is a more realistic intervention.

Implementation

Implementation is the part of the nursing process that nurses do best. Being at the bedside of the resident providing care is one of the most rewarding aspects of being a nurse. Implementation means putting the plan of care into action. Along with providing the nursing care that has been outlined in the resident's nursing care plan, the LPN continues to collect data that can be used to update and revise the plan of care.

Many interventions from the plan of care are assigned to CNAs; this is another strong reason to have CNAs attend the care plan development meeting. If CNAs have an opportunity to provide input into the plan of care and if they are present when it is discussed and developed, they will be more likely to carry out the interventions than if they are merely told what to do or handed a care plan to read.

Because nursing assistants on all shifts cannot attend the care plan meeting, a major challenge for the LPN is communicating the plan of care back to all CNAs. Various communication techniques can be used. Some facilities provide nursing assistants with written assignments that list all of the interventions for each resident. Many facilities place the plan of care in a book and make it available to the staff. Very often, however, the book is rarely consulted. Meeting regularly with nursing assistants to discuss the plan of care, giving each CNA written assignments with information on the plan of care, and using primary CNAs who care for the same residents each day ensure the implementation of the plan of care. These actions make it a working document rather than a useless piece of paper completed only to comply with regulations.

Another difficult aspect of implementation is that it must be documented. Charting is an important part of implementing the plan of care. Documentation of interventions requires recording not only that the intervention was done but also the resident's responses to the intervention. An entry such as the following provides no information about the resident's response to the treatment:

12/16/06 1420 Wet to dry saline packing to coccyx ulcer

A better picture is given in the following chart:

12/16/06 1420 Wet to dry saline packing to coccyx pressure ulcer. Ulcer is 3 × 2 cm and 1.5 cm deep. Ulcer margins are pink,

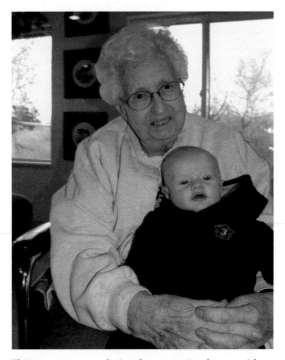

This woman was admitted to a nursing home with limited mobility, weakness, mild confusion, and heart failure. Her stated goal was to be strong enough to hold her great-grandchildren and to sit up and talk to her grandchildren, who ranged in age from 15 to 43. The MDS indicated several other goals to implement for her optimum health. As you can see, her priority goal as well as those identified through the MDS were met.

and there is granulation tissue evident. Small amount of yellow serous drainage on old packing. Resident complained of pain when old packing was removed and new packing inserted. Two small (6-mm) scabs on left buttocks from tape irritation. No redness or drainage noted.

Every visit with the resident is an opportunity to reassess nursing diagnoses and their implementation. Following is a simple model that can be used to document the nursing process with nursing interventions and resident responses:

- *Assessment*—What the nurse observed and assessed. Includes:
  - Objective measurements (blood pressure, laboratory values)
  - What the resident did (response to nursing intervention)
  - What the resident said

- *Action*—What the nurse did (nursing interventions): treatments, turning the resident, giving a medication, increasing the oxygen flow rate, hanging a tube feeding, inserting a catheter
- *Plan*—What the nurse plans to do: call the physician, call the family, reassess with the next treatment, refer resident to social services

The assessment-action-plan charting format is simple, yet it sets up a framework for documenting the nursing process in a narrative format.

CNAs also may be involved in documentation and may provide information for the LPN's documentation. For example, nursing assistants can complete flow sheets, which include interventions from the plan of care and activities from the resident's day. Flow sheets can be used to document such interventions as ADLs, walking programs, bowel and bladder training programs, and dietary intake and feeding programs. Results and trends from the flow sheets can be incorporated into the LPN's regular progress charting.

Evaluation

Evaluation is the final step in the nursing process. The main purpose of evaluation is to decide if the resident has met the identified goals and to assess the outcomes of the nursing care provided. Remember how, in the discussion of implementation, the importance of assessing the resident and documenting the resident's responses to care was emphasized? The chart and resident assessments are reviewed as part of evaluation.

When goals have been stated in measurable terms, the LPN should be able to review all of the data and decide whether the goal has been met, has been partially met, or remains unmet. This is a straightforward look at the resident's response to the nursing interventions. The evaluation of goal achievement needs to be documented in a monthly summary, in a quarterly review, or in the nursing notes.

Evaluation also requires that the nurse review the nursing process. This review helps to keep the plan of care up-to-date and reflects changes in the resident's health status. It also is an opportunity to decide which nursing interventions were ineffective (Box 4.3).

The reassessment of the resident and the plan of care in evaluation really address the dynamic strength of the nursing process.

> **BOX 4.3** **Significant Change in Resident's Status**
>
> Decrease in level of functioning in two or more activities of daily living
> Decrease or increase in the ability to walk or to use hands to grasp small objects
> Decline in health status that is unresponsive to treatment
> Changes in behavior or mood that cause daily problems in assisting the resident to achieve goals

Although the nursing process follows specific, organized steps, no step excludes collecting more data. Data collection is done by assessing the resident, updating goals and interventions, and conducting an ongoing evaluation of the outcome of the care that is provided. Nurses seem to use the nursing process even when they do not identify it as such. Consider the following example.

> *Mary Jones always was incontinent during the 1:00 a.m. rounds. The nursing staff decided to toilet her at 12:30 a.m.*

In this example, the nursing staff assessed incontinence as a problem. Their unstated goal was, "the resident will not be incontinent at 1:00 a.m. rounds." Their intervention was to toilet the resident 30 minutes before she was usually incontinent. After toileting the resident at 12:30 a.m., the resident would be checked for urinary incontinence at 1 a.m. If she was not incontinent, the goal would be achieved, and the staff would continue to toilet the resident at 12:30 a.m. to maintain that outcome. If the resident was toileted at 12:30 a.m. and she still was incontinent at 1:00 a.m., the staff may decide to toilet the resident at midnight. The care plan and charting examples provided in Figure 4.2 demonstrate the use of evaluation.

As this example shows, evaluation is ongoing and occurs daily, not just at the mandatory reassessment intervals. Evaluation does not occur only when the quarterly assessment is due. Would you continue to carry out an intervention that was not working for 3 months until the quarterly review was due? Many people help you evaluate the plan of care each day. Residents give you information through their behavior and by telling you if an intervention is helping or not. Families tell you about changes they notice. Nursing assistants frequently note subtle changes in residents and may alter interventions to accommodate the change in the residents.

Nursing Diagnosis Problems Addressed	Goals Outcomes of Care	Nursing Interventions	Evaluation
Physical Mobility, impaired related to musculoskeletal impairment as manifested by inability to transfer and ambulate without assistance	Resident will increase ambulation with walker in PT to independent use with minimal supervision in 90 days	■ Assess and document: Orthostatic BPs (lying/sitting/standing) ROM and strength of legs and arms Walking ability with walker and amount of assistance needed ■ Have walker in resident's reach at all times and use for all transfers and walking in room ■ Physical therapy for quad-strengthening exercises and ambulation with walker ■ Put on jogging pants for daily physical therapy	

DOCUMENTATION

October 11, 2006, 1:45 p.m.: Resident is transferred from bed to wheelchair with assistance of one. Uses walker to steady himself when standing. Ambulates with hold-on assistance from physical therapist using a walker. Ambulated two steps without hold-on assistance before becoming unsteady. Orthostatic BPs lying—138/82, sitting—110/80, standing—106/76, complained of being light-headed when he sat up. Dizziness passed in 5 minutes. Instructed to move slowly from lying–sitting–standing positions and not to move to another position until any dizziness or light-headedness passes. Will review medications and fluid intake for possible causes of orthostatic hypotension.

FIGURE 4.2 Sample care plan.

Making daily changes in the actual care given is common. Translating these changes into the written plan of care is less common. For the sake of communication and consistency among all staff, it is very important to ensure that the written plan of care is updated to reflect the actual care you want to be given.

COMPUTERS AND THE NURSING PROCESS

Increasingly, nursing facilities throughout the United States are installing computers to help nursing staff complete the MDS assessment and care plans. The LPN may be asked to enter MDS data directly on the computer or to complete the written form while another nurse enters the assessment data on the computer for all residents. Many different kinds of software are available that can be used by nurses to complete the MDS, RAPs, and care plans. Each software program is different, and generally no one program will do everything that you want it to do.

If you have never worked on a computer before, you may be fearful of using it for your assessment and care plans. Completing the MDS and the care plan on the computer has many benefits, however, that warrant overcoming your fears. One of the most time-consuming portions of the MDS is computing the triggers—that is, identifying the potential problem areas that need to be assessed further through the RAPs. Most MDS software packages compute the triggers in a matter of seconds. Completing the interdisciplinary care plan on the computer saves the nurse from a great deal of handwriting and lends itself to regular updating without further lengthy handwriting. Some software packages print out nursing assistant forms that include all the interventions from the plan of care assigned to the nursing assistant. These forms can be used as assignment sheets that communicate the plan of care to the CNA.

CONCLUSION

As an LPN, you have major responsibilities for delivering meaningful nursing care to residents in long-term care facilities. Your responsibilities include the management of care given by nursing assistants, working with the IDT, completing documents required by the federal government, and delivering excellent care to the frail and vulnerable people in your care. It is essential that you understand and become highly skilled in the content of this chapter. Best wishes as you proceed to meet that objective!

Resident Admission

December 1, 2006, 1 p.m.: Mr. B., 82-year-old white widowed man, is admitted to Room 112 of Quality Care Health Facility from Mercy Hospital via ambulance accompanied by daughter-in-law. Admitted with diagnosis of fractured left wrist, multiple hematomas and abrasions, Alzheimer's disease, diabetes mellitus, and a history of CHF. Dr. Ben Johnston notified of admission and verified orders. Dietary notified of 2 g sodium/no concentrated sweets diet. Medication orders faxed to the pharmacy:

   furosemide (Lasix) 40 mg qd for CHF and
      COPD
   digoxin (Lanoxin) 0.125 mg qd for CHF
   potassium chloride (K-tabs) 2 tabs qd for
      CHF
   glipizide (Glucotrol) 5 mg q a.m. for diabetes
   oxazepam (Serax) 20 mg qhs for insomnia
   haloperidol (Haldol) 1 mg bid for agitation
   ducosate (Dulcolax) sodium suppository qd
      prn constipation
   acetaminophen (Tylenol) gr 10 q4h prn
      pain
   hydrocolloid gel (DuoDerm) to open area on
      coccyx change qod
   mupirocin (Bactroban) to abrasions bid
   nystatin (Mycostatin) ointment to perineal
      rash bid 3 to 10 days
   Ace wrap and splint to left wrist at all times
   Return to clinic in 2 weeks

Son has durable power of attorney for financial and health-care decisions and has signed the advanced directive form for "Do Not Resuscitate." Resident has a living will, and his wishes are known to his family.

   Daughter-in-law reports that he has no known allergies, wears bifocals and reads large-print *Reader's Digest* occasionally, has upper and lower dentures, does not use a hearing aid, and has minimal difficulty hearing unless in a noisy room. Uses a cane to ambulate. Height, 5'9"; weight, 124 lb.

   Mr. B. is alert and oriented to self and daughter-in-law but states that it is 1936, that the season is winter, that the month is September, and that he is in Denver. Since his wife died 6 months ago, he has been living with his son and his family. His daughter-in-law has been his principal caregiver. Caring for Mr. B. has been quite stressful at times. He does not strike out but repeatedly asks the same questions over and over, even when the question has been answered. His daughter-in-law took a leave of absence from her job because Mr. B. could no longer stay in the house alone without becoming very anxious. He would call friends on the phone repeatedly and ask for his deceased wife. He would often go for walks and get lost.

   Mr. B. was admitted to Mercy Hospital after he had fallen on an uneven sidewalk four blocks from home and sustained a concussion, multiple facial hematomas, abrasions on his right arm and shoulder, a fractured left wrist, and a large hematoma on his left hip. His daughter-in-law had been in the basement folding laundry when Mr. B. left the house. The family is expressing much guilt over the decision to place Mr. B. in a long-term care facility, but they admit that he would be safer there.

   Mr. B. is able to walk with his cane but favors the left hip when he stands and is very unsteady. He forgets where he is and cries out for help. He is able to dress himself but must have supervision to remind him of what he is doing. Mr. B. is able to feed himself but has not been eating and has lost a significant amount of weight in the past 3 months. Mr. B. has been generally continent of his bladder and bowel except while in the hospital, where he was incontinent of both.

   Mr. B. was an accountant before he retired, and he would often spend hours with a paper and pencil "doing the books." He has always enjoyed classical music and was quite an accomplished pianist. He had season tickets to the ballet and the opera and would go often before his wife died 6 months ago.

   CHF = congestive heart failure; COPD = chronic obstructive pulmonary disease; bid = twice daily; prn = as needed; q a.m. = every morning; qod = every other day; q4h = every 4 hours; qhs = before bedtime, every hour of sleep.

Continued on page 66

Physical Assessment

General Appearance: Thin white man

Head and Neck:

White hair. Scalp dry with multiple areas of white dry flaking. Face symmetrical. Two 5-cm hematomas on left cheek and jaw; 2-cm hematoma on left forehead. Skin also is dry. Eyes are clear with no drainage, conjunctivae pink, pupils are equal at 5 mm and react briskly to light, consensual, and accommodative. No drainage from nose; patient is able to breathe through both nostrils. No drainage from ears. Did not appropriately respond when asked in a whisper to raise his arm. Oral mucous membranes are pink and dry. No denture irritation noted. No saliva pooling noted between gum and cheek. Tongue pink with no coating; remains at midline when extended from mouth. Throat dry with no pharyngeal drainage or redness noted; no cervical lymph nodes palpable; no thyroid nodules or enlargement palpated.

Chest:

Symmetrical chest movements. Breath sounds clear throughout except for expiratory crackle in base of left lower lobe that cleared with cough. Apical pulse: 78 and regular. No extra heart sounds noted. Back has multiple waxy, light brown to medium brown, 2- to 3-cm, flat, raised lesions. Moderate kyphosis of spine.

Abdomen and Buttocks:

Large (8×12 cm) hematoma over left hip and left lower abdominal area. Hard stool in rectum. Active bowel sounds in all quadrants. Abdomen soft. No masses palpable. Stage 2 pressure ulcer 2-×1.5-cm over coccyx that is oozing serous drainage. Three small fluid-filled vesicles in gluteal fold of right buttocks.

Genitourinary:

Normal male genitalia. Urinary meatus reddened. Urine dark amber and foul-smelling. Fiery red rash noted on inner aspects of both upper thighs and scrotum.

Extremities:

Full range of motion (ROM) of shoulders, elbows, right wrist, and fingers. Left wrist is splinted with a rigid plastic splint and wrapped with an Ace bandage that he is constantly unwrapping. Radial and brachial pulses strong and equal bilaterally. Healing abrasions noted over lateral aspect of left upper arm and left shoulder. Limited ROM of both hips with complaints of pain with movement of left hip. Full ROM of both knees and ankles. Femoral and popliteal pulses strong and equal bilaterally. Left pedal pulse weak and 1+ pitting edema noted in left ankle. Right pedal pulse strong and right ankle edematous with no pitting noted. Homans' sign not present bilaterally, and no complaints of calf tenderness to palpation. Eschar 1 cm in size noted along medial nail of the left great toe. No drainage noted, but there is slight redness around the eschar.

December 6, 2:00 p.m.: Mr. B. was found in another resident's room, pulling clothes out of the closet. This is a daily occurrence. Mr. B. cannot explain why he is in the other resident's room and does not know the way back to his room. He yells at his roommate to get out and yells randomly at other residents in the facility. When he is in his room, he cries for help but does not have any requests or needs when the staff members answer. He went 3 days without having a bowel movement and was incontinent of stool in the hallway 30 minutes after being given a suppository. Mr. B. attends activities when asked to go, but he often leaves the activity early. He naps for 1 to 2 hours in the afternoon and is awake frequently at night, when he has to be reminded to stay in bed. He was found one night stuck between the side rails and incontinent of urine.

The MDS for Mr. B. is shown in Figure 4.3.

Discussion

Use the following nursing diagnoses to organize your assessment data and develop a nursing care plan for Mr. B. Be prepared to submit your care plan in class. Following each nursing diagnosis, you will find possible problems you can address.

1. Nursing Diagnosis: *Self-Care Deficit* related to confusion manifested by inability to perform ADLs independently secondary to Alzheimer's disease and fractured wrist.
   ADL Function/Rehabilitation Potential
   Visual Function
2. Nursing Diagnosis: *Injury, high risk* for related to altered mobility as manifested by unsteadiness and wandering, secondary to hip injury and Alzheimer's disease.
   Falls
   Behavior Problems
3. Nursing Diagnosis: *Nutrition, altered: less than body requirements* related to lack of appetite as manifested by significant weight loss in last 30 days secondary to Alzheimer's disease.
   Nutritional Status
   Dehydration/Fluid Maintenance
4. Nursing Diagnosis: *Urinary Elimination, altered* and *Incontinence* related to confusion mobility as manifested by not going to the bathroom to void secondary to Alzheimer's disease.
   Urinary Incontinence and Indwelling Catheter

5. Nursing Diagnosis: *Thought Processes, altered* related to inaccurate interpretation of environment as manifested by inability to state season and date, inability to remember names of staff members, and inability to follow commands secondary to Alzheimer's disease and possible use of antipsychotic and sedative medication.
   Delirium
   Cognitive Loss/Dementia
   Communication
   Mood State
   Behavior Problem
   Psychotropic Drug Use
   Psychosocial Well-being
6. Nursing Diagnosis: *Skin Integrity, impaired* related to a fall and being restrained in bed during hospitalization manifested by hematomas, abrasions, blisters, and stage 2 coccyx pressure ulcer.
   Pressure Ulcer
7. Nursing Diagnosis: *Constipation* related to decreased fluid intake as manifested by bowel movements hard and difficult to pass and use of suppository secondary to Alzheimer's disease, altered nutrition intake, and dehydration.
   Dehydration and Fluid Maintenance
   Nutritional Status

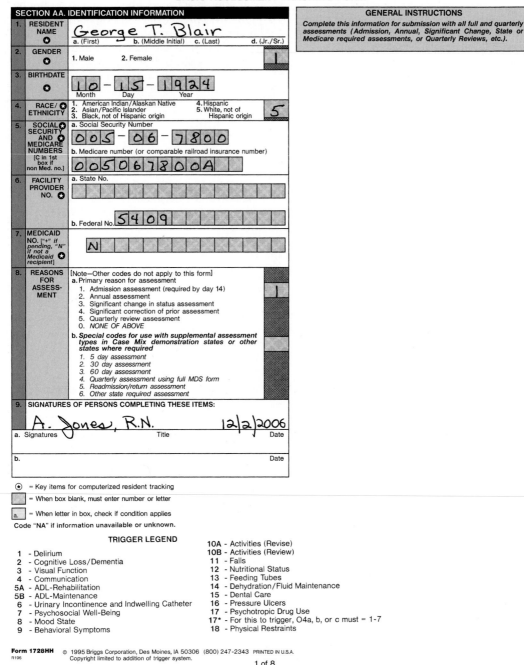

Numeric Identifier__ 784393

MINIMUM DATA SET (MDS) — *VERSION 2.0*
FOR NURSING HOME RESIDENT ASSESSMENT AND CARE SCREENING
BASIC ASSESSMENT TRACKING FORM

SECTION AA. IDENTIFICATION INFORMATION		GENERAL INSTRUCTIONS

1. RESIDENT NAME ✪ George T. Blair
a. (First)   b. (Middle Initial)   c. (Last)   d. (Jr./Sr.)

Complete this information for submission with all full and quarterly assessments (Admission, Annual, Significant Change, State or Medicare required assessments, or Quarterly Reviews, etc.).

2. GENDER ✪   1. Male   2. Female |1|

3. BIRTHDATE ✪ |1|0| — |1|5| — |1|9|2|4|
Month   Day   Year

4. RACE/ ✪ ETHNICITY
1. American Indian/Alaskan Native
2. Asian/Pacific Islander
3. Black, not of Hispanic origin
4. Hispanic
5. White, not of Hispanic origin |5|

5. SOCIAL✪ SECURITY AND ✪ MEDICARE NUMBERS [C in 1st box if non Med. no.]
a. Social Security Number
|0|0|5| — |0|6| — |7|8|0|0|
b. Medicare number (or comparable railroad insurance number)
|0|0|5|0|6|7|8|0|0|A|

6. FACILITY PROVIDER NO. ✪
a. State No. | | | | | | | | | | | | | | |
b. Federal No. |5|4|0|9| | | | | | | | | | |

7. MEDICAID NO. ["+" if pending, "N" if not a Medicaid ✪ recipient]
|N| | | | | | | | | | | | | |

8. REASONS FOR ASSESS-MENT
[Note—Other codes do not apply to this form]
a. Primary reason for assessment
1. Admission assessment (required by day 14)
2. Annual assessment
3. Significant change in status assessment
4. Significant correction of prior assessment
5. Quarterly review assessment
0. *NONE OF ABOVE* |1|

b. *Special codes for use with supplemental assessment types in Case Mix demonstration states or other states where required*
1. 5 day assessment
2. 30 day assessment
3. 60 day assessment
4. Quarterly assessment using full MDS form
5. Readmission/return assessment
6. Other state required assessment

9. SIGNATURES OF PERSONS COMPLETING THESE ITEMS:
A. Jones, R.N.   12/2/2006
a. Signatures   Title   Date
b.   Date

✪ = Key items for computerized resident tracking

▨ = When box blank, must enter number or letter

|a.| = When letter in box, check if condition applies

Code "NA" if information unavailable or unknown.

TRIGGER LEGEND

1 - Delirium
2 - Cognitive Loss/Dementia
3 - Visual Function
4 - Communication
5A - ADL-Rehabilitation
5B - ADL-Maintenance
6 - Urinary Incontinence and Indwelling Catheter
7 - Psychosocial Well-Being
8 - Mood State
9 - Behavioral Symptoms

10A - Activities (Revise)
10B - Activities (Review)
11 - Falls
12 - Nutritional Status
13 - Feeding Tubes
14 - Dehydration/Fluid Maintenance
15 - Dental Care
16 - Pressure Ulcers
17 - Psychotropic Drug Use
17* - For this to trigger, O4a, b, or c must = 1-7
18 - Physical Restraints

Form 1728HH © 1995 Briggs Corporation, Des Moines, IA 50306 (800) 247-2343 PRINTED IN U.S.A.
R196   Copyright limited to addition of trigger system.

1 of 8

FIGURE 4.3 Sample minimum data set.

Resident **George Blair**   Numeric Identifier **784393**

MINIMUM DATA SET (MDS) — *VERSION 2.0*
FOR NURSING HOME RESIDENT ASSESSMENT AND CARE SCREENING
BACKGROUND (FACE SHEET) INFORMATION AT ADMISSION

SECTION AB. DEMOGRAPHIC INFORMATION

1. DATE OF ENTRY
Date the stay began. Note — Does not include readmission if record was closed at time of temporary discharge to hospital, etc. In such cases, use prior admission date.

1 2 – 0 1 – 2 0 0 6
Month   Day   Year

2. ADMITTED FROM (AT ENTRY)
1. Private home/apt. with no home health services
2. Private home/apt. with home health services
3. Board and care/assisted living/group home
4. Nursing home
5. Acute care hospital
6. Psychiatric hospital, MR/DD facility
7. Rehabilitation hospital
8. Other

1

3. LIVED ALONE (PRIOR TO ENTRY)
0. No   1. Yes   2. In other facility

0

4. ZIP CODE OF PRIOR PRIMARY RESIDENCE

8 4 4 0 3

5. RESIDENTIAL HISTORY 5 YEARS PRIOR TO ENTRY
(**Check all settings** resident lived in during 5 years prior to date of entry given in item AB1 above.)

Prior stay at this nursing home	a.
Stay in other nursing home	b.
Other residential facility — board and care home, assisted living, group home	c.
MH/psychiatric setting	d.
MR/DD setting	e.
NONE OF ABOVE	f. ✓

6. LIFETIME OCCUPATION(S)
(Put "/" between two occupations)

a c c o u n t a n t

7. EDUCATION (Highest level completed)
1. No schooling
2. 8th grade/less
3. 9-11 grades
4. High school
5. Technical or trade school
6. Some college
7. Bachelor's degree
8. Graduate degree

7

8. LANGUAGE (Code for correct response)
a. Primary Language
0. English   1. Spanish   2. French   3. Other

0

b. If other, specify

9. MENTAL HEALTH HISTORY
Does resident's RECORD indicate any history of mental retardation, mental illness, or developmental disability problem?
0. No   1. Yes

0

10. CONDITIONS RELATED TO MR/DD STATUS
(**Check all conditions** that are related to MR/DD status that were manifested before age 22, and are likely to continue indefinitely.)

Not applicable — no MR/DD (Skip to AB11)	a.
MR/DD with organic condition	
Down's syndrome	b.
Autism	c.
Epilepsy	d.
Other organic condition related to MR/DD	e.
MR/DD with no organic condition	f.

11. DATE BACKGROUND INFORMATION COMPLETED

1 2 – 0 2 – 2 0 0 6
Month   Day   Year

☐ = When box blank, must enter number or letter

[a.] = When letter in box, check if condition applies

Code "NA" if information unavailable or unknown.

SECTION AC. CUSTOMARY ROUTINE

1. CUSTOMARY ROUTINE
(In year prior to DATE OF ENTRY to this nursing home, or year last in community if now being admitted from another nursing home)

(**Check all that apply.** If all information UNKNOWN, check last box only)

CYCLE OF DAILY EVENTS

Stays up late at night (e.g., after 9 pm)	a.
Naps regularly during day (at least 1 hour)	b.
Goes out 1+ days a week	c.
Stays busy with hobbies, reading, or fixed daily routine	d.
Spends most of time alone or watching TV	e.
Moves independently indoors (with appliances, if used)	f. ✓
Use of tobacco products at least daily	g.
NONE OF ABOVE	h.

EATING PATTERNS

Distinct food preferences	i.
Eats between meals all or most days	j.
Use of alcoholic beverage(s) at least weekly	k.
NONE OF ABOVE	l. ✓

ADL PATTERNS

In bedclothes much of day	m.
Wakens to toilet all or most nights	n. ✓
Has irregular bowel movement pattern	o.
Showers for bathing	p.
Bathing in PM	q.
NONE OF ABOVE	r.

INVOLVEMENT PATTERNS

Daily contact with relatives/close friends	s. ✓
Usually attends church, temple, synagogue (etc.)	t.
Finds strength in faith	u.
Daily animal companion/presence	v.
Involved in group activities	w.
NONE OF ABOVE	x.
UNKNOWN — Resident/family unable to provide information	y.

END

SECTION AD. FACE SHEET SIGNATURES
SIGNATURES OF PERSONS COMPLETING FACE SHEET:

A. Jones, R.N.   **12/2/2006**
a. Signature of RN Assessment Coordinator   Date

b. Signatures	Title	Sections	Date
c.			Date
d.			Date
e.			Date
f.			Date
g.			Date

NOTE: Normally, the MDS Face Sheet is completed once, when an individual first enters the facility. However, the face sheet is also required if the person is reentering this facility after a discharge where return had not previously been expected. It is **not** completed following temporary discharges to hospitals or after therapeutic leaves/home visits.

Form 1728HH © 1995 Briggs Corporation, Des Moines, IA 50306 (800) 247-2343 PRINTED IN U.S.A.
Copyright limited to addition of trigger system.

2 of 8   MDS 2.0   10/18/94N

FIGURE 4.3 (Continued)

(Continued)

Resident **George Blair**   Numeric Identifier **784393**

MINIMUM DATA SET (MDS) — *VERSION 2.0*
FOR NURSING HOME RESIDENT ASSESSMENT AND CARE SCREENING
FULL ASSESSMENT FORM
(Status in last 7 days, unless other time frame indicated)

SECTION A. IDENTIFICATION AND BACKGROUND INFORMATION

1. RESIDENT NAME
George T. Blair
a. (First) b. (Middle Initial) c. (Last) d. (Jr./Sr.)

2. ROOM NUMBER `112`

3. ASSESSMENT REFERENCE DATE
a. Last day of MDS observation period
`12` – `14` – `2006`
Month Day Year
b. Original (0) or corrected copy of form (enter number of correction) `0`

4a. DATE OF REENTRY
Date of reentry from most recent temporary discharge to a hospital in last 90 days (or since last assessment or admission if less than 90 days)
`_ _` – `_ _` – `_ _ _ _`
Month Day Year

5. MARITAL STATUS
1. Never married 3. Widowed 5. Divorced
2. Married 4. Separated
`3`

6. MEDICAL RECORD NO. `784393`

7. CURRENT PAYMENT SOURCES FOR N.H. STAY
(Billing Office to indicate; check all that apply in last 30 days)
Medicaid per diem — a.
Medicare per diem — b. ✔
Medicare ancillary part A — c.
Medicare ancillary part B — d.
CHAMPUS per diem — e.
VA per diem — f.
Self or family pays for full per diem — g.
Medicaid resident liability or Medicare co-payment — h.
Private insurance per diem (including co-payment) — i.
Other per diem — j.

8. REASONS FOR ASSESSMENT
[Note—If this is a discharge or reentry assessment, only a limited subset of MDS items need be completed]
a. Primary reason for assessment
1. Admission assessment (required by day 14)
2. Annual assessment
3. Significant change in status assessment
4. Significant correction of prior assessment
5. Quarterly review assessment
6. Discharged—return not anticipated
7. Discharged—return anticipated
8. Discharged prior to completing initial assessment
9. Reentry
0. NONE OF ABOVE
`1`
b. Special codes for use with supplemental assessment types in Case Mix demonstration states or other states where required
1. 5 day assessment
2. 30 day assessment
3. 60 day assessment
4. Quarterly assessment using full MDS form
5. Readmission/return assessment
6. Other state required assessment

9. RESPONSIBILITY/ LEGAL GUARDIAN
(Check all that apply)
Legal guardian — a.
Other legal oversight — b.
Durable power of attorney/health care — c. ✔
Durable power of attorney/financial — d. ✔
Family member responsible — e.
Patient responsible for self — f.
NONE OF ABOVE — g.

10. ADVANCED DIRECTIVES
(For those items with supporting documentation in the medical record, check all that apply)
Living will — a. ✔
Do not resuscitate — b. ✔
Do not hospitalize — c.
Organ donation — d.
Autopsy request — e.
Feeding restrictions — f.
Medication restrictions — g.
Other treatment restrictions — h.
NONE OF ABOVE — i.

SECTION B. COGNITIVE PATTERNS

1. COMATOSE
(Persistent vegetative state/no discernible consciousness)
0. No 1. Yes (If yes, skip to Section G)
`0`

2. MEMORY
(Recall of what was learned or known)
a. Short-term memory OK—seems/appears to recall after 5 minutes
0. Memory OK 1. Memory problem 2
`1`
b. Long-term memory OK—seems/appears to recall long past
0. Memory OK 1. Memory problem 2
`1`

☐ = When box blank, must enter number or letter.
a. = When letter in box, check if condition applies
Code "NA" if information unavailable or unknown.

3 of 8

MDS 2.0 10/18/94N

---

3. MEMORY/ RECALL ABILITY
(Check all that resident was normally able to recall during last 7 days)
Current season — a.
Location of own room — b.
Staff names/faces — c.
That he/she is in a nursing home — d.
NONE OF ABOVE are recalled — e. ✔

4. COGNITIVE SKILLS FOR DAILY DECISION-MAKING
(Made decisions regarding tasks of daily life)
0. INDEPENDENT—decisions consistent/reasonable
1. MODIFIED INDEPENDENCE—some difficulty in new situations only 2
2. MODERATELY IMPAIRED—decisions poor; cues/ supervision required 2
3. SEVERELY IMPAIRED—never/rarely made decisions 2, 5B
`3`

5. INDICATORS OF DELIRIUM— PERIODIC DISORDERED THINKING/ AWARENESS
(Code for behavior in the last 7 days.) [Note: Accurate assessment requires conversations with staff and family who have direct knowledge of resident's behavior over this time.]
0. Behavior not present
1. Behavior present, not of recent onset
2. Behavior present, over last 7 days appears different from resident's usual functioning (e.g., new onset or worsening)
a. EASILY DISTRACTED—(e.g., difficulty paying attention; gets sidetracked) 2 = 1, 17* `1`
b. PERIODS OF ALTERED PERCEPTION OR AWARENESS OF SURROUNDINGS—(e.g., moves lips or talks to someone not present; believes he/she is somewhere else; confuses night and day) 2 = 1, 17* `1`
c. EPISODES OF DISORGANIZED SPEECH—(e.g., speech is incoherent, nonsensical, irrelevant, or rambling from subject to subject; loses train of thought) 2 = 1, 17* `0`
d. PERIODS OF RESTLESSNESS—(e.g., fidgeting or picking at skin, clothing, napkins, etc.; frequent position changes; repetitive physical movements or calling out) 2 = 1, 17* `0`
e. PERIODS OF LETHARGY—(e.g., sluggishness; staring into space; difficult to arouse; little body movement) 2 = 1, 17* `0`
f. MENTAL FUNCTION VARIES OVER THE COURSE OF THE DAY—(e.g., sometimes better, sometimes worse; behaviors sometimes present, sometimes not) 2 = 1, 17* `0`

6. CHANGE IN COGNITIVE STATUS
Resident's cognitive status, skills, or abilities have changed as compared to status of 90 days ago (or since last assessment if less than 90 days)
0. No change 1. Improved 2. Deteriorated 1, 17* `2`

SECTION C. COMMUNICATION/HEARING PATTERNS

1. HEARING
(With hearing appliance, if used)
0. HEARS ADEQUATELY—normal talk, TV, phone
1. MINIMAL DIFFICULTY when not in quiet setting 4
2. HEARS IN SPECIAL SITUATIONS ONLY—speaker has to adjust tonal quality and speak distinctly 4
3. HIGHLY IMPAIRED/absence of useful hearing 4
`1`

2. COMMUNICATION DEVICES/ TECHNIQUES
(Check all that apply during last 7 days)
Hearing aid, present and used — a. ✔
Hearing aid, present and not used regularly — b.
Other receptive comm. techniques used (e.g., lip reading) — c.
NONE OF ABOVE — d.

3. MODES OF EXPRESSION
(Check all used by resident to make needs known)
Speech — a. ✔
Writing messages to express or clarify needs — b.
American sign language or Braille — c.
Signs/gestures/sounds — d. ✔
Communication board — e.
Other — f.
NONE OF ABOVE — g.

4. MAKING SELF UNDERSTOOD
(Expressing information content—however able)
0. UNDERSTOOD
1. USUALLY UNDERSTOOD—difficulty finding words or finishing thoughts 4
2. SOMETIMES UNDERSTOOD—ability is limited to making concrete requests 4
3. RARELY/NEVER UNDERSTOOD 4
`1`

5. SPEECH CLARITY
(Code for speech in the last 7 days)
0. CLEAR SPEECH—distinct, intelligible words
1. UNCLEAR SPEECH—slurred, mumbled words
2. NO SPEECH—absence of spoken words
`0`

6. ABILITY TO UNDERSTAND OTHERS
(Understanding verbal information content—however able)
0. UNDERSTANDS
1. USUALLY UNDERSTANDS—may miss some part/ intent of message 2, 4
2. SOMETIMES UNDERSTANDS—responds adequately to simple, direct communication 2, 4
3. RARELY/NEVER UNDERSTANDS 2, 4
`2`

7. CHANGE IN COMMUNICATION/ HEARING
Resident's ability to express, understand, or hear information has changed as compared to status of 90 days ago (or since last assessment if less than 90 days)
0. No change 1. Improved 2. Deteriorated 17*
`0`

FIGURE 4.3 (Continued) Sample minimum data set.

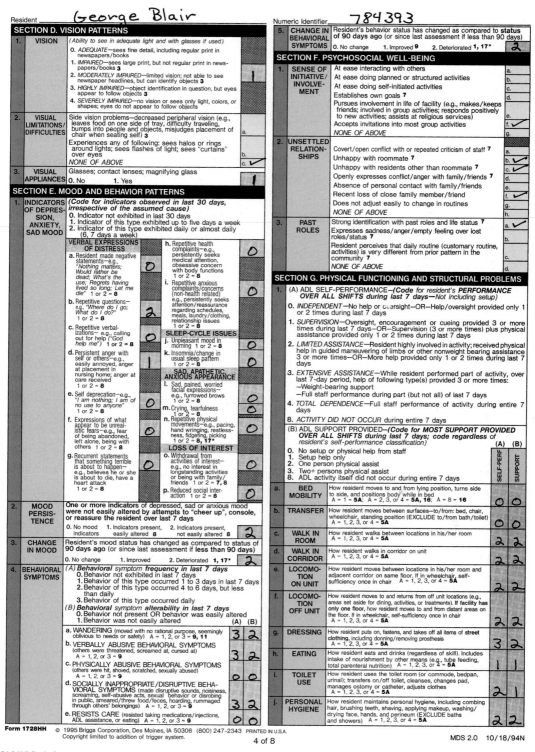

Resident _George Blair_   Numeric Identifier _784393_

SECTION D. VISION PATTERNS

1.	VISION	*(Ability to see in adequate light and with glasses if used)*	
		0. *ADEQUATE*—sees fine detail, including regular print in newspapers/books	
		1. *IMPAIRED*—sees large print, but not regular print in newspapers/books **3**	
		2. *MODERATELY IMPAIRED*—limited vision; not able to see newspaper headlines, but can identify objects **3**	
		3. *HIGHLY IMPAIRED*—object identification in question, but eyes appear to follow objects **3**	1
		4. *SEVERELY IMPAIRED*—no vision or sees only light, colors, or shapes; eyes do not appear to follow objects	

2.	VISUAL LIMITATIONS/ DIFFICULTIES	Side vision problems—decreased peripheral vision (e.g., leaves food on one side of tray, difficulty traveling, bumps into people and objects, misjudges placement of chair when seating self) **3**	a.	
		Experiences any of following: sees halos or rings around lights; sees flashes of light; sees "curtains" over eyes	b.	
		NONE OF ABOVE	c. ✓

3.	VISUAL APPLIANCES	Glasses; contact lenses; magnifying glass	
		0. No 1. Yes	1

SECTION E. MOOD AND BEHAVIOR PATTERNS

1.	INDICATORS OF DEPRESSION, ANXIETY, SAD MOOD	*(Code for indicators observed in last 30 days, irrespective of the assumed cause)*
		0. Indicator not exhibited in last 30 days
		1. Indicator of this type exhibited up to five days a week
		2. Indicator of this type exhibited daily or almost daily (6, 7 days a week)

VERBAL EXPRESSIONS OF DISTRESS

a. Resident made negative statements—e.g., "Nothing matters; Would rather be dead; What's the use; Regrets having lived so long; Let me die" 1 or 2 = **8**   `0`

b. Repetitive questions—e.g., "Where do I go; What do I do?" 1 or 2 = **8**   `2`

c. Repetitive verbalizations— e.g., calling out for help ("God help me") 1 or 2 = **8**   `0`

d. Persistent anger with self or others—e.g., easily annoyed, anger at placement in nursing home; anger at care received 1 or 2 = **8**   `1`

e. Self deprecation—e.g., "I am nothing; I am of no use to anyone" 1 or 2 = **8**   `0`

f. Expressions of what appear to be unrealistic fears—e.g., fear of being abandoned, left alone, being with others 1 or 2 = **8**   `0`

g. Recurrent statements that something terrible is about to happen—e.g., believes he or she is about to die, have a heart attack   `0`

h. Repetitive health complaints—e.g., persistently seeks medical attention, obsessive concern with body functions 1 or 2 = **8**   `0`

i. Repetitive anxious complaints/concerns (non-health related)—e.g., persistently seeks attention/reassurance regarding schedules, meals, laundry/clothing, relationship issues 1 or 2 = **8**   `0`

SLEEP-CYCLE ISSUES

j. Unpleasant mood in morning 1 or 2 = **8**   `0`

k. Insomnia/change in usual sleep pattern 1 or 2 = **8**   `0`

SAD, APATHETIC, ANXIOUS APPEARANCE

l. Sad, pained, worried facial expressions—e.g., furrowed brows 1 or 2 = **8**   `0`

m. Crying, tearfulness 1 or 2 = **8**   `0`

n. Repetitive physical movements—e.g., pacing, hand wringing, restlessness, fidgeting, picking 1 or 2 = **8, 17***   `0`

LOSS OF INTEREST

o. Withdrawal from activities of interest—e.g., no interest in longstanding activities or being with family/friends 1 or 2 = **7, 8**   `0`

p. Reduced social interaction 1 or 2 = **8**   `0`

2.	MOOD PERSISTENCE	One or more indicators of depressed, sad or anxious mood were not easily altered by attempts to "cheer up," console, or reassure the resident over last 7 days	
		0. No mood 1. Indicators present, 2. Indicators present, indicators easily altered **8** not easily altered **8**	2

3.	CHANGE IN MOOD	Resident's mood status has changed as compared to status of 90 days ago (or since last assessment if *less than 90 days*)	
		0. No change 1. Improved 2. Deteriorated **1, 17***	2

4.	BEHAVIORAL SYMPTOMS	*(A) Behavioral symptom frequency in last 7 days*
		0. Behavior not exhibited in last 7 days
		1. Behavior of this type occurred 1 to 3 days in last 7 days
		2. Behavior of this type occurred 4 to 6 days, but less than daily
		3. Behavior of this type occurred daily
		(B) Behavioral symptom alterability in last 7 days
		0. Behavior not present OR behavior was easily altered
		1. Behavior was not easily altered

		(A)	(B)
a. WANDERING (moved with no rational purpose, seemingly oblivious to needs or safety) A = 1, 2, or 3 = **9, 11**		3	2
b. VERBALLY ABUSIVE BEHAVIORAL SYMPTOMS (others were threatened, screamed at, cursed at) A = 1, 2, or 3 = **9**		3	2
c. PHYSICALLY ABUSIVE BEHAVIORAL SYMPTOMS (others were hit, shoved, scratched, sexually abused) A = 1, 2, or 3 = **9**		0	0
d. SOCIALLY INAPPROPRIATE/DISRUPTIVE BEHAVIORAL SYMPTOMS (made disruptive sounds, noisiness, screaming, self-abusive acts, sexual behavior or disrobing in public, smeared/threw food/feces, hoarding, rummaged through others' belongings) A = 1, 2, or 3 = **9**		3	2
e. RESISTS CARE (resisted taking medications/injections, ADL assistance, or eating) A = 1, 2, or 3 = **9**		0	0

Form 1728HH   © 1995 Briggs Corporation, Des Moines, IA 50306 (800) 247-2343 PRINTED IN U.S.A.
Copyright limited to addition of trigger system.

5.	CHANGE IN BEHAVIORAL SYMPTOMS	Resident's behavior status has changed as compared to **status** of 90 days ago (or since last assessment if less than 90 days)	
		0. No change 1. Improved **9** 2. Deteriorated **1, 17***	2

SECTION F. PSYCHOSOCIAL WELL-BEING

1.	SENSE OF INITIATIVE/ INVOLVEMENT	At ease interacting with others	a.	
		At ease doing planned or structured activities	b.	
		At ease doing self-initiated activities	c.	
		Establishes own goals **7**	d.	
		Pursues involvement in activities of facility (e.g., makes/keeps friends; involved in group activities; responds positively to new activities; assists at religious services)	e.	
		Accepts invitations into most group activities	f. ✓
		NONE OF ABOVE	g.

2.	UNSETTLED RELATIONSHIPS	Covert/open conflict with or repeated criticism of staff **7**	a.	
		Unhappy with roommate **7**	b. ✓
		Unhappy with residents other than roommate **7**	c. ✓
		Openly expresses conflict/anger with family/friends **7**	d.	
		Absence of personal contact with family/friends	e.	
		Recent loss of close family member/friend	f.	
		Does not adjust easily to change in routines	g.	
		NONE OF ABOVE	h.

3.	PAST ROLES	Strong identification with past roles and life status **7**	a. ✓
		Expresses sadness/anger/empty feeling over lost roles/status **7**	b.
		Resident perceives that daily routine (customary routine, activities) is very different from prior pattern in the community **7**	c.
		NONE OF ABOVE	d.

SECTION G. PHYSICAL FUNCTIONING AND STRUCTURAL PROBLEMS

1.	(A) ADL SELF-PERFORMANCE—*(Code for resident's PERFORMANCE OVER ALL SHIFTS during last 7 days—Not including setup)*
	0. *INDEPENDENT*—No help or oversight—OR—Help/oversight provided only 1 or 2 times during last 7 days
	1. *SUPERVISION*—Oversight, encouragement or cueing provided 3 or more times during last 7 days—OR—Supervision (3 or more times) plus physical assistance provided only 1 or 2 times during last 7 days
	2. *LIMITED ASSISTANCE*—Resident highly involved in activity; received physical help in guided maneuvering of limbs or other nonweight bearing assistance 3 or more times—OR—More help provided only 1 or 2 times during last 7 days
	3. *EXTENSIVE ASSISTANCE*—While resident performed part of activity, over last 7-day period, help of following type(s) provided 3 or more times: —Weight-bearing support —Full staff performance during part (but not all) of last 7 days
	4. *TOTAL DEPENDENCE*—Full staff performance of activity during entire 7 days
	8. *ACTIVITY DID NOT OCCUR* during entire 7 days
	(B) ADL SUPPORT PROVIDED—*(Code for MOST SUPPORT PROVIDED OVER ALL SHIFTS during last 7 days; code regardless of resident's self-performance classification)*
	0. No setup or physical help from staff
	1. Setup help only
	2. One person physical assist
	3. Two+ persons physical assist
	8. ADL activity itself did not occur during entire 7 days

			(A) SELF-PERF	(B) SUPPORT
a.	BED MOBILITY	How resident moves to and from lying position, turns side to side, and positions body while in bed A = 1 = **5A**; A = 2, 3, or 4 = **5A, 16**; A = 8 = **16**	0	0
b.	TRANSFER	How resident moves between surfaces—to/from: bed, chair, wheelchair, standing position (EXCLUDE to/from bath/toilet) A = 1, 2, 3, or 4 = **5A**	0	0
c.	WALK IN ROOM	How resident walks between locations in his/her room A = 1, 2, 3, or 4 = **5A**	2	2
d.	WALK IN CORRIDOR	How resident walks in corridor on unit A = 1, 2, 3, or 4 = **5A**	2	2
e.	LOCOMOTION ON UNIT	How resident moves between locations in his/her room and adjacent corridor on same floor. If in wheelchair, self-sufficiency once in chair A = 1, 2, 3, or 4 = **5A**	2	2
f.	LOCOMOTION OFF UNIT	How resident moves to and returns from off unit locations (e.g., areas set aside for dining, activities, or treatments). If facility has only one floor, how resident moves to and from distant areas on the floor. If in wheelchair, self-sufficiency once in chair A = 1, 2, 3, or 4 = **5A**	2	2
g.	DRESSING	How resident puts on, fastens, and takes off all items of street clothing, including donning/removing prosthesis A = 1, 2, 3, or 4 = **5A**	3	2
h.	EATING	How resident eats and drinks (regardless of skill). Includes intake of nourishment by other means (e.g., tube feeding, total parenteral nutrition) A = 1, 2, 3, or 4 = **5A**	1	1
i.	TOILET USE	How resident uses the toilet room (or commode, bedpan, urinal); transfers on/off toilet, cleanses, changes pad, manages ostomy or catheter, adjusts clothes A = 1, 2, 3, or 4 = **5A**	2	1
j.	PERSONAL HYGIENE	How resident maintains personal hygiene, including combing hair, brushing teeth, shaving, applying makeup, washing/ drying face, hands, and perineum (EXCLUDE baths and showers) A = 1, 2, 3, or 4 = **5A**	2	2

4 of 8

MDS 2.0   10/18/94N

FIGURE 4.3 (Continued)

(Continued)

Resident **George Blair**   Numeric Identifier **784393**

2.	BATHING	How resident takes full-body bath/shower, sponge bath, and transfers in/out of tub/shower (EXCLUDE washing of back and hair). **Code for most dependent** in self-performance and support. A = 1, 2, 3 or 4 =**5A** **(A) BATHING SELF-PERFORMANCE** codes appear below. 0. Independent—No help provided **(A) (B)** 1. Supervision—Oversight help only 2. Physical help limited to transfer only 3. Physical help in part of bathing activity 4. Total dependence 8. Activity itself did not occur during entire 7 days (Bathing support codes are as defined in Item 1, code B above)		**3** **2**	

3.	TEST FOR BALANCE	(Code for ability during test in the **last 7 days**) 0. Maintained position as required in test 1. Unsteady, but able to rebalance self without physical support
	(See training manual)	2. Partial physical support during test; or stands (sits) but does not follow directions for test 3. Not able to attempt test without physical help
		a. Balance while standing	**2**
		b. Balance while sitting—position, trunk control 1, 2, or 3 = **17***	

4.	FUNCTIONAL LIMITATION IN RANGE OF MOTION	(Code for limitations during **last 7 days** that interfered with daily functions or placed resident at risk of injury)
		(A) RANGE OF MOTION	**(B) VOLUNTARY MOVEMENT**
	(see training manual)	0. No limitation 1. Limitation on one side 2. Limitation on both sides	0. No loss 1. Partial loss 2. Full loss

		(A)	**(B)**
a.	Neck	0	0
b.	Arm—Including shoulder or elbow	0	0
c.	Hand—Including wrist or fingers	1	2
d.	Leg—Including hip or knee	2	1
e.	Foot—Including ankle or toes	0	0
f.	Other limitation or loss	0	0

5.	MODES OF LOCOMOTION	(Check all that apply during **last 7 days**)
		Cane/walker/crutch a.	Wheelchair primary mode of locomotion	d.
		Wheeled self b.		
		Other person wheeled c.	NONE OF ABOVE	e.

6.	MODES OF TRANSFER	(Check all that apply during **last 7 days**)
		Bedfast all or most of time **16** a.	Lifted mechanically	d.
		Bed rails used for bed mobility or transfer b.	Transfer aid (e.g., slide board, trapeze, cane, walker, brace)	e.
		Lifted manually c.	NONE OF ABOVE	f.

7.	TASK SEGMENTATION	Some or all of ADL activities were broken into subtasks during **last 7 days** so that resident could perform them 0. No 1. Yes	**1**

8.	ADL FUNCTIONAL REHABILITATION POTENTIAL	Resident believes he/she is capable of increased independence in at least some ADLs **5A**	a.
		Direct care staff believe resident is capable of increased independence in at least some ADLs **5A**	b.
		Resident able to perform tasks/activity but is very slow	c.
		Difference in ADL Self-Performance or ADL Support, comparing mornings to evenings	d.
		NONE OF ABOVE	e.

9.	CHANGE IN ADL FUNCTION	Resident's ADL self-performance status has changed as compared to status of **90 days ago** (or since last assessment if less than 90 days) 0. No change 1. Improved 2. Deteriorated	**0**

SECTION H. CONTINENCE IN LAST 14 DAYS

1.	CONTINENCE SELF-CONTROL CATEGORIES **(Code for resident's PERFORMANCE OVER ALL SHIFTS)**
	0. **CONTINENT**—Complete control (includes use of indwelling urinary catheter or ostomy device that does not leak urine or stool) 1. **USUALLY CONTINENT**—BLADDER, incontinent episodes once a week or less; BOWEL, less than weekly 2. **OCCASIONALLY INCONTINENT**—BLADDER, 2 or more times a week but not daily; BOWEL, once a week 3. **FREQUENTLY INCONTINENT**—BLADDER, tended to be incontinent daily, but some control present (e.g., on day shift); BOWEL, 2-3 times a week 4. **INCONTINENT**—Had inadequate control. BLADDER, multiple daily episodes; BOWEL, all (or almost all) of the time

a.	BOWEL CONTINENCE	Control of bowel movement, with appliance or bowel continence programs, if employed 1, 2, 3 or 4 = **16**	**3**
b.	BLADDER CONTINENCE	Control of urinary bladder function (if dribbles, volume insufficient to soak through underpants), with appliances (e.g., foley) or continence programs, if employed 2, 3 or 4 = **6**	**3**

2.	BOWEL ELIMINATION PATTERN	Bowel elimination pattern regular—at least one movement every three days	a.	Diarrhea	c.
				Fecal impaction **17***	d.
		Constipation **17***	b. ✓	NONE OF ABOVE	e.

3.	APPLIANCES AND PROGRAMS	Any scheduled toileting plan	a.	*Did not use toilet room/ commode/urinal	f.
		Bladder retraining program	b.	Pads/briefs used **6**	g.
		External (condom) catheter **6**	c.	Enemas/irrigation	h.
		Indwelling catheter **6**	d.	Ostomy present	i.
		Intermittent catheter **6**	e.	NONE OF ABOVE	j.

4.	CHANGE IN URINARY CONTINENCE	Resident's urinary continence has changed as compared to status of **90 days ago** (or since last assessment if less than 90 days) 0. No change 1. Improved 2. Deteriorated	**2**

SECTION I. DISEASE DIAGNOSES

Check only **those diseases that have a relationship** to current ADL status, cognitive status, mood and behavior status, medical treatments, nursing monitoring, or risk of death. (Do not list inactive diagnoses)

1.	DISEASES	(If none apply, CHECK the NONE OF ABOVE box)			
		ENDOCRINE/METABOLIC/ NUTRITIONAL		Hemiplegia/Hemiparesis	v.
		Diabetes mellitus	a. ✓	Multiple sclerosis	w.
		Hyperthyroidism	b.	Paraplegia	x.
		Hypothyroidism	c.	Parkinson's disease	y.
		HEART/CIRCULATION		Quadriplegia	z.
		Arteriosclerotic heart disease (ASHD)	d.	Seizure disorder	aa.
		Cardiac dysrhythmias	e.	Transient ischemic attack (TIA)	bb.
		Congestive heart failure	f. ✓	Traumatic brain injury	cc.
		Deep vein thrombosis	g.	**PSYCHIATRIC/MOOD**	
		Hypertension	h.	Anxiety disorder	dd.
		Hypotension **17***	i.	Depression **17***	ee.
		Peripheral vascular disease **16**	j.	Manic depression (bipolar disease)	ff.
		Other cardiovascular disease	k.	Schizophrenia	gg.
		MUSCULOSKELETAL		**PULMONARY**	
		Arthritis	l.	Asthma	hh.
		Hip fracture	m.	Emphysema/COPD	ii.
		Missing limb (e.g., amputation)	n.	**SENSORY**	
		Osteoporosis	o.	Cataracts **3**	jj.
		Pathological bone fracture	p.	Diabetic retinopathy	kk.
		NEUROLOGICAL		Glaucoma **3**	ll.
		Alzheimer's disease	q. ✓	Macular degeneration	mm.
		Aphasia	r.	**OTHER**	
		Cerebral palsy	s.	Allergies	nn.
		Cerebrovascular accident (stroke)	t.	Anemia	oo.
		Dementia other than Alzheimer's disease	u.	Cancer	pp.
				Renal failure	qq.
				NONE OF ABOVE	rr.

2.	INFECTIONS	(If none apply, CHECK the NONE OF ABOVE box)			
		Antibiotic resistant infection (e.g., Methicillin resistant staph)	a.	Septicemia	g.
		Clostridium difficile (c. diff.)	b.	Sexually transmitted diseases	h.
		Conjunctivitis	c.	Tuberculosis	i.
		HIV infection	d.	Urinary tract infection in last 30 days **14**	j.
		Pneumonia	e.	Viral hepatitis	k.
		Respiratory infection	f.	Wound infection	l.
				NONE OF ABOVE	m.

3.	OTHER CURRENT OR MORE DETAILED DIAGNOSES AND ICD-9 CODES	Dehydration 276.5 = **14**	a.	Fx L wrist	814.00
			b.	Hematomas	924.8
			c.	Abrasions	919.0
			d.		··
			e.		··

SECTION J. HEALTH CONDITIONS

1.	PROBLEM CONDITIONS	(Check all problems present in last 7 days unless other time frame is indicated)			
		INDICATORS OF FLUID STATUS		Dizziness/Vertigo **11, 17***	f.
		Weight gain or loss of 3 or more pounds within a 7 day period **14**	a. ✓	Edema	g. ✓
				Fever **14**	h.
		Inability to lie flat due to shortness of breath	b.	Hallucinations **17***	i.
		Dehydrated; output exceeds input **14**	c.	Internal bleeding **14**	j.
				Recurrent lung aspirations in last 90 days **17***	k.
		Insufficient fluid; did NOT consume all/almost all liquids provided during last 3 days **14**	d. ✓	Shortness of breath	l.
				Syncope (fainting) **17***	m.
		OTHER		Unsteady gait **17***	n. ✓
		Delusions	e.	Vomiting	o.
				NONE OF ABOVE	p.

FIGURE 4.3 (Continued) Sample minimum data set.

2.	PAIN SYMPTOMS	(Code the highest level of pain present in the last 7 days)

a. FREQUENCY with which resident complains or shows evidence of pain
- 0. No pain (skip to J4)
- 1. Pain less than daily
- 2. Pain daily **2**

b. INTENSITY of pain
- 1. Mild pain
- 2. Moderate pain
- 3. Times when pain is horrible or excruciating **2**

3.	PAIN SITE	(If pain present, check all sites that apply in last 7 days)

Back pain	a.	Incisional pain	f.
Bone pain	b.	Joint pain (other than hip)	g. ✓
Chest pain while doing usual activities	c.	Soft tissue pain (e.g., lesion, muscle)	h.
Headache	d.	Stomach pain	i.
Hip pain	e.	Other	j.

4.	ACCIDENTS	(Check all that apply)

Fell in past 30 days 11, 17*	a.	Hip fracture in last 180 days 17*	c.
Fell in past 31-180 days 11, 17*	b.	Other fracture in last 180 days 17*	d. ✓
		NONE OF ABOVE	e.

5.	STABILITY OF CONDITIONS	
		Conditions/diseases make resident's cognitive, ADL, mood or behavior patterns unstable—(fluctuating, precarious, or deteriorating)	a.
		Resident experiencing an acute episode or a flare-up of a recurrent or chronic problem	b.
		End-stage disease, 6 or fewer months to live	c.
		NONE OF ABOVE	d. ✓

SECTION K. ORAL/NUTRITIONAL STATUS

1.	ORAL PROBLEMS		
		Chewing problem	a.
		Swallowing problem 17*	b.
		Mouth pain 15	c.
		NONE OF ABOVE	d. ✓

2.	HEIGHT AND WEIGHT	Record (a.) height in inches and (b.) weight in pounds. Base weight on most recent measure in last 30 days; measure weight consistently in accord with standard facility practice—e.g., in a.m. after voiding, before meal, with shoes off, and in nightclothes.

a. HT (in.) **6 9**   b. WT (lb.) **1 2 4**

3.	WEIGHT CHANGE	a. Weight loss—5% or more in last 30 days; or 10% or more in last 180 days 0. No 1. Yes 12	**1**
		b. Weight gain—5% or more in last 30 days; or 10% or more in last 180 days 0. No 1. Yes	**0**

4.	NUTRITIONAL PROBLEMS				
		Complains about the taste of many foods 12	a.	Leaves 25% or more of food uneaten at most meals 12	c. ✓
		Regular or repetitive complaints of hunger	b.	NONE OF ABOVE	d.

5.	NUTRITIONAL APPROACHES	(Check all that apply in last 7 days)			
		Parenteral/IV 12, 14	a.	Dietary supplement between meals	f.
		Feeding tube 13, 14	b.	Plate guard, stabilized built-up utensil, etc.	g.
		Mechanically altered diet 12	c.	On a planned weight change program	h.
		Syringe (oral feeding) 12	d.		
		Therapeutic diet 12	e. ✓	NONE OF ABOVE	i.

6.	PARENTERAL OR ENTERAL INTAKE	(Skip to Section L if neither 5a nor 5b is checked)

a. Code the proportion of total calories the resident received through parenteral or tube feedings in the last 7 days
- 0. None
- 1. 1% to 25%
- 2. 26% to 50%
- 3. 51% to 75%
- 4. 76% to 100%   **0**

b. Code the average fluid intake per day by IV or tube in last 7 days
- 0. None
- 1. 1 to 500 cc/day
- 2. 501 to 1000 cc/day
- 3. 1001 to 1500 cc/day
- 4. 1501 to 2000 cc/day
- 5. 2001 or more cc/day   **0**

SECTION L. ORAL/DENTAL STATUS

1.	ORAL STATUS AND DISEASE PREVENTION		
		Debris (soft, easily movable substances) present in mouth prior to going to bed at night 15	a.
		Has dentures or removable bridge	b. ✓
		Some/all natural teeth lost—does not have or does not use dentures (or partial plates) 15	c.
		Broken, loose, or carious teeth 15	d.
		Inflamed gums (gingiva); swollen or bleeding gums; oral abscesses; ulcers or rashes 15	e.
		Daily cleaning of teeth/dentures or daily mouth care—by resident or staff Not ✓ = 15	f. ✓
		NONE OF ABOVE	g.

SECTION M. SKIN CONDITION

1.	ULCERS (Due to any cause)	(Record the number of ulcers at each ulcer stage—regardless of cause. If none present at a stage, record "0" (zero). Code all that apply during last 7 days. Code 9 = 9 or more.) [Requires full body exam.]	Number at Stage
		a. Stage 1. A persistent area of skin redness (without a break in the skin) that does not disappear when pressure is relieved.	**0**
		b. Stage 2. A partial thickness loss of skin layers that presents clinically as an abrasion, blister, or shallow crater.	**1**
		c. Stage 3. A full thickness of skin is lost, exposing the subcutaneous tissues—presents as a deep crater with or without undermining adjacent tissue.	**0**
		d. Stage 4. A full thickness of skin and subcutaneous tissue is lost, exposing muscle or bone.	**0**

2.	TYPE OF ULCER	(For each type of ulcer, code for the highest stage in the last 7 days using scale in item M1—i.e., 0=none; stages 1, 2, 3, 4)	
		a. Pressure ulcer—any lesion caused by pressure resulting in damage of underlying tissue 1 = 16; 2, 3, or 4 = 12, 16	**2**
		b. Stasis ulcer—open lesion caused by poor circulation in the lower extremities	**0**

3.	HISTORY OF RESOLVED ULCERS	Resident had an ulcer that was resolved or cured in LAST 90 DAYS 0. No 1. Yes 16	

4.	OTHER SKIN PROBLEMS OR LESIONS PRESENT	(Check all that apply during last 7 days)	
		Abrasions, bruises	a. ✓
		Burns (second or third degree)	b.
		Open lesions other than ulcers, rashes, cuts (e.g., cancer lesions)	c. ✓
		Rashes—e.g., intertrigo, eczema, drug rash, heat rash, herpes zoster	d.
		Skin desensitized to pain or pressure 16	e.
		Skin tears or cuts (other than surgery)	f.
		Surgical wounds	g.
		NONE OF ABOVE	h.

5.	SKIN TREATMENTS	(Check all that apply during last 7 days)	
		Pressure relieving device(s) for chair	a.
		Pressure relieving device(s) for bed	b.
		Turning/repositioning program	c.
		Nutrition or hydration intervention to manage skin problems	d.
		Ulcer care	e. ✓
		Surgical wound care	f.
		Application of dressings (with or without topical medications) other than to feet	g. ✓
		Application of ointments/medications (other than to feet)	h.
		Other preventative or protective skin care (other than to feet)	i.
		NONE OF ABOVE	j.

6.	FOOT PROBLEMS AND CARE	(Check all that apply during last 7 days)	
		Resident has one or more foot problems—e.g., corns, calluses, bunions, hammer toes, overlapping toes, pain, structural problems	a.
		Infection of the foot—e.g., cellulitis, purulent drainage	b.
		Open lesions on the foot	c.
		Nails/calluses trimmed during last 90 days	d.
		Received preventative or protective foot care (e.g., used special shoes, inserts, pads, toe separators)	e.
		Application of dressings (with or without topical medications)	f.
		NONE OF ABOVE	g. ✓

SECTION N. ACTIVITY PURSUIT PATTERNS

1.	TIME AWAKE	(Check appropriate time periods over last 7 days) Resident awake all or most of time (i.e., naps no more than one hour per time period) in the:	
	10B only if BOTH N1a = ✓ and N2 = 0	Morning 10B	a. ✓
		Afternoon	b.
		Evening	c.
		NONE OF ABOVE	d.

(IF RESIDENT IS COMATOSE, SKIP TO SECTION O)

2.	AVERAGE TIME INVOLVED IN ACTIVITIES	(When awake and not receiving treatments or ADL care)	
		0. Most—more than 2/3 of time 10B	
		1. Some—from 1/3 to 2/3 of time	
		2. Little—less than 1/3 of time 10A	
		3. None 10A	**1**

3.	PREFERRED ACTIVITY SETTINGS	(Check all settings in which activities are preferred)			
		Own room	a.	Outside facility	d.
		Day/activity room	b. ✓	NONE OF ABOVE	e.
		Inside NH/off unit	c.		

4.	GENERAL ACTIVITY PREFERENCES (Adapted to resident's current abilities)	(Check all PREFERENCES whether or not activity is currently available to resident)			
		Cards/other games	a.	Trips/shopping	g.
		Crafts/arts	b.	Walking/wheeling outdoors	h.
		Exercise/sports	c.	Watching TV	i.
		Music	d. ✓	Gardening or plants	j.
		Reading/writing	e.	Talking or conversing	k.
		Spiritual/religious activities	f.	Helping others	l.
				NONE OF ABOVE	m.

MDS 2.0   10/18/94N

FIGURE 4.3 (Continued)

(Continued)

Resident **George Blair**   Numeric Identifier **784393**

5.	**PREFERS CHANGE IN DAILY ROUTINE**	*Code for resident preferences in daily routines* 0. No change 1. Slight change 2. Major change	
		a. Type of activities in which resident is currently involved *1 or 2 = 10A*	0
		b. Extent of resident involvement in activity *1 or 2 = 10A*	0

SECTION O. MEDICATIONS

1.	**NUMBER OF MEDICATIONS**	*(Record the number of different medications used in the last 7 days; enter "0" if none used)*	10
2.	**NEW MEDICATIONS**	*(Resident currently receiving medications that were initiated during the last 90 days)* 0. No 1. Yes	1
3.	**INJECTIONS**	*(Record the number of DAYS injections of any type received during the last 7 days; enter "0" if none used)*	0
4.	**DAYS RECEIVED THE FOLLOWING MEDICATION**	*(Record the number of DAYS during last 7 days; enter "0" if not used. Note—enter "1" for long acting meds used less than weekly)* (NOTE: For **17** to actually be triggered, O4a, b, or c MUST = 1-7 AND at least one additional item marked **17*** must be indicated. See sections B, C, E, G, H, I, J, and K.)	
		a. Antipsychotic *1-7 = 17* d. Hypnotic	a. 7 d. 7
		b. Antianxiety *1-7 = 11, 17* e. Diuretic *1-7 = 14*	b. 0
		c. Antidepressant *1-7 = 11,17*	c. 0

SECTION P. SPECIAL TREATMENTS AND PROCEDURES

1. **SPECIAL TREATMENTS, PROCEDURES, AND PROGRAMS**

a. **SPECIAL CARE**—Check treatments or programs received during the *last 14 days*

TREATMENTS		PROGRAMS	
Chemotherapy	a.	Ventilator or respirator	l.
Dialysis	b.	Alcohol/drug treatment program	m.
IV medication	c.	Alzheimer's/dementia special care unit	n.
Intake/output	d.	Hospice care	o.
Monitoring acute medical condition	e.	Pediatric unit	p.
Ostomy care	f.	Respite care	q.
Oxygen therapy	g.	Training in skills required to return to the community (e.g., taking medications, house work, shopping, transportation, ADLs)	r.
Radiation	h.		
Suctioning	i.		
Tracheostomy care	j.		
Transfusions	k.	NONE OF ABOVE	s. ✔

b. **THERAPIES**—Record the number of days and total minutes each of the following therapies was administered (for at least 15 minutes a day) in the *last 7 calendar days* (Enter 0 if none or less than 15 min. daily) [Note—count only post admission therapies]

(A) = # of days administered for **15 minutes** or more
(B) = total # of minutes provided in last 7 days

	DAYS (A)	MINUTES (B)
a. Speech-language pathology and audiology services	0	
b. Occupational therapy	0	
c. Physical therapy	0	
d. Respiratory therapy	0	
e. Psychological therapy (by any licensed mental health professional)	0	

2. **INTERVENTION PROGRAMS FOR MOOD, BEHAVIOR, COGNITIVE LOSS**

(Check all interventions or strategies used in *last 7 days*—no matter where received)

Special behavior symptom evaluation program	a.
Evaluation by a licensed mental health specialist in *last 90 days*	b.
Group therapy	c.
Resident-specific deliberate changes in the environment to address mood/behavior patterns—e.g., providing bureau in which to rummage	d.
Reorientation—e.g., cueing	e.
NONE OF ABOVE	f. ✔

3. **NURSING REHABILITATION/ RESTORATIVE CARE**

Record the NUMBER OF DAYS each of the following rehabilitation or restorative techniques or practices was *provided to the resident for more than or equal to 15 minutes* per day in the *last 7 days* (Enter 0 if none or less than 15 min. daily.)

a. Range of motion (passive)	0	f. Walking	
b. Range of motion (active)	0	g. Dressing or grooming	0
c. Splint or brace assistance	0	h. Eating or swallowing	0
TRAINING AND SKILL PRACTICE IN:		i. Amputation/ prosthesis care	0
d. Bed mobility	0	j. Communication	0
e. Transfer	0	k. Other	0

4.	**DEVICES AND RESTRAINTS**	*(Use the following codes for last 7 days:)* 0. Not used 1. Used less than daily 2. Used daily	
		Bed rails	
		a. —Full bed rails on all open sides of bed	2
		b. —Other types of side rails used (e.g., half rail, one side)	0
		c. Trunk restraint *1 = 11, 18, 2 = 11, 16, 18*	0
		d. Limb restraint *1 or 2 = 18*	0
		e. Chair prevents rising *1 or 2 = 18*	0
5.	**HOSPITAL STAY(S)**	Record the number of times resident was admitted to hospital with an overnight stay in *last 90 days* (or since last assessment if less than 90 days). *(Enter 0 if no hospital admissions)*	0
6.	**EMERGENCY ROOM (ER) VISIT(S)**	Record number of times resident visited ER without an overnight stay in *last 90 days* (or since last assessment if less than 90 days). *(Enter 0 if no ER visits)*	0
7.	**PHYSICIAN VISITS**	In the **LAST 14 DAYS** (or since admission if less than 14 days in facility) how many days has the physician (or authorized assistant or practitioner) examined the resident? *(Enter 0 if none)*	0
8.	**PHYSICIAN ORDERS**	In the **LAST 14 DAYS** (or since admission if less than 14 days in facility) how many days has the physician (or authorized assistant or practitioner) changed the resident's orders? Do not include order renewals without change. *(Enter 0 if none)*	0
9.	**ABNORMAL LAB VALUES**	Has the resident had any abnormal lab values during the *last 90 days* (or since admission)? 0. No 1. Yes	1

SECTION Q. DISCHARGE POTENTIAL AND OVERALL STATUS

1.	**DISCHARGE POTENTIAL**	a. Resident expresses/indicates preference to return to the community 0. No 1. Yes	0
		b. Resident has a support person who is positive toward discharge 0. No 1. Yes	0
		c. Stay projected to be of a short duration—discharge projected **within 90 days** (do not include expected discharge due to death) 0. No 2. Within 31-90 days 1. Within 30 days 3. Discharge status uncertain	0
2.	**OVERALL CHANGE IN CARE NEEDS**	Resident's overall self sufficiency has changed significantly as compared to status of **90 days ago** (or since last assessment if less than 90 days) 0. No change 1. Improved—receives fewer supports, needs less restrictive level of care 2. Deteriorated—receives more support	2

SECTION R. ASSESSMENT INFORMATION

1. **PARTICIPATION IN ASSESSMENT**

a. Resident:	0. No 1. Yes	0
b. Family:	0. No 1. Yes 2. No family	1
c. Significant other:	0. No 1. Yes 2. None	0

2. SIGNATURES OF PERSONS COMPLETING THE ASSESSMENT:

A. Jones, R.N. (O, P, Q, R)

a. Signature of RN Assessment Coordinator (sign on above line)

b. Date RN Assessment Coordinator signed as complete: **1 2 – 1 4 – 2006**
   Month   Day   Year

Other Signatures	Title	Sections	Date
c. J. Spencer, LPN	(A, B, C, D, J, K, L)		12/12/2006
d. M. Moeller, LPN	(G, H, I, M)		12/14/2006
e. S. Miller, TRT	(N)		12/14/2006
a. A. Schmidt, MSW	(E, F)		12/10/2006
f.			Date
g.			Date
h.			Date

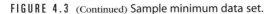

TRIGGER LEGEND

1 - Delirium	5B - ADL-Maintenance	10A - Activities (Revise)
2 - Cognitive Loss/Dementia	6B - Urinary Incontinence and Indwelling Catheter	10B - Activities (Review)
3 - Visual Function	7 - Psychosocial Well-Being	11 - Falls
4 - Communication	8 - Mood State	12 - Nutritional Status
5A - ADL-Rehabilitation	9 - Behavioral Symptoms	13 - Feeding Tubes

14 - Dehydration/Fluid Maintenance
15 - Dental Care
16 - Pressure Ulcers
17 - Psychotropic Drug Use
17* - For this to trigger, O4a, b, or c must = 1-7
18 - Physical Restraints

Form 1728HH © 1995 Briggs Corporation, Des Moines, IA 50306 (800) 247-2343 PRINTED IN U.S.A.
Copyright limited to addition of trigger system.

7 of 8

MDS 2.0 10/18/94N

FIGURE 4.3 (Continued) Sample minimum data set.

Resident's Name: George T. Blair	Medical Record No.: 784393

1. Check if RAP is triggered.

2. For each triggered RAP, use the RAP guidelines to identify areas needing further assessment. Document relevant assessment information regarding the resident's status.

- Describe:
  - —Nature of the condition (may include presence or lack of objective data and subjective complaints).
  - —Complications and risk factors that affect your decision to proceed to care planning.
  - —Factors that must be considered in developing individualized care plan interventions.
  - —Need for referrals/further evaluation by appropriate health professionals.
- Documentation should support your decision-making regarding whether to proceed with a care plan for a triggered RAP and the type(s) of care plan interventions that are appropriate for a particular resident.
- Documentation may appear anywhere in the clinical record (e.g., progress notes, consults, flowsheets, etc.).

3. Indicate under the Location of RAP Assessment Documentation column where information related to the RAP assessment can be found.

4. For each triggered RAP, indicate whether a new care plan, care plan revision, or continuation of current care plan is necessary to address the problem(s) identified in your assessment. The Care Planning Decision column must be completed within 7 days of completing the RAI (MDS and RAPs).

A. RAP Problem Area	(a) Check if Triggered	Location and Date of RAP Assessment Documentation	(b) Care Planning Decision—check if addressed in care plan
1. DELIRIUM	✓	Mood + behavior problems \ Admit notes \ Nsg notes	✓
2. COGNITIVE LOSS	✓	Poor STM + LTM \ Nsg. notes	✓
3. VISUAL FUNCTION	✓	Wears glasses \ Admit note	✓
4. COMMUNICATION	✓	Difficulty making needs \ Nsg. Known + following instruc \ note	✓
5. ADL FUNCTIONAL/ REHABILITATION POTENTIAL	✓	Assist ē ADL's \ Nsg. notes	✓
6. URINARY INCONTINENCE AND INDWELLING CATHETER	✓	Incont. of urine \ Admit note \ Nsg. note	✓
7. PSYCHOSOCIAL WELL-BEING	✓	Verbally abusive \ Nsg. note	✓
8. MOOD STATE	✓	Expressions of distress \ Nsg. note	✓
9. BEHAVIORAL SYMPTOMS	✓	Wandering + inapprop. behavior \ Nsg. notes	✓
10. ACTIVITIES			
11. FALLS	✓	Fell in last 2 wks \ Admit note	✓
12. NUTRITIONAL STATUS	✓	Wgt. loss, spec. diet \ Admit note \ Nsg note	✓
13. FEEDING TUBES			
14. DEHYDRATION/FLUID MAINTENANCE	✓	Constipation \ Nsg. note	✓
15. ORAL/DENTAL CARE			
16. PRESSURE ULCERS	✓	Coccyx pressure ulcer \ Admit note	✓
17. PSYCHOTROPIC DRUG USE	✓	Haldol bid + \ Admit note Oxazepam HS \ Nsg note	✓
18. PHYSICAL RESTRAINTS			

B. A. Jones, R.N.
1. Signature of RN Coordinator for RAP Assessment Process

A. Jones, R.N.
3. Signature of Person Completing Care Planning Decision

2. 1 2 – 1 4 – 2 0 0 6
   Month   Day   Year

4. 1 2 – 1 4 – 2 0 0 6
   Month   Day   Year

Form 1728HH © 1995 Briggs Corporation, Des Moines, IA 50306 (800) 247-2343 PRINTED IN U.S.A.
Copyright limited to addition of trigger system.
8 of 8   MDS 2.0   10/18/94N

FIGURE 4.3 (Continued)

(Continued)

RESIDENT ASSESSMENT PROTOCOL TRIGGER LEGEND FOR REVISED RAPS (FOR MDS VERSION 2.0)

Resident _____ Numeric Identifier _____

Key:
- ● = One item required to trigger
- ❷ = Two items required to trigger
- ★ = One of these three items (O4a, O4b, O4c), plus at least one other item (●★) required to trigger
- ●★ = Psychotropic Drug Use triggered only when at least one of the three items (O4a, O4b, O4c) identified by ★ also apply
- ⓐ = When both ADL triggers present, maintenance takes precedence

Proceed to RAP Review once triggered

MDS 2.0 ITEM AND DESCRIPTION		CODE	1 Delirium	2 Cognitive Loss/Dementia	3 Visual Function	4 Communication	5A ADL-Rehab Trigger A	5B ADL Maintenance Trigger B	6 Urinary Incont./Catheter	7 Psychosocial Well-Being	8 Mood State	9 Behavioral Symptoms	10A Activities Trig A (Revise)	10B Activities Trig B (Review)	11 Falls	12 Nutritional Status	13 Feeding Tubes	14 Dehydration/Fluid	15 Dental Care	16 Pressure Ulcers	17 Psychotropic Drug Use	18 Physical Restraints	ITEM
B2a	Short term memory	1		❷																			B2a
B2b	Long term memory	1		❷																			B2b
B4	Decision making	1,2		❷																			B4
B4	Decision making	3				●																	B4
B5a-B5f	Indicators of delirium	2	●																		●★		B5a-B5f
B6	Change in cognitive status	2	●																		●★		B6
C1	Hearing	1,2,3				❷																	C1
C4	Understood by others	1,2,3				❷																	C4
C6	Understand others	1,2,3			●	❷																	C6
C7	Change in communication	2				●															●★		C7
D1	Vision	1,2,3			●																		D1
D2a	Side vision problem	✓			●																		D2a
E1a-E1p	Indicators of depression, anxiety, sad mood	1,2									●												E1a-E1p
E1n	Repetitive movement	1,2																			●★		E1n
E1o	Withdrawal from activities	1,2									●												E1o
E2	Mood persistence	1,2									●												E2
E3	Change in mood	2			●																●★		E3
E4aA	Wandering	1,2,3										●	●										E4aA
E4bA-E4eA	Behavioral symptoms	1,2,3										❷											E4bA-E4eA
E5	Change in behavioral symptoms	1										●											E5
E5	Change in behavioral symptoms	2																			●★		E5
F1d	Establishes own goals	✓								●													F1d
F2a-F2d	Unsettled relationships	✓								❷													F2a-F2d
F3a	Strong id, past roles	✓								●													F3a
F3b	Lost roles	✓								●													F3b
F3c	Daily routine different	✓								●													F3c
G1aA	Bed mobility	1					●																G1aA
G1aA	Bed mobility	2,3,4					●													●			G1aA
G1aA	Bed mobility	8																		●			G1aA
G1bA-G1jA	ADL self-performance	1,2,3,4					❷																G1bA-G1jA
G2A	Bathing	1,2,3,4					❷																G2A
G3b	Balance while sitting	1,2,3																			●		G3b
G6a	Bedfast	✓																		●			G6a
G8a,b	Resident, staff believe capable	✓					●																G8a,b
H1a	Bowel incontinence	1,2,3,4																		●			H1a
H1b	Bladder incontinence	2,3,4							●														H1b
H2b	Constipation	✓																			●★		H2b
H2d	Fecal impaction	✓																			●★		H2d
H3c,d,e	Catheter use	✓							●														H3c,d,e
H3g	Use of pads/briefs	✓							●														H3g
I1i	Hypotension	✓																			●★		I1i
I1j	Peripheral vascular disease	✓																		●			I1j
I1ee	Depression	✓																			●★		I1ee
I1jj	Cataracts	✓			●																		I1jj
I1ll	Glaucoma	✓			●																		I1ll
I2j	UTI	✓													●								I2j
MDS 2.0 ITEM AND DESCRIPTION		**CODE**	1	2	3	4	5A	5B	6	7	8	9	10A	10B	11	12	13	14	15	16	17	18	**ITEM**

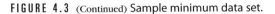

Form 1729HH BRIGGS, Des Moines, IA 50306 (800) 247-2343 PRINTED IN U.S.A.
R398

MDS 2.0 RAP TRIGGER LEGEND
MDS 2.0 10/18/94N

FIGURE 4.3 (Continued) Sample minimum data set.

RESIDENT ASSESSMENT PROTOCOL TRIGGER LEGEND FOR REVISED RAPS (FOR MDS VERSION 2.0)

Key:
- ● = One item required to trigger
- ② = Two items required to trigger
- ✷ = One of these three items (O4a, O4b, O4c), plus at least one other item (●✷) required to trigger
- ●✷ = Psychotropic Drug Use triggered only when at least one of the three items (O4a, O4b, O4c) identified by ✷ also apply
- ⓐ = When both ADL triggers present, maintenance takes precedence

Proceed to RAP Review once triggered

Column legend:
1 = Delirium · 2 = Cognitive Loss/Dementia · 3 = Visual Function · 4 = Communication · 5A = ADL-Rehabilitation · 5B = ADL-Maintenance (Trigger A ⓐ / Trigger B ⓑ) · 6 = Urinary Incontinence and Indwelling Catheter · 7 = Psychosocial Well-Being · 8 = Mood State · 9 = Behavioral Symptoms · 10A = Activities Trigger A (Revise) · 10B = Activities Trigger B (Review) · 11 = Falls · 12 = Nutritional Status · 13 = Feeding Tubes · 14 = Dehydration/Fluid Maintenance · 15 = Dental Care · 16 = Pressure Ulcers · 17 = Psychotropic Drug Use · 18 = Physical Restraints

MDS 2.0 ITEM	DESCRIPTION	CODE	1	2	3	4	5A	5B	6	7	8	9	10A	10B	11	12	13	14	15	16	17	18	ITEM
I3	Dehydration diagnosis	276.5																⊙					I3
J1a	Weight fluctuation	✓																⊙					J1a
J1c	Dehydrated	✓																⊙					J1c
J1d	Insufficient fluid	✓																⊙					J1d
J1f	Dizziness	✓													●						●✷		J1f
J1h	Fever	✓																●					J1h
J1i	Hallucinations	✓																			●✷		J1i
J1j	Internal bleeding	✓																●					J1j
J1k	Lung aspirations	✓																			●✷		J1k
J1m	Syncope	✓																			●✷		J1m
J1n	Unsteady gait	✓													⊙						●✷		J1n
J4a,b	Fell	✓											⊙		⊙						●✷		J4a,b
J4c	Hip fracture	✓																			●✷		J4c
K1b	Swallowing problem	✓																			●✷		K1b
K1c	Mouth pain	✓																	●				K1c
K3a	Weight loss	1														⊙							K3a
K4a	Taste alteration	✓														⊙							K4a
K4c	Leave 25% food	✓														⊙							K4c
K5a	Parenteral/IV feeding	✓														●	●						K5a
K5b	Feeding tube	✓															●	●					K5b
K5c	Mechanically altered	✓														●							K5c
K5d	Syringe feeding	✓														●							K5d
K5e	Therapeutic diet	✓														⊙							K5e
L1a,c,d,e	Dental	✓																	●				L1a,c,d,e
L1f	Daily cleaning teeth	Not ✓																	●				L1f
M2a	Pressure ulcer	2,3,4														⊙				⊙			M2a
M2a	Pressure ulcer	1																		●			M2a
M3	Previous pressure ulcer	1																		●			M3
M4e	Impaired tactile sense	✓																		●			M4e
N1a	Awake morning	✓											②										N1a
N2	Involved in activities	0											②										N2
N2	Involved in activities	2,3									●												N2
N5a,b	Prefer change in daily routine	1,2									●												N5a,b
O4a	Antipsychotics	1-7																			⊛		O4a
O4b	Antianxiety	1-7													●						✷		O4b
O4c	Antidepressants	1-7													●						✷		O4c
O4e	Diuretic	1-7																⊙					O4e
P4c	Trunk restraint	1													●							●	P4c
P4c	Trunk restraint	2													●					●		●	P4c
P4d	Limb restraint	1,2																				●	P4d
P4e	Chair prevents rising	1,2																				●	P4e

MDS 2.0 10/18/94N

FIGURE 4.3 (Continued)

Select the best answer to each question.

1. The nursing process is:

    a. A type of standardized care plan

    b. A framework for providing nursing care

    c. A procedure that registered nurses use to make care assignments

    d. An instinctive method of providing care

2. The steps in the nursing process are:

    a. Admission, inpatient care, and discharge

    b. Assessment, intervention, and documentation

    c. Assessment, nursing diagnosis, planning, intervention, and evaluation

    d. Admission, physical examination, interview, nursing history, and planning

3. Nursing diagnoses differ from medical diagnoses because they:

    a. Address the problems of the older person

    b. Are written in language that nurses understand

    c. Are standardized for any person who is receiving nursing care

    d. Are designed to address the medical treatment plan

4. When setting priorities during the planning stage of the nursing process, it is important to consider:

    a. The needs of the physician

    b. The needs of the family

    c. The needs of the nursing staff

    d. The needs of the resident

5. Evaluation of the nursing care plan is documented by means of:

    a. The nurse's notes

    b. The resident's care plan

    c. The physician's orders

    d. Revising the admission note

5 Legal and Ethical Considerations Regarding Older Adults

Mary Ann Anderson
Alicebelle Rubotzky

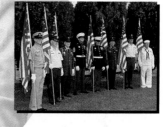

Learning Objectives

After completing this chapter, the student will be able to:

1. Compare and contrast the terms *legal* and *ethical*.
2. Define the term *liability* and discuss the impact it can have on your career.
3. Define the guiding principles of a restraint-free environment.
4. Outline the role of the licensed practical nurse (LPN) in using advanced directives and informed consent.
5. Describe the legal definition of elder abuse and the LPN's role in reporting it.
6. Express an understanding of the ethical responsibility of working with older adults in meeting their sexual needs.
7. Explain the HIPAA law and the significance it has for your nursing practice.

INTRODUCTION

Health-care decisions that are made daily across the United States are based on the legal and ethical definitions of health care. Advances in technology, increased resources, newer drug therapies, and other modalities of treatment continue to bring with them ethical and legal problems and solutions to the health-care system that are unprecedented. While the legislators and ethics committees of the United States debate the merits of treatment approaches, health-care providers deliberate every day regarding their own direct care role and often wonder if it is one of help or hindrance.

As a licensed practical nurse (LPN), you will be involved in making ethical and legal decisions that potentially are very complex. This chapter will assist you in understanding ethical and legal issues that relate specifically to the challenges facing older adults and their care.

ETHICS

Ethics is the study of moral actions and values. It is based on the principles of conduct that govern individuals and groups. Many people envision ethics as dealing with principles and moral concepts that determine what is good or bad behavior. The problem with this concept is determining who decides what is good and what is bad. Always ask yourself, "Is this decision one for the older adult, the nurse, the family, or an outside group like an ethics committee?"

A broader definition of ethics considers the value system of a person and the relationship of those values in determining what is good for an individual or group. It is important for LPNs to understand their own value systems and the ethical framework underlying the work performance that springs from them. The personal values of all the people involved in making health-care decisions for older adults form the most important aspect of the nurse's delivery of ethical health care.

Patient Care Partnership

The Patient's Bill of Rights was a document adopted by the American Hospital Association (AHA) in 1973. It was a single-page document that listed the ethical behavior that was seen as appropriate and proper for care of patients in a hospital. The AHA has updated and added content to the original Patient Bill of Rights and

refers to the new document (a booklet) as the Patient Care Partnership. By federal law, each nursing home must have available a similar document that discusses the rights of residents. Other organizations, such as the American Nurses' Association, American Dental Association, and National Respiratory Therapy Association, have ethical codes that guide the practice of each professional and are consistent with the Patient Care Partnership. Professional organizations publish standards of care that identify an ethical and legal model of practice. These models are often used in legal cases to determine the acceptable level of care.

The Patient Care Partnership is based on every individual's right to make decisions regarding health-care treatment. It is designed to serve as a model that defines acceptable behavior toward individuals in your care. All work done with persons of every age and condition should be based on the principles in the AHA booklet. The new document stresses access to health care and coverage. It is clear in not allowing racial or ethnic disparities. It covers billing and collection policies, and it defines the right of every person to be a partner in health-care decisions and delivery. The vision statement of the AHA is as follows:

> "Our vision is of a society of healthy communities where all individuals reach their highest potential for health."

Please read and review the Patient Care Partnership. You should be able to access a copy from your work setting if you work in a hospital. Your faculty person may have copies available, or you may need to purchase one from the AHA.

You can also access information by going to AHA's website at www.aha.org and searching for "Patient Care Partnership" (currently, the exact web address for the document is: http://www.aha.org/aha/issues/Communicating-With-Patients/pt-care-partnership.html). The Patient Care Partnership should be the foundation for the work you do with elderly people. It has special significance when dealing with the older adults who may be struggling with the stress of a new situation, limited short-term memory, or chronic disease.

The Law

The legal system is based on rules and regulations that guide society in a formal and binding manner. These regulations are human-made rules capable of being changed by the legislative and judiciary systems of the United States, whose officials are elected and appointed as representatives of the public. The law gives you, as a health-care provider, a general foundation for guiding your work; it may or may not complement your personal value system.

Ideally, the care you give is ethical and legal. It is possible, however, for a legal approach to care to seem unethical to you because it conflicts with your value system. This is when ethical-legal dilemmas occur. For example, the law recognizes the right of a competent person to refuse therapy. All individuals have that right regardless of the agreement or disagreement of the health-care system with the decision. An older adult has the right to refuse to have a pace-maker replaced. Such replacement is essentially a benign procedure with minimal risk, and not to have it done amounts to a death sentence. It is the person's right to accept or refuse the therapy, however. The values of the health-care provider do not change the principles of the law.

Another example is provided by Dr. Jean Watson in her theory the "science of human caring" and is explained in detail in her book *Nursing: Human Science and Human Caring— A Theory of Nursing* (Watson, 1985). In her book, Watson emphasizes the importance of valuing persons as individuals and avoiding objectifying them. She explains that a nurse gives legal care when going into a person's room to perform a complicated dressing change. The nurse assesses the wound site, plans what will be done, removes the old dressing, and replaces it with a new dressing. (The dressing then is evaluated for effectiveness, right? I hope you recognize the use of the nursing process

here.) The law does not indicate that the nurse needs to talk to the person or to explain the procedure or the healing process. For that care to be ethical, the nurse must take the time to talk to the person, however, and treat the person as a human being rather than an object with a wound to dress. Another simple example is that of bathing persons with dementia. Federal law requires that persons in nursing homes be kept clean. It is possible for a nursing assistant to give a resident a bath that is abusive by allowing no protection of modesty, by not waiting for the water to warm, or by being verbally abusive. This situation could be described as a legal, but unethical, bath.

In the midst of the time pressures of the complex world of health care, one must be careful to define legal and ethical care. Nurses experience legal and ethical issues in their work every day. It is important to be able to distinguish between ethics and the law.

Laws can be developed and passed on national, state, and local levels. Nurses are influenced mostly by national (federal) laws and state laws. Examples of federal laws include the Patient Self-Determination Act of 1990, which requires asking people if they have living wills, durable power of attorney, or advance directives. There also is the Health Insurance Portability and Accountability Act (HIPAA), which includes regulations about patient privacy. This law was enacted in April 2003.

Nurse practice acts are state laws that tell the requirements for licensure and the limits of nursing practice. Every nurse needs to be familiar with the nurse practice act in the state where he or she is practicing. Nurse practice acts differ from state to state, so if you practice in more than one state, you need to know the differences.

Each hospital, home care agency, and nursing home has its own policies and procedures that must be in compliance with the state and federal laws. An employee of each health-care organization is a representative of that agency and is expected to follow all of the rules and regulations. Failure to do that is a reason for being terminated from a job. If an employee believes that laws are being broken by the agency's rules and regulations, there is a citizen's duty to report this to the agency authorities, such as a supervisor, or the legal authorities, such as the Department of Health, or both. This type of situation can lead to a serious legal and ethical dilemma. It is best to be certain of your facts before you take on such a serious risk. Consult a person who knows more about

A comparison of ethics and the law

Ethics	The Law
Study of moral actions and values	Rules and regulations that guide society in a formal and binding manner
Principles of conduct that govern individuals and groups; generally complement your personal values	Provides a binding foundation of rules that will guide your work; it may not complement your personal values
Critical to examine and understand your own value system in order to give ethical care	Must understand and apply the law to every nursing care situation

Note: The highest level of nursing, that of holistic caring, can be given only when both ethical and legal care are administered.

the law than you do. You also can consult a textbook, speak with an attorney, or do a Web search before you take any action.

LEGAL LIABILITY

Nurses do not commit wrongful acts deliberately, yet they are at risk every day for making a mistake for which they are liable. The term *liability* means that you are legally and morally responsible for an action taken. There are risky behaviors that can increase the possibility of making an error, increasing your risk of liability. These risks are apparent when the following occur:

1. Working when you are physically or emotionally exhausted
2. Working with inadequate staff
3. Not having the necessary equipment available to meet patient or resident needs
4. Not following the policies and procedures of the institution
5. Practicing beyond the scope of the nurse practice act
6. Allowing an impaired nurse or certified nursing assistant (CNA) to work without reporting him or her

The responsibility of the mistakes that can occur during any of the above-listed situations is a serious one and requires your best effort at all times to avoid it.

When I was a student and practicing nurse at St. Benedict's Hospital, working without adequate staff (#2 in the list) was not a problem. If I needed more help, one call to the convent brought as many nurses as anyone could need. There never was a nursing shortage because

PRIORITY SETTING 5.1

The priority for this chapter is for you always to identify the nurse practice act for the state where you are practicing nursing as well as the rules and regulations at your place of employment. You are responsible for knowing the law and the policies that determine your practice. No one else can assume that responsibility for you.

those dedicated women—who were licensed nurses—were only a phone call away, but I realize they were the "good old days!" With today's emphasis on lowering health costs, registered nurses (RNs) have been replaced by LPNs, and the care pool has been filled with CNAs. I am not discrediting any health-care worker because *everyone* is valuable. Some analysts have noted, however, that the increase in the number of medical and nursing errors over the past several years correlates with the decrease in the number of licensed nurses being employed. Whatever the reason for the increase in nursing errors, the reality is that the nurse administering the erroneous care is legally liable for whatever happens.

Not only are you liable for your own actions, but you also are liable for any personnel working under your supervision. You could be arrested, go to court, and stand trial if you or the personnel you were supervising commit a nursing error. If found guilty, you would be fined, go to jail, or go to prison. Even if you are found innocent, you will be hurt by the experience: There will be an attorney to pay; your reputation as a professional caregiver will be damaged; and you will have lost some of your salary because you were in jail, awaiting trial, or attending the trial. I am not trying to scare you, but it is crucial for you to understand the seriousness of allowing bad situations to continue while putting the persons in your care, the persons you are supervising, and yourself in danger.

If there is a situation that puts anyone in your work environment at risk, do something to improve that situation. You are the licensed person, and not only do you want the situation to be changed, but also you could be liable for the situation itself. If any situation is present that could cause a medical or nursing error—including, but not limited to, the six previously listed risky behaviors and negligence, malpractice, and omission, which are discussed next—you need to work through the chain of command until the problem is solved. Working through the chain of command means going to your charge nurse, your nurse manager, and, if there is no resolution, the administrator. As you are probably a nursing student at the beginning of your career, I understand that the very thought of going to a hospital or nursing home administrator might be intimidating. It would be nice if you and your charge nurse and nurse manager went to the administrator together, but in a risky situation, you must do whatever it takes, and I strongly suggest doing it before a patient injury occurs.

It is difficult to confront a serious problem, but your ethics will guide you, and I predict you would not be the only nurse troubled by the problem. Gather your resources and, in a patient and professional way, work with your nurse manager, the unlicensed staff, and any others who can support you in making the work environment a safe and risk-free place to practice nursing.

ACTS OF NEGLIGENCE, MALPRACTICE, AND OMISSION

Two legal terms that are important to nurses are *negligence* and *malpractice*. Negligence is the failure of anyone to use care and caution to prevent harm to other people. Malpractice is the negligence on the part of a professional person in providing care to another person. Negligence and malpractice can occur if a medical professional fails to be cautious in doing something or fails to do something that needed to be done; the latter situation is called *omission*.

Every person is ethically and legally responsible and accountable for his or her own actions. Professional people who are licensed to care for others because they have special education, knowledge, and experience are held to a higher standard than other people. For example, as a nurse, you have a duty to protect and advocate for the people in your care as well as provide physical and emotional care for them.

Negligence is failure to exercise adequate care. The determination of negligence is based on the level of performance that is expected of an LPN as determined by the state nurse practice act, the policies and procedures for the facility where the LPN works, and what is considered safe and prudent care by other LPNs. For example, if you start an intravenous (IV) procedure, even in an emergency situation, and you are not IV-certified, you have broken the law as outlined in the nurse practice act, and you are liable for your behavior even if there is a good outcome from your actions. Why? Because you broke the law. Even if the outcome is good, you could be sued.

As a licensed nurse, you are liable for any acts of negligence and malpractice that you perform. If you are working on a team with CNAs, you are responsible or liable for their actions as well.

I remember being the charge nurse on a hospital-based nursing home unit when a patient was transferred from the intensive care unit (ICU). It was very unusual to have a transfer directly from ICU, but it was a busy day, and I simply accepted the patient. He was an elderly man who had fallen out of bed and had a bruise and gash on his forehead. I asked an experienced and trusted CNA to get him settled into his bed and to let me know when he was settled so that I could come in and do his admission assessment. The unit was full, and I had blood running. Although there were two LPNs working with me, neither of them could legally work with the blood except to observe it. I checked on the blood and the resident receiving the blood (ethical care!). Then I headed to the room with the man from ICU. Before I got to the room, someone met me and said to come quickly. The man was being walked to the restroom, lost consciousness, and fell, hitting his head again. I was horrified that the CNA had not used the wheelchair to move him! Although this case did not go to court, I was liable for the negligence of the CNA. The physician was called, and when he got to the floor, he asked for " ... the stupid person who had let his patient fall!" The CNA walked up to him, but I got there in time to say, "I am responsible." It was the truth; I was legally liable for the CNA's actions.

The situation with the CNA was one of negligent care. If a nurse is accused of malpractice and is being investigated and tried in a court of law, how do judges and juries know the difference between good care, malpractice, and negligent care?

The legal system looks at what is the action that is expected from a reasonable and prudent person under the same circumstances. A prudent, responsible nurse is someone who is careful, thoughtful, and wise about his or her actions. This person also is a professional who renews nursing knowledge by reading, attending workshops and conferences, and simply "keeping up" with the profession. This is something I strongly recommend that you do.

Sometimes there is a small group of nurses who work together, cut corners, and neglect to follow rules unless someone in authority is watching. Such nurses are not prudent and responsible. A court would not use their behavior as a standard of care. Instead, the court would use expert witnesses, laws, agency rules, current textbooks, and standards of care published by professional organizations to show what a reasonable, prudent nurse would do under the circumstances.

Four conditions are needed to have malpractice or negligence:

1. A duty to the client
2. A failure to meet that duty or a breach of duty
3. An injury or negative outcome caused by not meeting that duty (causation)
4. Actual harm or damages suffered by the person who is receiving care

When these four criteria are met, the nurse is legally liable, or responsible, for the action in a court of law.

Many other nursing issues are closely related to meeting the criteria of the law. One additional issue is the concept of omission. Omission occurs when you omit something that is either ordered or expected as a normal part of treatment for a person. Classic examples of omission involve treatment or medication. Omission also could involve failure to notify a supervisor or physician of a situation with a patient. Many lawsuits are based on omissions of care. Even though the act is something you did not do rather than something you did do, you are liable for your behavior.

Many issues within the realm of nursing are profoundly affected by ethical and legal concepts. The purpose of this chapter is to discuss issues closely associated with nursing care of older adults, such as the use of restraints, advanced directives, informed consent, and elder abuse.

USE OF RESTRAINTS

The long-practiced tradition of using restraints was an accepted aspect of nursing care of elderly adults until the 1980s. Nursing leaders joined other health-care professionals in drafting legislation and working with legislators to introduce and pass federal laws for reforming care of elderly adults in the United States. In 1987, the nursing home reform legislation was added to the Omnibus Reconciliation Act (OBRA) and became the law that was instrumental in dramatically changing and improving care of elderly residents in long-term care facilities. Gradually, states wrote and passed their own laws that reinforced the federal law and added improvements for the states. One very dramatic change was the reduction of the use of restraints and the gradual implementation of a restraint-free environment in the care of elderly residents.

Nurses who continue to use restraints often believe they are a means of preventing falls and wandering episodes. Evidence never did support that falls are prevented by restraints. Older adults who were restrained to prevent wandering often were seriously injured because of the restraint. Frequently, their injuries were worse than if they had been wandering and fallen. When restraints were used in large numbers, the injuries and deaths caused by the restraints outnumbered the injuries and deaths caused by wandering, even though the restraints were applied carefully and correctly. Most restraint deaths were from asphyxiation from crushing the trachea on a side rail or vest restraint or from obstruction of breathing owing to being pressed against the mattress between the bed and the side rail.

The legal system considers the use of restraints as well as the threat of using restraints as unlawful imprisonment. Anything that restricts a person's movement is considered a restraint. These items include side rails, protective vests, wheelchairs with trays, safety belts, and geriatric chairs. People fight and strongly resist being tied and shackled, which can cause death, severe injuries, skin excoriation, bruising, and pressure ulcers. These hard lessons were the reasons nurses took such strong political action in the late 20th century to "untie the elderly."

In the remote and rare situation when a restraint seems essential, the decision should be made with the interdisciplinary team (IDT) and by law must include informing the family. In hospitals, it sometimes is necessary to restrain a patient to maintain lifesaving procedures such as a tracheostomy, urinary catheter, or intravenous tubing (IV). A physician's order for application of a short-term restraint requires the nurse to make careful observation and to perform periodic removal, skin care, and range of motion exercises. In an emergency, when it is necessary to protect the older adult or others from danger, a nurse may apply restraints without a physician's order or the IDT assessment and decision making. The circumstances and the observation and care given need to be documented carefully. In all instances, the least-confining restraint should be used.

Other Considerations

The staff in either a hospital or a nursing home should have some common strategies for managing confused older people. There may need to be a policy of placing mattresses on the floor or of lowering the bed near the floor to keep a night wanderer from falling out of bed. If wandering occurs more frequently at night or in the late afternoon, these are the times the staff should be increased so that residents can be closely monitored. At present in most facilities, evening and night shifts are times of minimal staffing, however. There are numerous devices available to assist with this problem, including alarmed doors, wristband alarms, and bed alarm pads. With these devices, the older adult has freedom of movement, but the staff is immediately alerted when the older person is moving.

Implementing a restraint-free environment requires the education of everyone on staff, including ancillary people, to the principles of working there. Along with the education program, it is important to assist staff to focus on their personal values regarding care for the elderly person. This should help in establishing desirable approaches to care. A restraint-free environment is an innovative care strategy that also requires thought by bright and creative people who feel a commitment to the rights of all people, especially older adults.

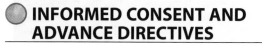

INFORMED CONSENT AND ADVANCE DIRECTIVES

Informed Consent

Another very similar legal and ethical concern is the concept of *informed consent*. The Patient Care Partnership clearly outlines a person's right to information before giving consent to treatment. The law says that there needs to be a signature

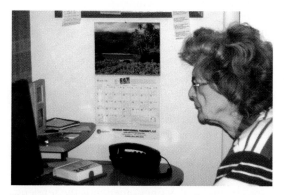

This woman is 82 years old and is proficient at using Facebook and e-mail. She gets a great deal of enjoyment out of them both. Also, she is an example of someone who is breaking one of the stereotypes of the elderly. The stereotype is that older persons do not like or know how to use technology. Do not let any negative stereotypes determine the degree of legal or ethical rights for older persons.

on the consent form. The ethical aspect of this situation is that the older adult and others have the right to all the information available on the treatment or procedure for which consent is being given.

As the nurse, you will assume the role of patient advocate. The physician is responsible for obtaining the consent by clearly informing the patient of all possible outcomes of the procedure and any alternatives to treatment that are available. A complete explanation of the procedure is essential. Would you stop a patient from going to surgery if, as you were assisting him or her onto the cart, the patient asked, "Tell me again, what is it the doctor is going to do?" Legal and ethical knowledge says that you should.

There are better ways to manage this type of situation than to postpone the scheduled surgery. One is simply to be sure ahead of time that the patient has the information needed to make decisions about the health and treatment plan. This situation can become challenging when the patient is a frail elderly person who is experiencing behavior that ranges from forgetfulness to dementia. Is it enough just to get the signature when you know the person will not remember the instructions? The answer to that is no, it is not enough.

You would need to ask yourself if you value the patient and his or her rights as outlined in the Patient Care Partnership. Do you value the principle behind the informed consent rule? It is hoped that you do. The work may involve reporting the forgetfulness or dementia to the nursing manager. In a nursing home environment, it would be important to share that information at the IDT meeting. Talking to the family may be something you do or that is delegated to the social worker. The priority is to ensure that the elderly person has complete information when asked to make a decision regarding health care.

Some older adults have a medical power of attorney entrusted to a family member or friend. If so, that is the person who should understand the procedure and sign the consent form. The elderly person also should be well informed even though the person may not remember the information. When elderly people do not have family members to assume this responsibility, the court appoints a legal guardian. The guardian is responsible for all legal documents.

Advance Directives

There are several legal and moral concerns with the issue of advanced directives. An advance directive is a legal document made and signed by a competent adult regarding life-sustaining issues and other concerns related to terminal care. In 1990, Congress passed the Patient Self-Determination Act that requires all health-care institutions that receive federal funding (Medicare and Medicaid) to ask patients, on admission, if they have an advance directive. This could be a living will or a durable power of attorney, which gives another person the legal responsibility to make terminal care decisions. If there is an advance directive, it is to be noted in the medical record. When the directive is noted, the patient's wishes should be followed.

States have various laws regarding the use of a living will, and family members may have different ideas as to what the patient's terminal care should be. The best advice you can have for this complicated issue is to know the policies for the facility where you work and the laws of your state. You also may want to discuss this issue with a more experienced nurse before you have to deal with it. Dying is such a personal and permanent issue for each person. It is important for you to know what to do and how to manage the multiple situations that can occur by being prepared.

⬤ ELDER ABUSE

Occurrences of elder abuse are increasing in the United States. It is estimated that 5% of older adults are abused each year, most often by a close family member. Abuse exists in family homes, nursing homes, and hospitals. It is done by family members, paid caregivers, and strangers. It seems to be a consequence of life in Western society, which moves faster and faster, with more and more demands. Into this scenario comes an increasing number of older people who, as a natural consequence of aging, move more slowly and experience mental changes that require patience from caregivers. The United States has never had so many older citizens, and society does not seem adequately prepared to adapt to them and their needs.

Because of this lack of emphasis on understanding and meeting the needs of elderly adults, caregivers tend to experience burnout. Accompanying this phenomenon is the tendency to abuse the elder for causing the feelings of burnout and frustration. Elder abuse is the most extreme and destructive form of ageism that can be demonstrated.

Elder abuse is also against the law, and every state in the United States has laws that say that is true. As a licensed nurse, it is your responsibility to determine what the law is in your state and the policies and procedures for handling abuse in the organization where you work. Whatever the particulars of the law are, it will state that you are responsible, under the law, to report all suspected cases of elder abuse.

Elder abuse can occur in many forms, including the following:

- Inflicting pain or injury
- Withholding food, money, medication, or care
- Confinement; physical or chemical restraint
- Theft or intentional mismanagement of assets
- Sexual abuse
- Threatening to do any of the above

The composite picture of the person most likely to be abused is a woman, 75 years old, who lives with a relative. She is physically, financially, or socially dependent on others. For LPNs who work in home care or in day-care centers, this description should be kept in mind. Do any of the people in your care have unexplained bruises or other markings? Do they seem unusually hungry or frightened? Are they unwilling to talk about their family member, or do they act fearful when you mention the family member responsible for their care? Any of these behaviors could be indications of abuse, and they deserve your attention.

If you are an LPN in a nursing home or hospital, it is critical to be alert for staff members who treat older people in negative and degrading ways. If a confused person is even more confused or is screaming and crying after receiving "care" from a particular staff member, be on the alert. Another cue is when residents have more bruises after a particular staff member has worked than at other times. Residents who are complaining of things being lost may be victims of theft. An older adult should not have a fearful countenance when a family or staff member comes near; be on the lookout for such behavior.

All cases of suspected abuse must be reported to the proper authorities. In all settings, it is proper for you, the LPN, to report suspected abuse to your supervisor. If nothing is done to prevent the behaviors that seemed suspicious to you, it is an ethical and a legal mandate that you find the proper avenue for reporting your information to a legal authority. You can determine the proper protocol for reporting abuse by reviewing the abuse laws in your state and the policies and procedures in your work setting that govern this situation.

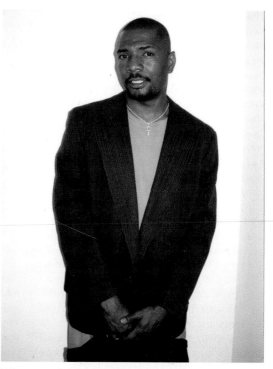

Whenever there is a question about elder abuse, immediately contact the social worker or ombudsman at the facility where you work. This social worker specializes in elder abuse investigation.

In most situations, the elderly person is moved to a safer environment, or the employee who was performing the acts of abuse is put on probation, terminated, or arrested. If the abuse is occurring in the home, the situation becomes very complex. A family that allows elder abuse is obviously dysfunctional. Perhaps the abuse is occurring because of parental abuse of the child when the child, now turned caregiver, was younger. Perhaps it is simply a response to the distress of caring for an aging parent. Sometimes, the abused elder does not want to be moved out of the situation because of concern over being moved into a nursing home or other facility. This is a choice that the older person is allowed to make. In most situations, the family members will be required to receive counseling in an effort to alter abusive behavior.

SEXUAL NEEDS

Another ageist concept in our society is that old people are asexual. Biologically, this is simply not true. Sexual needs are as basic as eating and socializing. The aging process does not remove that need from the physiological schema of older adults. The question is, how do you provide for the fulfillment or manage the needs of older adults for whom you are responsible?

Older people need love, too. I recall attending a conference many years ago in which the presenter, a music therapist, made the statement that every person needs 14 hugs a day. I do not believe that she had any scientific data to validate her point, but when she said it, I believed her! She continued to say that most of society finds old people very unlovable and unhuggable. I immediately began a lifelong quest to provide as many hugs to older people as I could give in a lifetime. Older people in our society are touch starved; often people do not readily touch or hug them. Does this flash of unscientific insight bring to your awareness that you can do something positive about meeting this need for older adults in your care? It would be very exciting to see a care plan that said: 14 hugs a day evenly distributed over 24 hours.

A myth that needs to be dispelled is that "dirty old men" are reaching and grabbing inappropriate parts of the female body. This unkind stereotyping is generally directed at an older, confused man. Instead of restraining or isolating that individual, you should assess him from a professional level.

An example of an intervention with an older man whose wife recently died could be sitting with him and asking, "You miss your wife, don't you?" to provoke a discussion of his sexual feelings. After your discussion with this man, you may learn strategies that will help him manage his sexual feelings in a more appropriate manner. Perhaps he needs a picture of his deceased wife that he can keep with him at all times, for instance, in the dining room or when he is in the hallway in his wheelchair. It may take something as simple as teaching the nursing assistants to point to the picture of his wife and ask him to tell them about her to ward off his confused attempts at meeting his sexual needs. Perhaps the solution is more complex, and the nursing assistants need to be taught how to stop his inappropriate behavior in a respectful manner that recognizes sexual needs as normal and confusion as a reality. It is your responsibility, in an ethical framework, to determine the approaches and strategies that would provide for effective management of the sexual needs of the older people in your care.

Another problem that occurs sometimes is masturbation. Masturbation is a normal sexual outlet for people. Teenagers generally masturbate as part of their sexual experimentation. Adults often masturbate as part of their sexual relationships with other individuals. It is not abnormal for older people to masturbate. It is something they have either done intermittently or worked hard at suppressing throughout their lives. It is not wrong for an older adult to masturbate; however, because of different levels of cognitive ability, an older person may be participating in this activity in an inappropriate place. Masturbating in the dayroom or in any environment in front of others is inappropriate behavior. If this should occur, it is your responsibility gently and kindly to stop the activity and take the person to his or her room. It is appropriate to leave the person alone there to do as he or she wishes. This approach is an effective one to use if the person is acting out for attention or is forgetful or confused. If you walk into an older adult's room and the person is masturbating, just excuse yourself and close the door.

Often in nursing home settings, there is controversy about allowing married couples to room together or to have time for conjugal visits. Sometimes it is unwise to have couples room together because one may need more care than the other, and the stronger person becomes worn out trying to administer to every need of the ill or degenerating spouse. Abusive behavior brought on because of dementia could be another reason. Only reasons that would jeopardize the health of one or both of the people involved are valid, however, for keeping a married couple separated. It is normal for married people to live together, and it is normal for married people to have sex together.

Another situation that can occur is unmarried, consenting adults having an intimate relationship. You have the ethical and legal responsibility of protecting demented, developmentally disabled, or mentally ill persons from the sexual advances of others. If that person does not have the ability to make day-to-day decisions, the person doesn't have the ability to make the normal, everyday decision to have an intimate relationship. As a licensed nurse, you are responsible for protecting such a person from what could be defined as sexual abuse.

What about elderly residents who are not cognitively impaired? Counselors do not go around the halls of high schools or universities to keep teenagers and young adults from holding hands or kissing. Why does society think it is necessary to do that for older adults? Sexual feelings and expressions are a normal part of living, even if one is old, handicapped, or

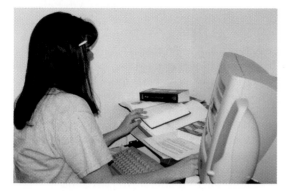

It is your responsibility as a licensed nurse to learn the laws in the state where you practice. This generally requires study through books or on the Internet, but do it you must. The excuse of "I didn't know" is unacceptable in any situation when you have broken the law or violated the nurse practice act.

confused. Every dependent human being has the right to expect protection from sexual abuse, but every human being also has the right to express sexual feelings within the framework of society's norms.

 ## CONFIDENTIALITY

An underlying rule of professional health care is confidentially. Every individual in the health-care system deserves perfect confidentiality regarding his or her personal information. That includes age, weight, diagnosis, family matters, and any other item of personal living for the individual. No patient has only one caregiver, however. That means information has to be communicated verbally and in written format to others on the health-care team for effective care

to be delivered to the person who is ill. That type of professional sharing is critical and needs to happen in an efficient manner. There is always the possibility, however, of a discussion at lunch or break with a colleague regarding someone or a procedure that is interesting. When you engage in such conversations, you are breaking the law.

The U.S. government developed the Health Insurance Portability and Accountability Act (HIPAA) as a strong effort to protect individuals' personal medical information. Confidentiality always has been an aspect of professional nursing; however, the HIPAA law brings the requirement of confidentiality in professional behavior to the forefront of practice. The law allows patients access to their medical records, provides a method for making formal complaints to the government when patients believe their confidentiality has been abused, and gives patients control over how their personal information may be used.

Maintaining confidentiality of information for every patient in your care is an essential moral behavior. It also is a legal responsibility.

 ## CONCLUSION

This chapter covers several diverse topics that have legal and ethical ramifications in giving care to older adults. Every topic is important and needs to be addressed by you as a gerontological nurse. Older people have rights, and when these people come into the health-care system, you, the licensed nurse, are the unofficial advocate for them. Their legal and ethical rights are your responsibility. The concepts explained in this chapter should help to provide you with a strong foundation for fulfilling that role.

As the 11–7 charge nurse on a 20-bed unit at Cherry Dale Nursing Home, you have had concerns over the staffing on your shift. Often, you have found the nursing assistants restraining residents for their own good without telling you. You have discussed the problem with the nursing assistants and have taught them about the restraint-free environment at Cherry Dale. Despite your efforts, there still is one "old-time" nursing assistant who does not follow the facility's rules and regulations and ignores your instructions.

This is your first charge nurse position as an LPN. You recognize that the nursing assistants see you as an inexperienced nurse. This is especially true of the older nursing assistant. During your first 6 weeks on the job, you believe you have made progress in earning the trust you need from the nursing assistants. One or two are still restraining residents at night without telling you, however.

You discussed this problem with your nurse manager, and she simply told you that you were a charge nurse now, and it was your responsibility to follow the policies of the facility. The policy indicates that restraints are not used unless there is a documentable situation that risks the life of the older adult, such as displacement of a nasogastric tube or intravenous needle.

What are the ethical and legal ramifications regarding your current dilemma? How will you resolve the problem?

Discussion

Because you are the licensed nurse responsible for what occurs on your shift, you are legally and ethically accountable for the behavior of the nursing assistants who work with you. Because they are violating facility policy, it is as if you were actually performing the act.

It is unethical and illegal to restrain people without following the criteria discussed in this chapter. When the restraint of older adults occurs, and it breaks the rules and regulations of the facility, your legal accountability is compounded. It is important that you realize that the law is being broken every time the residents are restrained. It does not matter if you know about it or not. The point is that, as the charge nurse, you should know about it. Reporting the situation to your supervisor does not release you from responsibility either. She gave you clear instructions as to what to do; you are to follow the facility's policy regarding restraints. The ethical problems of restraining residents are as serious as the legal ones.

Solution

There is more than one approach that could resolve this problem. The truth is that you may have to use them all before you find an appropriate solution.

Make it clear to all the nursing assistants that the law is being broken and the act of restraining residents on your shift is a criminal offense. Next,

- Use the experience and wisdom of the nursing assistants to process different solutions to the problem of residents wandering or potentially falling at night. The nursing assistants will appreciate being asked to assist in solving the problem rather than being told what to do. Try all ideas that do not go against the policy of the institution, the law, or your ethical standards.
- Share your creative solutions with the nurse manager. Let her know how prudent and safe the care is on your shift. (Remember that prudent and safe care is the care that most LPNs would give in the same situation.) You also should build a case for additional staffing on your shift, if that is the problem.
- Document the unique approaches of care you use on your shift, and share them with the other shifts by means of verbal report and the nursing care plan.

Select the best answer to each question.

1. Ethics is the study of moral actions and values. One of the dilemmas within ethical thinking is concern over:

   a. Who decides what is right and what is wrong

   b. Whoever pays the bill deciding what is ethical

   c. Ethical and legal behavior being the same

   d. The rules of ethical behavior changing daily

2. If you were not IV certified and you were to find a client bleeding and in need of immediate fluids to save his life, one of the following defines your legal role. Mark the correct answer.

   a. Under the Good Samaritan Act, you are required to do all you can to save the person's life, so you would start IV fluids and call the physician.

   b. Call the RN and have her handle it. After all, she has the advanced license.

   c. Call an ambulance for immediate transport.

   d. Administer first aid, leave a nursing assistant with the resident, and call the physician or the RN.

3. The legal concept of omission in care applies when:

   a. The physician has missed a diagnosis, and you have omitted treatment for it because nothing was ordered.

   b. You have intentionally or unintentionally missed an antibiotic dose.

   c. Residents are given baths only every other day.

   d. The RN does not work the weekend.

4. A restraint-free environment consists of an environment in which:

   a. Many of the residents fall or wander, but they do not sue the facility because they want to be without restraint.

   b. Mattresses are placed on the floor so that residents will not fall out of bed.

   c. The least-restrictive device is used on each resident.

   d. Restrictive devices are not used for any reason.

5. Elder abuse is a growing concern in modern society. Which of the following statements is correct?

   a. It is against the law to threaten abuse as well as to perform abusive acts.

   b. Elder abuse includes inflicting pain or injury but not confining an older person.

   c. Elder abuse is likely to happen to a male client, older than age 85, who lives with a relative.

   d. It is the legal responsibility of the RN to report all suspected cases of elder abuse; this is not the responsibility of the LPN.

6 Promoting Wellness

Mary Ann Anderson

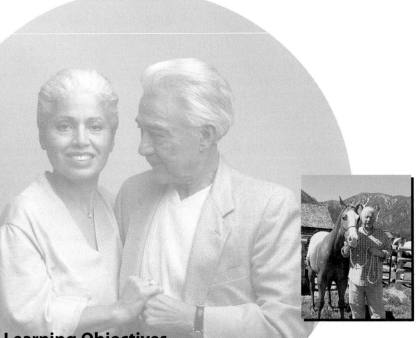

Learning Objectives

After completing this chapter, the student will be able to:

1. Recognize aging as a normal process of living rather than a disease process.
2. Describe the role nurses play in health-promotion and disease-prevention activities for older people.
3. Describe key health-promotion and disease-prevention activities appropriate for older people.
4. Understand the importance motivation plays in an older person's ability to participate in health-promotion and disease-prevention activities.

INTRODUCTION

One of the positive aspects of being a gerontological nurse is the variety of ways you are able to work with older people. The role of the licensed practical nurse (LPN) is crucial in the care of elderly persons. You are the person who gives direct care to most older people who seek out health-care services. Many nurses think only of care given in a nursing home when they consider gerontological nursing, yet you have learned that only 5% of people older than age 65 are nursing home residents. Where do the others live, and what type of nursing care do they need?

Many older adults need your knowledge and support to stay healthy. To help these individuals, you need skills and knowledge in holistic health promotion and wellness. Health is the absence of illness. Most elderly persons have multiple chronic illnesses, however, for which there is only management, not cure. Can they ever be well? Yes, if you consider the concept of holistic wellness. When considered holistically, health implies " . . . a wholeness and harmony of body, mind and spirit" (Eliopolous, 2010). That will be the focus of wellness used in this chapter.

The search for eternal youth has a long history. People have died in their search for the Fountain of Youth, and others have killed for what they thought would prevent them from aging. The legends surrounding the "forever young" concept are taking on a new reality and meaning for the aging society in the United States because people are living to be older than ever before (remember the older-than-85-years age group and the elite-old?). The modern version of the legend of the Fountain of Youth is embodied in the concept of health promotion. The focus is on living longer and healthier, an opportunity offered to today's society that has not existed previously.

The older people of the United States are generally healthier than those of previous generations. This change is due to improved nutrition, sanitation, immunizations, and overall safety in work environments and everyday life. Today's older people have benefited from improved health care as well. People older than age 65 constitute 12% of the population, yet they use slightly more than one-third of U.S. expenditures for health care. The remarkable advances in surgery, pharmacology, and the technology available for diagnosis and treatment have made tremendous contributions to the prolonging of life for older people.

Some elderly people complain about getting old. They have not found the Fountain of Youth and are upset about it! It is important to acknowledge that diminished eyesight and hearing are normal processes of aging, as is weight gain and the common "enemy" arthritis. Aging is associated with losses of friends and family because of death or nursing home placement; the loss of income is also a problem for some older people, as are the acute and chronic diseases that tend to accompany the aging process. Yet, the objective of wellness defined by harmony between the body, mind, and spirit can occur if individuals strive for gerotranscendence as they age. When aging individuals achieve this developmental stage, they are able to accept the naturally occurring losses of the aging experience. They also have plans for their future and have strong relationships with supportive and caring people.

Can you see how important these characteristics are to health and wellness? It can make the difference between good to excellent or poor quality of life. *Remember:* the objective is not to run a marathon or never to experience illness. Rather, the objective is harmony between the body, mind, and spirit.

Our society emphasizes age-related changes and common health problems as diseases experienced by older people, when actually they are normal consequences of aging. Not enough attention has been given to the positive side of aging and the beneficial effects of health-promotion activities to prevent disease and to slow the effects of chronic disease. Do you think that this lack of attention is another form of ageism? If so, what can you do about it as a nurse?

Current health-care concepts emphasize vitality and independence for older people as a primary concern. Regardless of age, as people laugh more, walk more, eat better, relax more, and think better of themselves and their relationships, they move beyond the neutral point of good health. Many of the complaints associated with the aging process, such as joint stiffness, weight gain, fatigue, loss of bone mass, and loneliness, can be prevented or managed by basic health-promotion activities. One does not have to be free of disease to experience the benefits of health and wellness.

Most health-promotion activities focus on exercise, stress management, nutrition, and dealing with substance abuse. In addition, it is important that wellness activities for older adults include relationships and self-care.

ILLNESS/WELLNESS AS A CONTINUUM

If you think of health as a continuum with illness on one end and health on the other, you can understand better the importance of health promotion. By using a holistic approach to examine the continuum, you focus your attention on the person's previous experience with life, existing support systems (e.g., family, church), and personal strengths. The point is that everyone wants health, and holistic health-promotion activities are the way to achieve that goal.

Physicians and nurses traditionally focus on working with patients who are on the illness end of the continuum or who have symptoms of disease or disability. As a person's health improves, traditional medicine becomes less involved in helping the person reach optimal well-being. In contrast, health-promotion efforts primarily are focused on the opposite, or wellness, side of the continuum.

In more recent years, nurses have begun to use health-promotion efforts even when dealing with people on the illness side of the continuum. Special exercise and nutrition programs have been designed for cardiac rehabilitation, exercise and weight-lifting programs for chair-bound persons, and weight management programs for older persons. The remainder of this chapter focuses on health-promotion activities on the illness and the wellness sides of the health continuum.

Motivation

If you, as a nurse, want to be successful in promoting healthy choices in older people, you need to understand the importance of individual motivation. Desire must be present on the part of an older adult to make a change. It is critical to explore what motivates an older person to eat right, exercise, and avoid unhealthy behaviors on an individual basis. This is true for all people, even yourself.

As a part of human behavior, motivation is the incentive or drive that causes a person to act. Incentive to take action is based on needs and desires that are internal and external to the person. An older person may have an incentive to exercise three times a week if it helps the individual experience less discomfort or immobility from arthritis. For some people, the incentive may need to be more than physical wellness. A need also may exist for a mental wellness experience, such as that derived from socialization with others while exercising, such as in a water aerobic class or with a group doing mall walking.

The nursing challenge is to assist older adults in identifying their own incentives for participation in health-promotion and disease-prevention activities. This information allows the nurse to have greater insight into ways to promote health and lessens the frustration experienced from what are often incorrectly referred to as *noncompliant patients*. Compliance occurs only if the individual can personally identify a need or desire to exercise, eat correctly, reduce stress, or make other changes necessary for improved wellness. This is motivation experienced by people in an individual way. Often, assisting to identify the motivation is one way that you, the LPN, can help an older adult.

Incentives

Studies have disclosed some of the reasons (incentives) for older people to participate in health-promotion behaviors, such as the following:

- A belief that activities improve fitness and health
- The enjoyment of socialization

- A belief that activities help maintain independence
- A desire to feel good and have fun

Knowledge about why a person participates in health promotion (or the incentives for doing so) can be determined through a caring and focused interview. After personal incentives have been identified, you can reinforce them in health-promotion activities. In addition to understanding individual motivation, you need to help individuals plan their short-term and long-term goals for making health changes. The secret to success in health behavior is to help the older adult choose personal goals with care and then learn to enjoy achieving them.

Health-Promotion Activities

When older adults have identified an area of health, they have an incentive to maintain or improve their health. The challenge is to locate a properly designed activity. Many current health-promotion activities are biased for youth and have excluded older adults by design. Four reasons underscore why the current focus on health-promotion activities is often inappropriate for older people:

1. The focus frequently is on life extension or on reducing the risks of premature death. If a person stops smoking, reduces fat intake, and exercises, the risk of a heart attack at an early age is reduced. For elderly people who have already lived beyond the average life expectancy, life extension may not be as important as quality of life. Stopping smoking, reducing fat intake, and exercising are important at any age, but for different reasons. The focus must be on health-promotion benefits specific to an older person.

2. Emphasis is often placed on advancing "youthfulness" and preventing aging. Older people recognize that they do not fit the image of youth and have already experienced some results of aging. This does not mean self-image and appearance are not important to older people, but that the image needs to match the older person's self-perception.

3. Health-promotion programs focus on preventing chronic disease. Remember that 50% of older people already have three chronic diseases. When these programs focus on management of the symptoms of the disease rather than on its prevention, more older adults have a reason to participate.

4. A focus on self-responsibility for health fails to consider the limitations imposed by personal circumstances. An individual who has a need and desire to walk daily for exercise may live in an unsafe neighborhood. An older adult may have a desire to eat a healthy diet but may be unable to afford the proper food. The external environment may pose barriers to older people that are difficult to overcome. These problems need careful attention.

As you, the LPN, look at the key areas of health promotion for older people, your goal must be to design, plan, and provide activities that are sensitive to individual needs and responsibility. Properly designed health-promotion activities should be:

- Accessible (transportation, time of day, location)
- Enjoyable and social (mental and physical wellness)
- Reasonable (focus on the right activity for the right reason)
- Sensitive to needs of older people (hearing, vision, functional level)

Health-promotion strategies must be based on the belief that the individual is the only one who can choose a path to a healthy life. Consequently, you, the nurse, must be sure that health-promotion activities are individually designed so that the pathways exist.

CRITICALLY EXAMINE THE FOLLOWING

Reread the four reasons listed in the text. Look at them through the lens of your new knowledge of ageism. Discuss what you have identified as ageist thinking. Answer the questions listed and be prepared to share your thinking in class.

1. What do you identify as ageist thinking?
2. Evaluate each "reason," and list one "real-world" solution to the ageist thinking you identified. A response for Reason 2 could be: I have laugh lines around my eyes. I am going to make the comment, as often as I can, that "I love my laugh lines because they are a measure of the fun I have had over the past 35 years. I want to grow old so I have 35 more years of fun!"

Identifying "real-world" thinking is a challenge to your traditional thinking. Spend some time with this assignment and identify things that you really are willing to do.

REGULAR EXAMINATIONS

Before excellent health-promotion activities can be designed for an individual, physical examinations of most body systems need to be completed. An annual physical examination is important in terms of maintaining health and promoting wellness. Many older adults need to be seen more frequently because of the chronic diseases that generally accompany old age. Some older people avoid making such appointments because they have limited funds to pay the co-pay, they lack convenient transportation, or they do not recognize that there is something that can be treated. Some people think that being ill is part of being old, so they accept their condition and do not seek treatment.

Regular visits to the physician can help prevent acute conditions and are an asset for managing chronic diseases. Regular blood work as an indicator of overall health is critical, as are examinations for colon, breast, cervical, and prostate cancers. The physician's visit is the time to obtain immunizations such as annual flu shots, tetanus immunizations (every 10 years), and pneumonia immunization.

Medications should be monitored for effectiveness and drug interactions. Encourage your elderly patients to bring a list of all medications, including over-the-counter (OTC) drugs, with them when visiting the physician. The physician needs to know every medication taken to avoid problems.

Feet often are a problem and may necessitate regular visits to a podiatrist to manage care of aging thickened toenails, bunions, corns, and calluses. Vision should be checked annually to monitor for glaucoma, cataracts, and other eye problems. Dental visits ideally should be twice a year and annually for people who wear dentures. Denture wearers still need to see a dentist because everyone should have an annual oral examination to check for mouth cancer. Audiology examinations do not need to be done unless there is a hearing problem. The benefits of regular examinations of the body are to prevent, treat, and monitor physical conditions. Yet problems do occur even with careful attention to health-promoting activities. Chronic diseases are a common problem.

CHRONIC DISEASE

As an LPN giving care to older adults, you need to understand the promotion of wellness in the

---

holistic sense. This concept needs to go beyond the vision of physically well, older people living in their own homes independently. More than 80% of older adults experience at least one chronic disease condition, and 50% report three chronic disease conditions. People older than 85 years experience increased difficulty with home management activities and are more likely to depend on assistance in their living situations. Regardless of age, living arrangement, or health condition, the goal for health promotion should be to assist older adults in reaching a state of optimal health—the legendary Fountain of Youth.

The most common health problems of older adults are associated with chronic diseases. The most frequent chronic conditions include arthritis, hypertension, heart conditions, hearing impairments, and dementia. Because of these

conditions, older people visit physicians more often, are hospitalized more frequently, take more prescription and OTC drugs, and experience more functional problems than younger people. The focus of many medical treatment interventions in the United States is on *curing* acute conditions. Chronic illnesses, which are the predominate illnesses of older adults, cannot be cured, but instead require management with a focus on caring. It is important to understand that chronic diseases do not have a cure; instead, they need to be managed.

Treatment Strategies

Management of chronic conditions involves treating symptoms and maximizing the strengths of an older person. You need to understand the aging process and older adults in general and advocate and lobby for what they need. For an older adult who has arthritis and who is in severe pain, it is important to treat the symptom of pain. If pain is minimized, the person is better able to stay active and prevent the further disabling effects of immobility. Nurses are the key people to recognize the symptom (pain) and administer the prescribed treatment (medication). As a gerontological nurse, you must go one step further and consider the impact of the disease and its treatment on the older person's ability to perform activities of daily living (ADLs), which include personal care, dressing, and eating. In addition, instrumental activities of daily living (IADLs), which are often more difficult, need to

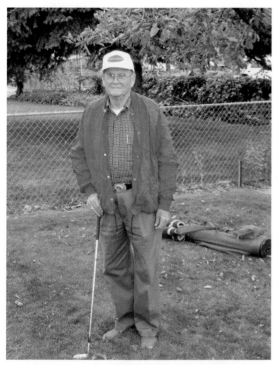

Although coronary artery disease generally is not considered a chronic disease, for this 72-year-old man, it is. He was diagnosed and scheduled for surgery 22 years ago. The blood work done before surgery indicated that he had leukemia, however, which disqualified him from heart surgery. Since then he has lived his life in slow motion. He still goes golfing but rides a cart and sometimes elects to skip a difficult hole. He does his yard work but does the mowing over a 3-day period each week. This man has adapted to what has become, for him, a chronic disease.

be considered. IADLs are activities such as shopping, doing the laundry, and cleaning the house. So consider:

What could be done to prevent the onset of pain?
What would be the side effects of the pain medication?
How has the older person coped with pain in the past? Would the same approach be effective now?

An LPN must recognize the importance of good health and its correlation with functional independence among older people. Understanding does not always make it clear, however, what kind of activities would promote health and prevent development of further secondary conditions that result in dependency.

NUTRITION

With advancing age, a person's general health is determined to a great extent by the effects of dietary patterns over the years. Staying physically and mentally active is important to all older adults. They need to understand the role proper nutrition plays in their lives, even in later years.

As bodies age, four changes occur that affect what a person needs to have optimal nutrition:

1. The body's rate of metabolism slows and no longer needs the same amount of energy and food to do the same amount of work. Older adults often comment that they have not changed how they are eating and exercising, but they are now gaining weight. As people age, lean body mass decreases, and body fat increases. This may result in weight gain and can lead to obesity.
2. The senses of taste and smell may be less keen. Some or all of an elderly person's teeth may need to be replaced by dental appliances. As a result, older people may find themselves eating different foods and drinking less fluid.
3. Social aspects of eating are important. As people age, they retire, their families grow up and move, and their spouses and friends die. This results in changes in the socialization of eating. One of the most difficult adjustments seems to be cooking for one and eating alone.
4. Environmental factors greatly influence nutritional habits of older adults. Lack of transportation to food stores and restaurants, inability to manage reading labels and shopping, and insufficient money to buy healthy food can be major barriers to eating properly.

Poor dietary habits contribute to many diseases that occur in older persons. Chronic diseases, such as heart disease and cancer, can be slowed—and for some people, prevented—by avoiding obesity and decreasing the amount of fat in one's diet. Studies from the American Heart Association (2007) suggest that high cholesterol levels increase the risk for atherosclerosis. The American Cancer Society found marked increases in the incidence of cancer of the uterus, gallbladder, kidney, stomach, colon, and breast associated with obesity.

Osteoporosis affects 25% of women older than 60. The loss of bone mass and bone strength as a result of this disease leads to broken hips, arms, and legs and to back injuries. Osteoporosis is often referred to as a "silent" disease. Few signs or symptoms appear until a bone breaks. Adding calcium to the diet, participating in a regular exercise regimen, and avoiding alcohol and smoking are key prevention strategies.

Other chronic problems that are frequent complaints of older people include constipation, urinary incontinence, and arthritis. Nutrition plays a role in each of these conditions. More information on nutrition is provided in Chapter 7.

Although one-on-one teaching may be easier, group learning that incorporates an opportunity for socialization and fun is much more likely to result in positive outcomes. You, as the LPN, may want to organize a group of elderly people in the community to participate in learning nutrition principles. One of the principles that should be taught is the food pyramid (see Chapter 7). This information, which is new to some people, replaces the basic four concepts that most older people were taught.

Health-promotion activities aimed at altering a lifetime of eating habits must be reasonable, and the benefits need to be made apparent. Nurses should clearly understand what motivates the individual. In addition, nurses must be aware of the unique nutritional needs and problems that accompany later years.

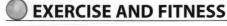 EXERCISE AND FITNESS

In the 1970s, the fitness movement in the United States began. In the late 1970s and early 1980s, society begin to stress the importance of fitness for older adults. Studies continue to emphasize the benefits of exercise and its importance to total health for all ages. The body's responses to

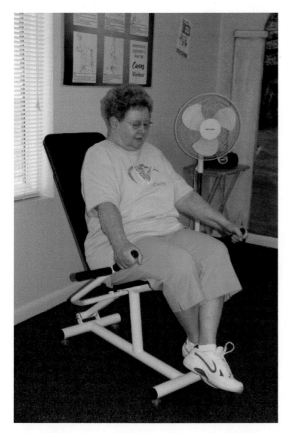

This woman comes to Curves, a women's exercise club, three times a week to maintain her strength. This type of program has assisted her in losing weight as well as in being stronger. Besides, she says, it is fun to socialize with the people there.

exercise are fundamentally the same throughout life. Exercise stimulates the mind, maintains fitness, prevents or slows progression of some diseases, helps to establish social contacts, and generally improves quality of life.

Fatigue and lack of energy, poor sleeping habits, and poor circulation are common reports of older adults. These problems often result in inactivity. Inactivity leads to muscle wasting and weakening of the bones. This vicious circle results in disabling conditions and functional dependency. If exercise could be packed into a pill, it would be the most widely prescribed and beneficial medicine in the world. Chronic conditions such as heart disease, diabetes, osteoporosis, arthritis, obesity, and depression all have been shown to improve or experience a slowing of progression with regular physical activity.

Physiologically, a regular exercise program can build and maintain muscle strength and endurance and can improve the capacity of the heart, circulatory system, and lungs. The commonly heard phrase "use it or lose it" is the overall theme for exercise and fitness in a person's later years. Exercise programs for people older than 60 should emphasize a regular routine of exercise to expand and increase strength, flexibility, and endurance. Such exercise programs can be developed for individuals with a wide range of conditions, from wheelchair-bound or bedbound frail elderly people to physically active individuals. By-products of a good fitness program include increased energy, buildup of lean body mass, and increased self-esteem.

Strengthening

Strengthening exercises help build and maintain muscle condition by moving muscles against resistance. Simple strengthening exercises are needed to promote activity without tiring a person too easily. Muscle strength is also crucial to the support of joints and can help prevent problems related to arthritis. Improving muscle strength is a primary objective in slowing the progression of osteoporosis. Patients confined to bed lose bone mass very quickly. It can be restored, however, when exercise is resumed. Something as simple as doing range-of-motion exercises while holding a soup can makes a difference in strength for most older adults.

As a nurse, you must be aware of the impact a short-term illness can have on an older person. Something as commonplace as the flu can cause significant weakness and inactivity. Weak muscles lead to falls, which cause hip fractures and other injuries. If older adults are unaware of the importance of strengthening exercises, no incentive can return them to the normal level of function.

Strength-building exercises are important for a person with diabetes because the exercises help regulate glucose metabolism by increasing muscle mass. The greater the muscle mass, the greater the glycogen level in the muscles, and the more energy will be available in reserve for periods of exertion.

Flexibility

Flexibility exercises involve slow stretching motions. Medical and fitness experts agree that stretching is the most important part of an exercise program designed to prevent injuries, reduce muscle tension, and maintain range of motion. As a result of the normal aging process, muscles tend to lose elasticity, and tissues around the joints thicken. Flexibility exercises can delay or reverse this process by preventing muscles from becoming short and tight.

All stretching motions should be done gradually and slowly, without any sudden force or jerking motion. You should encourage a variety of stretching exercises for different parts of the body, including arms, shoulders, back, chest, stomach, buttocks, thighs, and calves. All exercise routines should include warm-up and cooldown with 5 to 15 minutes of stretching exercises. As the older person's range of motion increases, the individual will be able to reach, turn, and move in all directions with more grace and less pain.

Endurance

Endurance-building or aerobic exercises improve the function of the heart, lungs, and blood vessels. A frequent report from older people is "feeling tired." Endurance-building

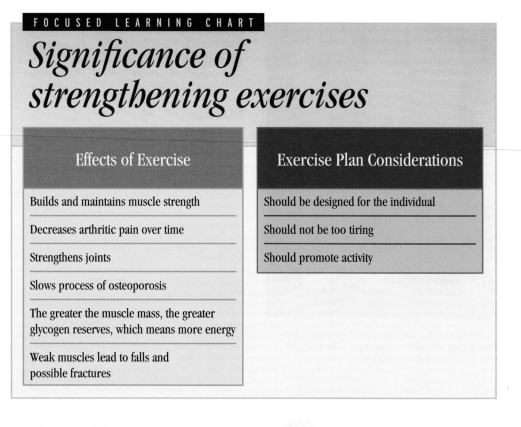

FOCUSED LEARNING CHART

Significance of strengthening exercises

Effects of Exercise	Exercise Plan Considerations
Builds and maintains muscle strength	Should be designed for the individual
Decreases arthritic pain over time	Should not be too tiring
Strengthens joints	Should promote activity
Slows process of osteoporosis	
The greater the muscle mass, the greater glycogen reserves, which means more energy	
Weak muscles lead to falls and possible fractures	

exercises help strengthen the heart to pump blood and the lungs to exchange oxygen and increase the elasticity of blood vessels. These functions are a vital part of fitness and feeling good. Walking, cycling, and swimming or water aerobics are excellent all-around exercises.

As stated earlier, the basic components of an exercise routine for older people include strengthening, flexibility, and endurance. In addition, attention must be given to breathing during exercising. Breathing is a vital part of an exercise program. As a person concentrates on the exercise, it is easy to forget to breathe. The correct breathing technique is to breathe out during vigorous effort or exertion and breathe in as the muscles relax.

Roll breathing is also a good way to reduce tension and to induce relaxation. As a result of changes related to aging, some older people experience a general loss of elasticity of the chest muscles and some postural changes. These gradual changes often affect the way they breathe. This is especially true for frail and bed-bound elderly adults. The roll-breathing exercises outlined in Box 6.1 encourage deep breathing and are very helpful as a relaxation technique and a component of an exercise program.

A last comment on exercise is a caution for older adults who have not been exercising on a regular basis, who are frail, or who have cardiovascular problems. Anyone with heart problems or high blood pressure, who is overweight, or who has been told to be cautious in personal activity level should have an exercise program prescribed by a physician.

Physical fitness is one component of life that enables people to live it to its fullest. As a nurse, you have a responsibility to understand and teach the importance of exercise and fitness to elderly patients. Remember to think holistically. What environment is best for the older person, who is there to be a support person, what is the incentive to make change? If you know these things and assist in making a plan that uses them, the program will be more successful.

Stress

Stress motivates people to act, forces them to think under pressure, and challenges them to be creative and resourceful human beings. The key is to be able to strike a balance between too much stress and not enough, between positive stress (*eustress*) and stress that is harmful (*distress*). As with all areas of health promotion, it is never too late to improve a technique. Failure

---

BOX 6.1 **Roll Breathing**

The object of roll breathing is to develop full use of the lungs. It can be practiced in any position but is best learned lying down, with the knees bent.

1. Place your left hand on your abdomen and your right hand on your chest. Notice how your hands move as you breathe in and out.
2. Practice filling your lower lungs by breathing so that your left hand goes up and down while your right hand remains still. Always inhale through your nose and exhale through your mouth.
3. When you have filled and emptied your lower lungs 8 to 10 times with ease, add the second step to your breathing: inhale first into your lower lungs as before but then continue inhaling into your upper chest. As you do so, your right hand will rise and your left hand will fall a little as your stomach is drawn in.
4. As you slowly exhale through your mouth, make a quiet, relaxing whooshing sound as first your left hand and then your right hand falls. Exhale and feel the tension leaving your body as you become more and more relaxed.
5. Practice breathing in and out in this manner for 3 to 5 minutes. Notice that the movement of your abdomen and chest is like the rolling motion of waves, rising and falling in a rhythmic motion.

Roll breathing should be practiced daily for several weeks until it can be done almost anywhere, providing you with an instant relaxation tool anytime you need one. *Caution:* Some people get dizzy the first few times they try roll breathing. Get up slowly and with support.

Reprinted with permission from Kemper, D. W., Deneen, J. E., Giuffré, J. V. *Growing Younger Handbook* (2nd ed.). © Copyright 1992 HEALTHWISE, Incorporated, P.O. Box 1989, Boise, ID 83701. Copying of any portion of this material is not permitted without express written permission of HEALTHWISE, Incorporated.

---

to take a healthy approach to dealing with stress can greatly increase the risk of developing or worsening heart disease, cancer, and other chronic diseases.

For most older people, stress is related to three basic areas: environment, body, and mind. Environmental stressors are weather, crime, crowds, time pressures, and the demands of others. The human body can experience stress because of illness, accidents, drugs, lack of sleep, and normal changes related to aging. The mind can create stress for people because of negative attitudes and perceptions, boredom, despair, and hopelessness.

Regularly occurring events such as trips to the grocery store, pain from arthritis, and fear of the unknown conditions of retirement all may create stress for older people. Stress-related problems and symptoms include ulcers (stomach pain), high blood pressure (no symptoms), arthritis (joint pain and muscle tension), heart disease (chest pain and difficulty breathing), cancer (increased susceptibility), headaches (constant worry), circulatory problems (cold hands and feet), and backaches (muscle spasm and chronic pain).

One of the most important strategies for health promotion is to help older people recognize their personal reactions to stress and their bodies' physiological responses. Tools used to recognize stress include a stress log or journal of daily stressful situations, life change inventory, and stress control inventory.

After an individual has recognized personal stress and his or her response to it, several interventions are available to help relieve it. As a nurse, you should understand and be able to recommend appropriate stress-reducing activities. These activities may be divided into the two categories: quick relaxers and long-term stress management skills.

A quick relaxer is something a person can do in 2 or 3 minutes to relax and counteract symptoms of distress. One of the most important, yet difficult, skills for some older people is learning simply to relax. Learning how to relax helps older people sleep better, control blood pressure, lower cholesterol, reduce headaches, relieve depression, reduce or eliminate use of drugs and alcohol, and smile more. Examples of quick relaxers include roll breathing, progressive muscle relaxation, imagining a pleasant place or situation, eye relaxation, and exercise. The importance of exercise was discussed earlier in this chapter; however, it is worth emphasizing that exercise is the most natural way to relax. For the greatest calming effect, an elderly individual can combine fitness activities with breathing and other mental relaxation techniques.

For some older people, dealing with stress requires more than a few "stress-buster" quickie techniques. If stress causes continuous physical and mental discomfort that results in illness, learning how to deal with the source of stress needs to be a major goal. This assumes that the individual understands what is causing the stress.

Using the four stress management options listed here as a teaching tool is very helpful for many people. The four basic options are:

1. Attempt symptom relief (quick techniques).
2. Accept the stressor (change perception or attitude). *Example:* Your children frequently call you at the last minute to baby-sit your grandchildren. You may accept the stress and decide you really do not need much time to prepare, so say yes and enjoy! Another choice is to lovingly say no!
3. Alter the stressor (change or alter the source of stress so it is no longer there). *Example:* Make the decision that you will not be able to baby-sit unless they let you know 1 day ahead of time.
4. Avoid the stressor (remove yourself from the stressor). *Example:* Decide you will not be a babysitter for your grandchildren. After the source of stress has been pinpointed, the older person often can decide whether to accept, alter, or avoid it.

Stress management techniques may be unfamiliar to many older individuals, even though stress and recognition of stress have been buzzwords for some time. Teaching older people stress management can be done very successfully through either group or individual activities.

⬤ LIFESTYLES

Maintaining a healthy lifestyle at any age involves more than getting fit, eating right, and coping with stress. Other challenging issues that people of all ages encounter are relationships, possible alcohol and drug abuse, and lack of self-care.

Relationships

Human life is constantly defined and redefined by our ties to others. The term *relationship* means any significant bonding in which a person feels a strong sense of responsibility toward the physical and emotional welfare of others.

As people grow older, the reality is that all relationships eventually end. Whether through divorce from a spouse or death of a spouse, child, family member, friend, or pet, the loss redefines one's life. An individual's ability to

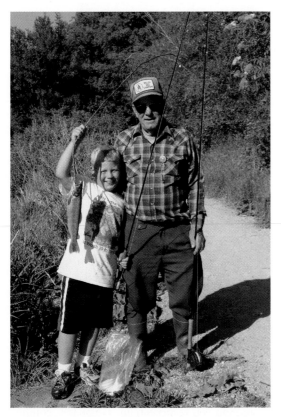

This 65-year-old man goes fishing with his youngest grandson two or three times a week. From Utah, they have traveled to Alaska and Washington to fish as well as to the many beautiful fishing places in their own locale. Fishing always has been part of this man's lifestyle, but now he has the added close relationship with his grandson.

years predicts how they will deal with these same stressors later.

As years pass, life changes can become increasingly complex. Older adults must deal with changes caused by retirement, which can have major impacts on home life, health, finances, and role changes. In addition, the loss of relationships may be frequent and numerous.

As a nurse, you have an opportunity to help older adults gain insight into loss and life change (see Chapter 11). Chapter 11 contains a section on the stages of grief that may be helpful to you in understanding reactions of older adults to loss. You need to assess the effect that loss has on a person's ability to function with day-to-day activities. As an LPN, you must ask questions and allow the older person to share concerns. Health-promotion activities that focus on mental wellness can provide an excellent opportunity for older adults to express the concerns they face. The American Association of Retired Persons (AARP) preretirement program offers a useful notebook that helps lead discussions about the myths, fears, and reality of change as one grows older.

deal with the process of grief over the losses can result in significant personal and health changes and changes in dealing with others. How strongly these changes affect the rest of one's life depends on how well the individual, and those involved the personal life of the individual, cope with the loss. How people have coped with change and crisis in younger

Alcohol, Drugs, and Aging

Abuse of alcohol and drugs among older men and women is a more serious problem than most people realize. Until more recently, older problem drinkers tended to be ignored by health professionals and the general public. The neglect occurred for the following reasons:

- The elderly population in the United States was small, and few older individuals were identified as alcoholics.
- Chronic problem drinkers (individuals who had abused alcohol off and on for most of their lives) often died before old age.
- Older people frequently have been able to hide drinking problems because they often are retired or have few social contacts.

POINT OF INTEREST

Throughout my 40-plus years of nursing, I always have been a gerontological nurse in my heart. I have had other jobs, but my interest is in elderly people. At some point in my career, I began referring to the elderly persons in my care as "wise and wonderful." It is a simple thing; I don't recall anything special that caused me to start using that term. It just happened because of the respect I developed for the wonderful, old "survivors" with whom I was privileged to work.

Some families may unknowingly accept or encourage drinking in older family members. They may have the attitude that drinking should be tolerated because older people have only a limited time left to live and should be allowed to enjoy themselves. Sometimes the alcohol consumption seems to be an insignificant amount to the family, and they blame the resulting impairment on aging.

The amount, time, and place of alcohol consumption have little significance. The critical issue that needs to be addressed is what alcohol does to an individual's quality of life and functional ability. Older problem drinkers seem to be of two types. The first type is the chronic abuser, who has used alcohol heavily throughout life. Approximately two-thirds of older alcoholics are in this group. The second type begins excessive drinking late in life, often in response to situational factors such as retirement, reduced income, declining health, or the deaths of friends and loved ones. In these cases, alcohol is first used for temporary relief but later becomes a problem.

The physical effects of alcohol are significant for older people. Alcohol impairs mental alertness, judgment, physical coordination, and reaction time. These problems mimic and exacerbate the deleterious effects of other chronic conditions (dementia, depression, and arthritis) and increase the risks of falls and other accidents.

As people age, they seem to become less tolerant of even small amounts of alcohol, and the effect of alcohol on the body may be unusual. For example, the effects of alcohol on the cardiovascular system may mask the pain of an oncoming heart attack. Older people are the greatest consumers of prescription and OTC drugs. The combined use of alcohol and drugs increases the likelihood of a toxic or lethal effect.

Treatment efforts for older alcoholics have not been fruitful. It is easy to overlook or accept problem drinking because the drinking seems to offer enjoyment or comfort. It is much harder to create social alternatives to the life events that lie behind alcoholism.

As a health professional, you may be tempted to rush over or omit assessment questions referring to alcohol intake. Because nurses often play a key role in recognizing alcohol and drug problems, you cannot afford to avoid such questions. You always should ask what the impact of this problem may be on the older person's ability to function. It becomes easy to see that the physical, mental, and social impact of drinking could contribute to alcohol dependency.

The primary health-promotion goal is helping older adults and their families recognize when alcohol is a problem. Second, straightforward information must be given to elderly adults regarding the effects of alcohol, especially in combination with drugs. The nurse needs to understand the older person's reason for drinking. Health-promotion activities that create alternatives should be made available to an older person with an alcohol problem.

Because of their critical importance, drug issues are discussed extensively in Chapter 20; however, emphasis on the problem of drug dependency and abuse is important. Drug abuse depends on the relationship of the individual to the drug in question. Harmful drug relationships are frequently termed *overmedication, dependency, abuse, problem usage,* and *habituation.* Regardless of the reason, if an older person misuses a drug or becomes dependent on it, the effects are similar to those of problem drinking. Physical and mental impairments resulting from prescribed or OTC drugs mimic disease states and increase the risk of falls, accidents, and dependency.

One role of health promotion is to offer education and screening regarding drug use. Promoting self-responsibility is the key component. Nurses must assess the impact of drug treatment on an older person's ability to complete ADLs. If a patient cannot afford a prescribed drug, he or she probably will not take the medication as ordered. If the older adult does not understand what outcomes are expected from the drug treatment, misuse of a drug may ensue by taking it for too long or taking too much of it.

● SELF-CARE—TAKING CHARGE

Older adults are best qualified to keep themselves healthy and to know when they are ill. As a nurse, you need to respect and explore what the older person reports as the problem. Do not take charge and deny an older adult responsibility for personal health and health management.

Self-care, self-help, and *self-maintenance* are terms often used interchangeably to describe various aspects of an individual's efforts to maintain optimal health and functionality. When an individual cannot assume responsibility for self, the patient has the nursing diagnosis, Self-Care Deficit. Most individuals with this diagnosis need medical or nursing intervention.

From a nursing perspective, the focus is frequently on ADLs, which are the most basic self-care activities engaged in by older adults. It is common to see dependence in at least some basic ADLs for older people. Surveys show that 18% of people older than 65 years who live in the community are dependent in at least one ADL. In nursing homes, the prevalence is 80%. In addition to ADLs, an older person needs to manage IADLs, such as selecting a physician and other health-care providers and knowing how and when to access the health-care system.

Regardless of whether an older adult is attempting to overcome a functional deficit in ADLs or IADLs, the same self-care skills are needed. Self-care involves the following:

1. Accepting personal responsibility for one's own health
2. Adopting healthy lifestyle habits with regard to fitness, relaxation, and nutrition
3. Learning how to make the changes you choose to accomplish the things you want to do

Can you understand how these three characteristics complement the concept of gerotranscendence? If you can't, discuss this with someone who is familiar with gerotranscendence, such as a classmate, and work to identify the relationships.

Accepting personal responsibility for health behaviors applies to the "why" of the decision more than the "what." *Self-responsibility* means that the older adult does not rely solely on spouse, children, physician, or nurse to determine "what to do to be healthy." The person must be allowed to think through the options and make each decision. This does not mean that a person should not seek the assistance of others, but rather that a need exists to work in partnership with the physician, nurse, or family (separately or together) to make the best decision.

The self-care concept emphasizes the need for encouraging individuals to take a more active role in maintaining or improving their health. Often, the patient does not understand this process, and it is not easy for older people to accomplish. Health-promotion strategies related to self-care must include helping the older adult understand how to be in charge of personal health decisions. Your efforts should be focused on enabling an older person to be a wise medical consumer and to know how and when to work and communicate as a partner with the health-care team.

Your role as a health professional is twofold. First, you must offer activities to develop self-care skills, such as one-on-one or group activities that teach how to be an informed medical consumer, and you must provide information on prevention and screening guidelines, such as for a mammogram or a prostate examination. Second, you must ensure that the environment enables the older adult to use the skills to make choices and assume self-responsibility. If an older adult wants to be a partner with the physician in a health decision, the physician should take the time to answer questions and ultimately let the treatment decision be made by the older adult. This same situation applies to nursing. If the older adult is expected to be involved in a self-care activity program, you, as a nurse, must be prepared to explain the benefits, procedures, and risks and be willing to let the older adult make the decision.

CONCLUSION

Until more recently, the needs of older adults often have been ignored in the health-promotion movement. Health professionals mistakenly assumed that elderly people had no interest in health-promotion programs. As the United States has become more and more a home to an aging society, these views have changed.

As a nurse, you must understand the importance of promoting holistic wellness to all older adults, regardless of the presence or absence of disease. Attainment of a disease-free existence is not a realistic goal. Health-promotion efforts should be directed toward maintaining functional independence for older people.

Older Americans need information about how to lead healthy lifestyles. When information and opportunities are provided, older people often are willing to make the changes necessary to improve their health. Exercising regularly, maintaining a nutritious diet, managing stress effectively, taking medications safely, avoiding overuse of alcohol, and recognizing self-care as a choice are all behaviors that improve health and the quality of life. Pursuit of high-level wellness in later years is the responsibility of the individual and society.

CASE STUDY

Mrs. C. is a 65-year-old widow who has lived alone since the death of her husband 2 years ago. She retired 1 year ago from her job of 25 years as a secretary. After retirement, she participated in a health-promotion and screening clinic at the senior center. After completing a lifestyle inventory and screening, the following problems were noted in the categories of health promotion:

Nutrition: 10 lb overweight

Exercise: Does no regular exercise

Stress: Cries easily, often unable to sleep at night, complains of fatigue and generally low energy

Relationships: Misses people at work, talks about missing deceased husband

Substance abuse: Takes an OTC sleeping pill and one glass of wine before bed

Self-care: Has not seen a physician since she had a hysterectomy 10 years ago; never had a mammogram and does not perform breast self-examination; cannot recall immunization history but is sure she has not had any in the past 10 years; has never had a flu shot or pneumococcal vaccine; recently had blood pressure taken at a drug store machine, which measured 150/92 mm Hg.

Discussion

1. List additional assessment data that should be known in each of the categories of health promotion.
2. How might you determine Mrs. C.'s greatest concern?
3. What part does Mrs. C.'s motivation play in developing a wellness plan?
4. What conditions or disease states might develop if Mrs. C. continues with no changes in her life?
5. What might be the first priority for Mrs. C.?

Solution

1. Additional information in each category might include:

   Nutrition
   What are her daily eating habits? What type and amount of food and fluids does she consume? Does she eat alone?

   Exercise
   What is her normal daily activity level? How does this differ from her daily activity level before retirement?

   Stress
   What is her perception of coping with changes such as death and retirement? Has she stated any other physical complaints, such as fatigue, headaches?

   Relationships
   What family or friends are important to her? In what social activities is she involved? Does she have any hobbies?

   Substance Abuse
   When did she begin drinking wine every evening? When did her sleeping problems begin? Has she always taken sleeping pills?

   Self-Care
   Does she have a primary care physician? Does she understand the importance of exercise and disease prevention? Does she know the danger of combining drugs and alcohol?

2. Asking Mrs. C., "What is your biggest worry or concern in your life at this time?" would be a beginning. Although the nurse may see many areas of concern, Mrs. C.'s own concerns are more critical.
3. If the nurse begins by focusing on what Mrs. C. considers most important, it is easier for Mrs. C. to understand her own motivation.
4. Some potential conditions include:
   Excess weight, which may lead or contribute to high blood pressure and physical limitation

Lack of exercise, which may contribute to weight gain but may also worsen arthritis and its effects on mobility

Emotional stress, which may lead to depression

Relationship concerns, which also may contribute to depression, isolation, and abuse of drugs and alcohol

Combination of alcohol and OTC sleeping pills, which may lead to further sleeping problems, alcohol and drug misuse, depression, injury, and further isolation

5. If Mrs. C. has not seen a physician for 10 years, she needs at least a baseline physical assessment. She has some significant conditions that need to be addressed, such as borderline high blood pressure, sleep problems, and weight gain. In addition, she should have a basic screening related to disease prevention.

Select the best answer to each question.

1. Incentives for older persons to participate in health-promotion behaviors include:

   a. The belief that they will find the Fountain of Youth

   b. The belief that activities will help them die well

   c. The belief that activities will help keep them independent

   d. The belief that it will please their physician

2. Health-promotion programs appropriate for older people should focus on:

   a. Maintaining functional abilities

   b. Advancing youthfulness

   c. Enhancing chronic illnesses

   d. Developing dependence on others for care

3. Basic components of an exercise routine for older people are:

   a. Strengthening, endurance, and flexibility

   b. Strengthening, dieting, and power walking

   c. Strengthening, dieting, and aerobics

   d. Strengthening, aerobics, and the food pyramid

4. Age-related changes that affect nutrition include:

   a. Increase in the ability to taste

   b. Increase in body fat

   c. Increase in lean body mass

   d. Increased metabolic rate because of aging thyroid

5. Older people with a drinking problem are often ignored because:

   a. They have many social opportunities to drink

   b. The amount of alcohol consumed may seem small

   c. The resulting impairment may seem to be age related

   d. So many older people drink

7

Nutrition for Older Adults

Judith Pratt

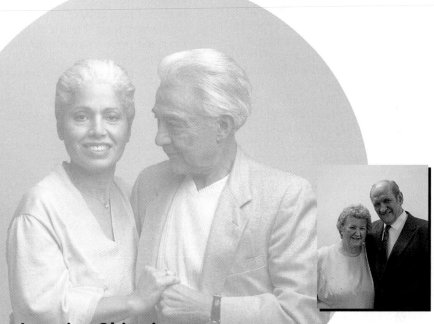

Learning Objectives

After completing this chapter, the student will be able to:

1. Perform a nutritional assessment on an older adult.
2. Make nutritional food choices by using the food pyramid as a guide.
3. Identify the influence carbohydrates, proteins, and fats have on maintaining a healthy body.
4. Identify the influence vitamins and minerals have on maintaining a healthy body.
5. Discuss therapeutic diets for older adults with special nutritional needs.
6. List four basic causes of electrolyte imbalance.

INTRODUCTION

A nutritious intake of food is essential at any age to achieve optimal health. Good nutrition is a major contributor to feeling well. Healthy eating provides the body with energy to do things, such as work or play. It promotes clear thinking, fights disease, and usually tastes good. I often think of children (and adults) in third world countries who go to bed hungry and wake up to nothing or very little to eat. It is appalling that so many people die of malnourishment in this world. Nurses are key to teaching and supporting older persons in their care to understand and use the vast nutritional choices available in the United States. Nutrition is a crucial behavior for positive health in every aspect of living.

The amount and type of food necessary to promote health generally changes as people age. Younger people can "get away" with eating donuts or candy, whereas older people generally cannot eat such things without a weight gain or an increase in their blood sugar. This is because of their slower metabolism and other normal aging physiology. Foods that contain carbohydrates, proteins, fats, vitamins, and minerals in the appropriate amounts must be included in dietary planning for older adults.

As a licensed practical nurse (LPN), you need to be aware of physical changes related to aging that affect food intake. Examples of these changes could be gastric disorders caused by normal gastrointestinal (GI) changes and chronic diseases or illnesses that impact nutritional requirements. In addition, certain foods and medications can cause adverse drug reactions. Older adults may have difficulty chewing or swallowing food because of disease or poor dentition. Sensory changes in seeing, smelling, and tasting foods may influence an older person's appetite. Loss of appetite also can occur as psychosocial changes bring on depression, dependency on others for meals, and changes in cognitive skills. As you perform nutritional assessments on older adults, you need to think about reasons why they may have nutritional deficits and ways you can assist them and their family in overcoming the problem.

NUTRITIONAL ASSESSMENT

The place where you work may or may not have a nutritional assessment tool, and assessment tools may vary from nursing home to hospital. In many facilities, a dietitian does the nutritional assessment, but that is not always true. You need to be mindful of the basics of a nutritional risk assessment so that you can perform one successfully wherever you are working. The basics are as follows (Tabloski, 2006):

1. Has an illness or the person's condition been responsible for a change in eating patterns?
2. Does the person eat fewer than two meals a day?
3. Does the person's diet include fruits, vegetables, meat, and milk products?
4. Does the person's diet frequently include alcoholic drinks?
5. Does the person have difficulty chewing or swallowing food (known as *dysphasia*)?
6. Does the person have the resources to purchase food?
7. Does the person eat alone most of the time?
8. Does the person take three or more medications, either prescribed or over-the-counter (OTC), each day?
9. Has the person lost or gained more than 10 lb in the past 6 months?
10. Is the person able to shop, cook, and feed himself or herself?

Any of these nutritional risks can lead to malnourishment and can compromise health. You need to report the nutritional risks you identify to your supervisor. Good nutrition is essential to good health. The reconciliation of the basic problems listed is critical to improved health.

The objective in gerontological nursing is the best health possible for the best possible quality of life. Good nutrition is a powerful tool in making that happen. Five vegetables and fruits a day can make a profound difference in an older person's life. First, there is more energy because of the increase in natural vitamins and minerals. There is more roughage, which results in regular bowel movements and the elimination of laxatives. Finally, well-prepared fruits and vegetables taste good and are colorful on the plate; this can stimulate appetite for many people.

MANAGING WEIGHT

Monitoring weight also is an effective tool in assessing nutritional status. You need to be attentive to any changes in an older adult's weight. If there is weight gain, perhaps the person needs to become more active. It also is wise to check for

The priority you need to set, to ensure good nutrition for the older adults in your care, is your commitment to their health. First, learn the information in this chapter. There is quite a bit of detail, but these are only the basics. They are the minimum you need to learn to be effective in promoting nutritional health. Then:

1. Apply the information to your own life.
2. Take a nonthreatening stand and work with team members to see that effective nutritional assessments are done on admission for all patients.
3. Support your nurse manager or volunteer to assist in putting the pertinent information from the assessments into the care plans.
4. Go further and put up signs so the staff will know what assistance and encouragement each person needs. Examples are: "Offer fluids or juice every 2 hours and record." "Cut up fresh fruit for Mrs. Jonas." "Stay and visit with Mr. Tanaki while he eats. Encourage him to eat more food." "Mr. Welling has a food journal at the desk. Please record all food consumed."

As a caring professional, you are one member of the health-care team who can work with others to identify and manage nutritional problems that exist with older adults.

edema because the weight gain could be caused by a greater physiological problem. If there is weight loss, this needs to be reported to the registered nurse (RN) to assess for possible causative factors.

Most of the common reasons older adults lose weight are related to the fact that they are older. Older adults generally have less mobility and may be unable to prepare meals efficiently or go shopping. Older people generally don't like to eat alone. Some elderly people are forgetful and may neglect to prepare meals.

Older adults often have a decreased income, so they may not have the money or transportation to obtain adequate food. I remember an elderly woman who attended a gerontological clinic and asked me if it was "OK" for her not to take her antihypertensive

medication so she could buy food. This is a serious problem because Medicare does not cover medications, so without a supplemental insurance, medications are very expensive for someone on a set income. A thorough and caring interview should reveal many of these problems and others that are age related.

There are several disease-related reasons why an older adult may lose weight. Are there changes in health that could cause weight loss, such as fever, infection, fracture, or a wound? Does the older adult have metabolic changes that affect food absorption, digestion, or elimination? Have you noticed the older adult experiencing chewing or swallowing difficulties, or an inability to self-feed or even to see the food? Perhaps the person is depressed, or maybe the food does not taste good. If you are doing home care, there could be reasons the older adult cannot purchase, prepare, or eat the food. Be sure to ask about any problems related to nutrition. Part of a good assessment would be to ask the older adult why, in his or her opinion, the weight loss is happening.

Reasons for weight gain can also be related to the process of aging. Weight gain is a problem for people of any age but seems worse for elderly persons who often have orthopedic conditions such as arthritis. First, the activity rate for older people generally is decreased. Did you know that the basal metabolic rate declines by 2% each decade of life? Unless people compensate for that normal physiological change by eating less, they gain weight. In addition, as the human body ages, it has less lean body mass, and an equal amount of increased fat tissue (adipose tissue). Because adipose tissue metabolizes more slowly than lean body mass, it does not burn calories as quickly.

TRACKING NUTRITIONAL INTAKE

During an illness, nutrition performs a vital role in the body's ability to heal. The critical foods—foods that provide energy and nutrients—are divided into three groups: carbohydrates, proteins, and fats. Each food group is necessary to maintain and repair the body during health and illness. It is important for you to have the knowledge to assess the inclusion of these food groups in a person's diet. This assessment can be done by evaluating if the person's diet includes a variety of fruits and vegetables and meats or other protein-rich foods, including bread and cereals. The assessment can be done by observing what the older adult is eating during mealtime or by keeping a food journal. You can discuss a food journal with the RN with whom you work. If you have observed a patient or resident eating minimal amounts of food or showing signs of listlessness, you should talk to the RN about the problem and perhaps suggest a food journal. A food journal is a designated place where the person removing the food tray writes down not only the percentage of the food eaten but also the actual food. Then someone, such as a dietitian, is assigned to determine if the person is eating enough calories and specific nutrients. Sometimes the journal needs to be kept for only 3 days. A week also is common. It is a great way to gather the detailed information needed to assist an older person with good nutrition. The dietitian is an excellent resource when there is a problem with someone not eating nutritious foods.

A review of the food groups, carbohydrates, proteins, and fats, can help you in your ability to assess and evaluate nutritional needs of older adults. Carbohydrates, proteins, and fats are found in various fruits and vegetables, meats, milk, and breads and cereal foods. It is important for older adults to eat a variety of foods with these nutrients to ensure that the body can maintain and repair itself.

NUTRITIONAL NEEDS OF OLDER ADULTS

Regardless of the health status of an older adult, he or she needs to have food that provides calories for energy and nutrients to maintain body functions. A person's food needs for optimal health change with age, physical activity, and health status. That is the reason scientists at Tufts University have modified the U.S. Department of Agriculture's MyPyramid to indicate the nutritional needs of people older than 70 years of age (Lichtenstein et al., 2008).

Anatomy of MyPyramid

One size doesn't fit all

USDA's new MyPyramid symbolizes a personalized approach to healthy eating and physical activity. The symbol has been designed to be simple. It has been developed to remind consumers to make healthy food choices and to be active every day. The different parts of the symbol are described below.

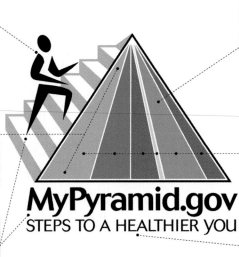

Activity
Activity is represented by the steps and the person climbing them, as a reminder of the importance of daily physical activity.

Moderation
Moderation is represented by the narrowing of each food group from bottom to top. The wider base stands for foods with little or no solid fats or added sugars. These should be selected more often. The narrower top area stands for foods containing more added sugars and solid fats. The more active you are, the more of these foods can fit into your diet.

Personalization
Personalization is shown by the person on the steps, the slogan, and the URL. Find the kinds and amounts of food to eat each day at MyPyramid.gov.

Proportionality
Proportionality is shown by the different widths of the food group bands. The widths suggest how much food a person should choose from each group. The widths are just a general guide, not exact proportions. Check the Web site for how much is right for you.

Variety
Variety is symbolized by the 6 color bands representing the 5 food groups of the Pyramid and oils. This illustrates that foods from all groups are needed each day for good health.

Gradual Improvement
Gradual improvement is encouraged by the slogan. It suggests that individuals can benefit from taking small steps to improve their diet and lifestyle each day.

MyPyramid.gov
STEPS TO A HEALTHIER YOU

USDA U.S. Department of Agriculture Center for Nutrition Policy and Promotion April 2005 CNPP-16
USDA is an equal opportunity provider and employer.

GRAINS   VEGETABLES   FRUITS   OILS   MILK   MEAT & BEANS

MyPyramid, the U.S. government's revised food guide pyramid, is an excellent resource in determining a nutritious diet for older adults. (From United States Department of Agriculture, Washington, D.C., 2005.)

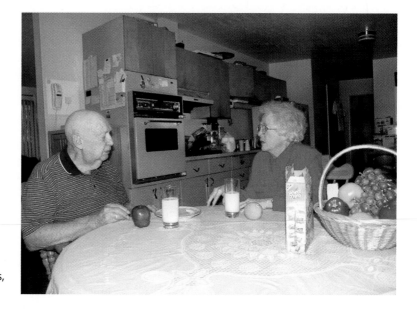

This couple has learned the value of healthy nutritious food. Their meals focus on fresh fruits and vegetables, sodium restriction, calcium intake through dairy products, and low-fat proteins.

The modified pyramid has two layers added to the base. One is water, indicating the importance of drinking the necessary eight glasses a day. The second base layer is exercise, which is crucial for healthy aging. In addition, this pyramid has a flag at the top to represent the need for dietary supplements because of the decreased absorption that accompanies the aging process. Another aspect of the modified pyramid is the outline of the nutrient-dense foods. Because most elderly people have to eat less food to maintain their appropriate weight (remember they lose 2% efficiency in their metabolism every decade and have decreased

lean mass), they need to eat foods filled with nutrients (nutrient-dense) rather than nutrient-poor foods. The nutrient-dense foods are highlighted on the pyramid and include vegetables, whole grains, lean meats, dry beans, and nuts. The modified pyramid is important to your knowledge base for teaching and supporting older people in their quest for nutritional health.

Imagine you are a certified nursing assistant (CNA) working two part-time jobs while you are in school pursuing your LPN education. You work 1 day a week for Sea Side Long Term Care Center and 1 day a week for Mountain Top Home Health. You enjoy working for both agencies and have received excellent evaluations from your supervisors. You have cared for the same people for 3 weeks now and have been part of the process of improving older adults' health with attention to good nursing care. You love what you are doing and enjoy applying what you are learning in school to the patients and residents.

You have been caring for Mrs. Salvador for the past 3 weeks. Mrs. Salvador is a 75-year-old Hispanic resident who has enjoyed good health until about 6 weeks ago. She was the sole caregiver for her husband, who had Alzheimer's disease for the last 5 years. Mr. Salvador died 2 months ago. Mrs. Salvador fell 6 weeks ago while visiting her husband's grave site. She fractured her left hip and her left elbow. A week after her surgery, Mrs. Salvador was transferred to Sea Side Long Term Care Center for physical therapy. She needs physical therapy before she will be able to care for herself at home. You noticed Mrs. Salvador has lost 4 lb since her

CRITICALLY EXAMINE THE FOLLOWING:

To help you to be effective in assessing the nutritional status of others, you need to evaluate your own eating patterns and nutritional condition. This will help you be more understanding of the potential difficulty of managing a nutritious menu for older people in your care. The United States Department of Agriculture has created a food guide, MyPyramid, that can assist you in analyzing your own eating patterns. Use the Internet and go to the www.mypyramid.gov Web site to see how you are doing. Do the self-evaluation. How would you assess your eating habits? What do you need to change to make your diet healthier? Write a 1-page summary of your nutritional evaluation and be prepared to submit it to your instructor.

admission to the unit. Consider the following questions you should ask when evaluating her weight loss:

1. Was Mrs. Salvador losing weight before her accident?
2. What questions should you consider that were in the nutritional assessment tool in this chapter?
3. Does Mrs. Salvador's diet include adequate amounts of carbohydrates, proteins, and fats to assist in her healing?
4. What information should you report to the RN?

Carbohydrate Foods

You can begin your assessment of Mrs. Salvador's diet by noting carbohydrate foods she is eating. There are two types of carbohydrates: complex and simple. Complex carbohydrates are those that the body breaks down slowly and that sustain energy over a longer period. Because Mrs. Salvador is recovering from surgery to repair her hip and elbow, her body requires more complex carbohydrates to replace the loss of reserved or stored carbohydrates called glycogen. Older adults are healthier when their bodies have a sufficient supply of glycogen reserves. Simple carbohydrates differ from complex carbohydrates in that they are easier for the body to digest and they provide a source of quick energy.

You need to know which foods provide carbohydrates that promote health. Carbohydrates come from grains, beans, nuts, milk, meat, fruits, and vegetables. Honey, molasses, sugar, and syrups also contain carbohydrates. You can assess Mrs. Salvador's carbohydrate intake by evaluating whether or not these foods have been included in her meals and if she has been eating them. The more carbohydrate foods are processed, the more the dietary fiber will be broken down, and some of the carbohydrate nutritional value will be lost. You need to encourage Mrs. Salvador to eat foods containing fiber to aid in her digestion and to maintain proper bowel function. Simple carbohydrates come from milk and foods high in sugar content, and they are a source of quick energy. These carbohydrates would be valuable for Mrs. Salvador before her physical therapy treatments. The food guide MyPyramid provides a visual representation of the sources of carbohydrates that need to be included in her diet. The food guide will be helpful to you in teaching Mrs. Salvador what she should be eating.

Protein Foods

Sources of food rich in proteins come from plants and animals. Plant sources of proteins come from grains and include breads, rice, cereals, and pasta. Dried beans and dark green, deep yellow, and starchy vegetables are considered good sources of plant proteins. Animal sources of proteins come from milk, cheese, yogurt, meat, fish, and poultry. Refer to the MyPyramid food guide for a visual representation of the sources of proteins that need to be included in a healthy diet. Frequent use of the food guide will assist you in mastering the information necessary to give meaningful nutritional care to the older people in your care.

You should assess the protein foods in Mrs. Salvador's diet. Proteins are the building blocks of the body. They are necessary for building and repairing body tissue and are important for Mrs. Salvador as she recovers from her accident and subsequent surgery.

Proteins are divided into structural and functional categories. Structural proteins contain the amino acids that make up the hair, muscles,

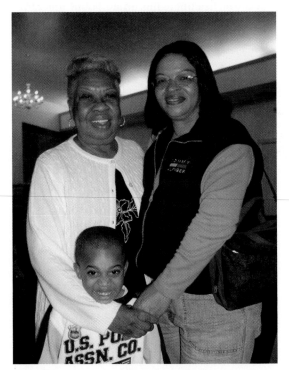

Most older adults eat healthier meals and eat more of the meal if they are eating with family members. This daughter and her son have dinner with grandma three times a week. This assures the grandma of good food and company. She says she really looks forward to these dinners.

tendons, and skin. Functional proteins help the body perform the activities that keep the body alive, such as moving oxygen through the circulatory system. Hemoglobin; insulin; and myosin, which is found in muscle tissue and is the reason the muscles can contract, are functional proteins. The body requires a supply of proteins to repair worn-out or damaged tissues and to build up new tissue. They also play an important part in maintaining the body's water balance in metabolic activities and the body's defense system (Nix, 2005).

When using the term *protein,* you need to remember the term *amino acids.* There are thousands of different proteins, and they all are made of various combinations of amino acids. The two classifications of amino acids are essential and nonessential. You should not confuse the terms *essential* and *nonessential* amino acids with their value to the body because both kinds of amino acids are important for good health. Nonessential amino acids refer to amino acids that the body can make itself. Essential amino acids are the amino acids that the body cannot make itself and must be part of the diet. Essential and nonessential amino acids are necessary for the body to function properly.

The terms *complete* and *incomplete proteins* refer to the foods that supply proteins to the body. A complete protein comes from animal sources and contains essential and nonessential amino acids. Incomplete proteins come from plant sources, but plants do not include both essential and nonessential amino acids. By eating different plant sources during the same meal, the body gets a supply of complete and incomplete proteins that provide the essential and nonessential amino acids for building, maintaining, and repairing the body. Think of eating beans and rice in the same meal. Each of these foods is an incomplete protein food. When they are eaten in the same meal, however, the body is able to use them as a complete protein. This way of obtaining protein for the body is used by millions of people who either like rice and beans instead of meat or cannot afford fresh meat to eat.

Age, gender, chronic diseases, fevers, infections, surgery, and traumatic injury are factors in determining the need for added protein for the body's maintenance and repair. The physician may order a laboratory test to measure the nitrogen level of a recovering older person to determine how well the body is maintaining its tissue. In malnutrition or an illness, the body may not have the proper nitrogen balance to support health. A positive balance of nitrogen indicates that there are adequate sources of protein for the body to use to build and repair tissues. A negative nitrogen balance indicates wasting of muscle tissues and impairment of body organs and their functions. As an example, a nitrogen imbalance would put Mrs. Salvador at risk for infections and other complications.

Laboratory tests of Mrs. Salvador's blood and urine samples measure nitrogen balance. Urine tests measure protein metabolism. An increase in nitrogen level indicates that excess body tissue is being broken down. A serum hemoglobin, hematocrit, or serum albumin measurement helps diagnose protein deficits (Nix, 2005).

When you are collecting urine for laboratory tests that contain the words *creatinine, albumin, transferrin, prealbumin,* or *retinol-binding protein,* you will know the urine is being tested for nitrogen balance. The RN will give you instructions on how the urine should be collected. The letters *BUN* on a laboratory request or report are related to nitrogen balance. Dietary adjustments may be ordered after the laboratory results have been reviewed by the physician. Monitoring Mrs. Salvador's dietary protein intake is crucial for managing her nitrogen balance.

Fat Foods

Fats are a group of foods that, when absorbed into the body, serve as a support and protection for the internal organs. Adipose (fat) tissue serves as a buffer or cushion from an external injury. Fats help to sustain the body's temperature. Certain vitamins—A, D, E, and K—are fat-soluble. The body must have foods containing fats to absorb these important vitamins. Some fat is required by the body to maintain health.

Fats are found in plants such as beans and nuts and in oils produced from plants. Fats also are found in meat, poultry, fish, shellfish, and eggs. The food guide MyPyramid provides a visual representation of the sources of fats that are heart healthy, are vital for a healthy body, and should be included in the diet. Mrs. Salvador requires fat in her daily diet because fat is required to maintain health, provides a way for fat-soluble vitamins to be effective, and serves as a support and protection for Mrs. Salvador's internal organs.

Remember that you are pretending to be a CNA who works for a nursing home and a home health facility. One day after your nutrition class, you realize that you are interested in the role played by nutrition in diets of older adults so that they can be healthy or improve their health after an illness or accident. You begin to think about the Rice family. You have been working with the Rice family for the past 2 months. Mr. Rice had a stroke 3 months ago and still needs help with bathing. The Rices have enjoyed your visits and requested your services when you are working at the home care service.

Mrs. Rice is interested in her husband's care and is always asking you questions about tips to help him return to better health. Mrs. Rice's care and concern are helping Mr. Rice to assist more in his own care. During your visits with the Rice family, you have been able to observe what foods are routinely being eaten. Mrs. Rice is interested in giving Mr. Rice nutritious meals. You have noticed, however, that Mrs. Rice includes many foods high in carbohydrates. Mrs. Rice has been overweight most of her adult life. She has not been able to leave home very often and seems to be gaining more weight. You have encouraged Mrs. Rice not to forget to take care of herself. You suggested she see her physician when she started complaining about being thirsty all the time and needing to urinate more frequently (classic symptoms of diabetes mellitus).

You recall information from your nutrition class that research and science indicated that too many carbohydrates in the diet can lead to vascular disease, type 2 diabetes, cancer, arthritis, obesity, and other chronic diseases. Is it possible that Mrs. Rice is at risk for any of these conditions? You know that excess carbohydrates are stored as fat in the body. Excess fat may lead to a change in the body's hormonal system that can suppress the immune system and leave the person at risk for an infection (Insel, Turner, & Ross, 2006). Do you think Mrs. Rice is at risk for an infection?

You understand that chronic diseases may be a result of an individual's personal nutritional history. Mrs. Rice has an appointment with her physician in 1 week. You suggest she keep a food journal of all the foods she eats for the next week and share it with her physician. A food journal is an excellent method by which to monitor carbohydrates, proteins, and fats that are included in the daily diet.

Vitamin Foods

Vitamins are classified as either water-soluble or fat-soluble. Water-soluble vitamins are absorbed in water. As mentioned earlier, fat-soluble vitamins require fats for the body to absorb them. The names of vitamins are taken from the alphabet, letters A through K. With one exception, which you will see shortly, vitamins are not produced by the body and must be extracted from foods (or nutritional supplements). The food guide MyPyramid provides a visual representation of the sources of foods containing vitamins that should be included in the diet.

Vitamin A is a fat-soluble vitamin that comes from animal and plant sources. Plant sources of vitamin A are dark green leafy vegetables and deep yellow or orange fruits and vegetables (Dudek, 2006). Vitamin A is necessary for good vision, hair, skin, gums, glands, and other body functions. Studies are ongoing to determine the role of vitamin A in cardiovascular diseases and cancers (Behan, 2006; Dudek, 2006; Nix, 2005). You should follow the research on the role of vitamin A in the diet and encourage the people in your care to eat foods that are rich in vitamin A. This information will help them improve or maintain their health. Vitamin A can be stored in the body's fat; a deficit in vitamin A may not be noted for some time. Some older adults take megadoses of vitamin A, which may become toxic. A symptom of excess vitamin A is a yellowish orange skin color. Always ask about the consumption of food supplements and carefully document what is being taken. This is especially important to do with vitamin A intake.

There are several classes of B vitamins, and they all are water-soluble. The B vitamins are listed as the B vitamin complex. Vitamin B_1 (thiamine) is necessary for the nervous system to function correctly and to help older adults have an appetite. Older adults who drink excess alcohol or have had a poor nutritional intake may need to have thiamine supplements. Foods rich in thiamine come from whole grains or enriched cereals, nuts, organ meats, and legumes (Behan, 2006; Dudek, 2006; Nix, 2005). Should you ask the Rices and Mrs. Salvador about their use of alcohol? If so, why? The answer is yes, you should, because it is part of a thorough nutritional assessment.

Riboflavin (vitamin B_2) is essential in building and maintaining healthy tissue. Riboflavin is necessary for wound healing as well. Foods rich in riboflavin are milk products, whole-grain and enriched breads and cereals, eggs, meats, and leafy green vegetables (Behan, 2006; Dudek, 2006; Nix, 2005). It is easy to understand why riboflavin in the diet is important for Mrs. Salvador and Mr. Rice, isn't it?

Niacin (vitamin B_3) is essential in maintaining a healthy nervous system and skin and in preventing dementia. This is a critical vitamin for someone like Mr. Rice because of his stroke, which is seriously affecting his nervous system. Foods rich in niacin are whole grains and enriched breads and cereals that are high in proteins. It is possible, however, for older people to have too much niacin in the diet. Symptoms of niacin toxicity are diarrhea, vomiting, gastric ulcers, and liver damage. Older people need to be assessed for vitamin supplements in their diets and encouraged to seek counsel concerning the consumption of megavitamins because of the multiple toxicity possibilities (Behan, 2006; Dudek, 2006; Nix, 2005).

Pyridoxine (vitamin B_6) assists in the metabolism and use of glycogen that has been stored as a fuel. Pyridoxine is required for brain activity and normal functioning of the central nervous system. Pyridoxine promotes healthy skin. Think about why pyridoxine would be important in maintaining and repairing Mrs. Salvador's and Mr. Rice's bodies at this time. Food sources of pyridoxine are eggs, whole-wheat products, peanuts, walnuts, and animal sources. Pyridoxine can be lost during processing of frozen foods, luncheon meats, and cereal foods. This is important for Mrs. Rice to know, and no one except you are there to teach her. Toxicity from pyridoxine can occur with the inclusion of megadoses from dietary supplements. The classic symptom of toxicity is lack of muscle coordination. An overdose of pyridoxine has the potential for nerve damage as well.

Cobalamin (vitamin B_{12}) is essential for the production of hemoglobin and for proper nervous system function. Anemia and GI and neurological changes can result from insufficient amounts of cobalamin. The best foods containing cobalamin are from animal sources. Older adults who do not eat many animal products may require a supplemental source of cobalamin. The people you care for may require medical interventions if their diets are low in food sources from animals (Behan, 2006; Dudek, 2006; Nix, 2005). Meals on Wheels is an excellent intervention from the community and may need to be considered.

Folate belongs to the B vitamin complex but was not given a number. Folic acid is the most stable form of folate. Folic acid is rarely found in foods but is a supplement in vitamins and in fortified foods. Folate is essential to the formation of body cells and hemoglobin. Folate can be found in green leafy vegetables, dried beans and peas, organ foods, and orange juice. Folate from foods cannot be used well by the body; foods enriched with folic acid should be included in the diet (Behan, 2006; Dudek, 2006; Nix, 2005).

More recent studies indicate that if women get adequate doses of vitamin B_6 and folic acids in their diets, they cut their risk of cardiovascular disease by 50%. In addition, a 9.3-year study of 579 older adults suggested that an intake of folate at or above the Recommended Daily Allowance is associated with a reduced risk of Alzheimer's disease (Corrada et al., 2005).

Vitamin C is next in the vitamin alphabet list. Vitamin C is also known as ascorbic acid. Vitamin C is water-soluble and is easily lost in cooking. Vitamin C cannot be stored by the

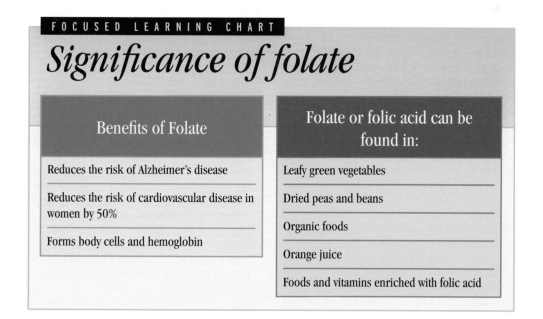

FOCUSED LEARNING CHART

Significance of folate

Benefits of Folate	Folate or folic acid can be found in:
Reduces the risk of Alzheimer's disease	Leafy green vegetables
Reduces the risk of cardiovascular disease in women by 50%	Dried peas and beans
	Organic foods
Forms body cells and hemoglobin	Orange juice
	Foods and vitamins enriched with folic acid

body, so there must be a daily intake of food containing vitamin C. The body needs vitamin C to build and repair body tissues and bones and to keep teeth and gums healthy. Lack of vitamin C causes wounds to fail to heal, bones to weaken, and muscles to degenerate and puts the older adult at risk for infections and falling. Many foods are good sources of vitamin C. Citrus fruits, strawberries, kiwi fruit, tomatoes, cantaloupe, and dark green vegetables are only a few of the fruits and vegetables that are rich in vitamin C (Behan, 2006; Dudek, 2006; Nix, 2005).

Vitamin D (cholecalciferol) is one of the fat-soluble vitamins. Cholecalciferol is not actually a vitamin because it is produced naturally by the body. The body can produce its own vitamin D if there is enough exposure to the sun. Few people have enough sun exposure, however, to produce sufficient vitamin D. Vitamin D is necessary for the absorption of calcium and phosphorus to maintain bone tissue and many other body functions. Without vitamin D, calcium cannot be absorbed. Older adults are at risk for vitamin D deficiencies if they are not eating enough fortified foods. Older women who have vitamin D deficiency are at risk for bone loss, which puts them at risk for fractures owing to osteoporosis. Vitamin D occurs naturally in very few foods. The sources of vitamin D are the sun, fish oils, and foods fortified with vitamin D. Excessive amounts of vitamin D supplements increase the risk of older adults absorbing more calcium than their bodies need. Increased calcium puts a strain on the kidneys and soft tissues of the body (Behan, 2006; Dudek, 2006; Nix, 2005).

Vitamin E (alpha-tocopherol) is a fat-soluble vitamin. Vitamin E provides protection for many body tissues and prevents red blood cells from being broken down. There is evidence that vitamin E aids in wound healing. Studies are ongoing to determine the role of vitamin E in preventing cancer and heart disease. Foods rich in vitamin E include peanut butter, nuts, seeds, wheat germ, and vegetable oils. Vegetable oils have been found to be the best sources of vitamin E. Leafy vegetables and animal sources also provide the body with vitamin E. Large doses of vitamin E may interfere with blood clotting; vitamin E is not toxic, however (Behan, 2006; Dudek, 2006; Nix, 2005).

Vitamin K is a fat-soluble vitamin. The main roles of vitamin K are blood-clotting functions, aiding in bone development, and regulating blood calcium. Foods that supply vitamin K are leafy vegetables, cabbage, broccoli, cauliflower, fruits, and animal sources. Vitamin K is extracted by bacteria in the intestine from food sources that contain vitamin K. Antibiotics that kill bacteria in the intestine may interfere with the production of vitamin K, and complications can occur. Hemorrhaging is a complication of vitamin K deficiency. You should report dark or bloody stools to the RN at any time, but you should be especially vigilant if the older person you are caring for is taking antibiotics. There are no studies to indicate toxicity to vitamin K (Behan, 2006; Dudek, 2006; Nix, 2005).

The food guide MyPyramid provides a visual representation of food sources that are rich in vitamins. Think about all the vitamins and how the body requires these vitamins to build, maintain, and repair itself.

Mineral Foods

Along with the necessity of vitamins in the diet, you need to recognize the importance of the minerals people require to maintain a healthy body. Minerals are inorganic substances that are found in nature and in the human body. The 54 inorganic substances, called elements, that have been identified can be found on a chemical periodic table; 25 of these elements, or minerals, are found in the human body. Minerals make up only a small part of the body but are found in all body tissues and fluids. Minerals are classified according to the amount needed to maintain a healthy body. Macrominerals, or major minerals, are needed in greater amounts than microminerals, also called trace minerals. Macrominerals and microminerals are essential for the body (Dudek, 2006; Nix, 2005). Included in the macrominerals are calcium, phosphorus, sodium, magnesium, chloride, and potassium. These minerals are known as electrolytes and can be lost as a result

CRITICALLY EXAMINE THE FOLLOWING:

Consider the body's need for vitamins in helping Mrs. Salvador recover from her accident and subsequent surgery. Make a list of the effects that insufficient nutrients could have on her body. Think of her actual problems rather than making a list of each vitamin and listing its symptoms when it is insufficient. Design a day's worth of meals with the foods that would assist her with healing. Include what you have learned from the previous sections on specific foods as well. Be prepared to share your menu plan with the class.

of vomiting, diarrhea, excessive sweating, or urination. The electrolytes must be kept in balance, or the older adult is at risk for complications. The food guide MyPyramid provides a visual representation of the sources of food that provide macrominerals and microminerals.

Calcium is the most prevalent mineral found in the body. Bones and teeth are composed primarily of calcium. In older adults, additional calcium is necessary for the maintenance of bones and teeth. Calcium also is required for many other body functions, including blood clotting, muscle and nerve activity, digestion, and maintenance of blood pressure. Ask yourself, "Should Mrs. Salvador and the Rices continue to eat foods that contain calcium?" They should simply because of their age. Calcium is best absorbed in connection with vitamin D. Calcium is found in milk and milk products, leafy vegetables, legumes, and fortified food products. Osteoporosis can occur if there is a calcium deficiency. Renal stones are a risk if the body has too much calcium. Mrs. Rice asked you if she or Mr. Rice should take a calcium supplement. This question should be referred to the RN and then the physician. There are many calcium supplements on the market, and Mrs. Rice needs to be advised as to whether a supplement is needed (Dudek, 2006; Nix, 2005).

After calcium, phosphorus is the most common mineral in the body. Phosphorus combines with calcium in the maintenance of bones. Phosphorus is found throughout the body and is required for metabolism and cell membrane maintenance. Phosphorus helps maintain the body's chemical balance and is necessary for some of the vitamins to be used by the body. Phosphorus is readily available because it is found in all meat products, grain products, fruits, and vegetables. Symptoms of low phosphorus levels are weakness, pain, and loss of appetite.

Mrs. Salvador and the Rices should not be deficient in phosphorus unless they have been consuming large quantities of antacids that contain aluminium hydroxide. The aluminium hydroxide reacts chemically with phosphorus and cancels out its usefulness to the body. Mrs. Rice told you she has been taking more antacids since Mr. Rice had his stroke. You need to encourage Mrs. Rice to tell her physician about her history of antacid use or get her permission to report it to the case manager (Dudek, 2006; Nix, 2005).

Mrs. Rice's history of being thirsty and her report of frequent urination is an indicator of diabetes. Magnesium deficiencies occur with alcohol abuse, renal disease, cardiovascular disease, diabetes, starvation, chronic diarrhea, and vomiting. Magnesium is necessary for energy, maintaining cell membranes, muscle activity, and metabolism. Sources of magnesium are whole grains, green leafy vegetables, dried peas and beans, nuts, and cocoa (Dudek, 2006; Nix, 2005). Ask yourself, "What symptoms should I be aware of that would indicate Mrs. Salvador or the Rices may have low magnesium levels?"

Sodium is responsible for maintaining the water balance in the body. Sodium is necessary for glucose activity and nerve and muscle functions. Sodium deficiency is rare unless an older adult has chronic diarrhea, vomiting, excessive sweating, or kidney disease. The body usually excretes excess sodium through the kidneys. Drinking fluids usually dilutes the sodium, but edema and hypertension may result if there is kidney impairment. Ask yourself, "Will Mrs. Rice's sodium level be affected by her frequent urination and her wanting to drink more water? Does Mrs. Rice have symptoms of edema?"

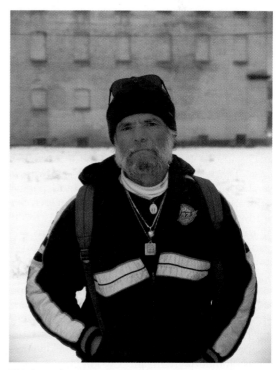

This homeless man has learned where to go for the best meals possible. Some restaurants (e.g., fast-food places) discard their uneaten food at specific times of the day. This assures their customers of fresh food. It also provides this man with a good burger that is reasonably fresh. He also goes to the Salvation Army for lunch and the homeless shelter for dinner. Most of his day is spent outdoors, even on cold days like this one.

Sodium is found in processed foods and is often added during cooking and at the table. To lower sodium levels, an older adult may be advised to limit salt intake and to reduce processed foods in the diet. Numerous foods contain sodium in various amounts. Mrs. Rice's physician may prescribe a diet to reduce her sodium intake.

Chloride, which is a form of chlorine, is found in the body's tissues and fluids. Despite the fact that the body contains only a small amount of chloride, this mineral is important in digestion and in maintaining water balance. Chloride partners with sodium (sodium chloride) in the diet. Chloride deficiency is rare. Too much chloride can result in hypertension and perhaps vomiting (Dudek, 2006; Nix, 2005).

Potassium is found in body fluids. Potassium is responsible for the functions of the nervous and musculoskeletal systems, metabolic activities, blood pressure, insulin release, and water balance. Why should the Rices be interested in potassium-rich foods? The best sources of potassium are unprocessed fruits and vegetables. Potassium is water-soluble and can be lost when cooked in water. Some foods may be rich sources of potassium but also contain high levels of sodium. Processed foods are often high in sodium but low in potassium. A dietitian is the best health professional to help you with a list of foods that are rich in potassium. An older adult who has a potassium deficiency may have muscle weakness and loss of appetite. Diuretics may cause potassium loss through the urine. A resident you were caring for a week ago was on a potassium replacement regimen, and part of your care plan was to monitor for cardiac symptoms, breathing problems, bloating, and overall muscle weakness and to report these signs and symptoms to the RN immediately if they were present (Dudek, 2006; Nix, 2005).

Minor minerals, which are called trace minerals, in the human body include iron, zinc, iodine, selenium, copper, manganese, chromium, molybdenum, and fluoride. Iron is responsible for producing hemoglobin and aiding in metabolism. Deficits in iron may reduce the effectiveness of the immune system, affect wound healing, and cause weakness and fatigue. Excess iron may increase risk of infections, organ damage, and joint disease. Foods rich in iron are fortified breads and cereals, red meat, and legumes (Dudek, 2006; Nix, 2005).

Zinc is essential for wound healing and insulin storage, and it aids in metabolic and immune functions. Zinc comes from animal sources, legumes, and whole grains. Deficits in zinc may cause abnormal glucose tolerance, impaired wound healing, weight loss, loss of night vision, and diarrhea. Too much zinc can cause anemia, vomiting, renal failure, malabsorption of calcium, dizziness, and muscle pain (Dudek, 2006; Nix, 2005). Why would zinc be important in Mrs. Salvador's and Mrs. Rice's diets?

Iodine is a component of the thyroid hormone, which regulates metabolism. An iodine deficiency can cause a thyroid goiter, weight gain, and lethargy. Why is it important for Mrs. Rice's physician to assess her thyroid? Excess iodine may cause an enlarged goiter. Sources of iodine are iodized salt, dairy products, breads, and seafood (Behan, 2006; Dudek, 2006; Nix, 2005).

Selenium aids in healing and in preventing disease, and it is essential to metabolic activities. A deficiency in selenium may cause heart disease. Excess selenium may cause nerve damage, nausea, and vomiting. Selenium comes from animal sources, seafood, and whole grains (Behan, 2006; Dudek, 2006; Nix, 2005). What specific foods should Mrs. Salvador and the Rices include in their diets to help in healing?

Copper partners with the body's iron to produce hemoglobin. Sources of copper are organ meats, seafood, nuts, legumes, and seeds. In a report that was being given at Sea Side last week, you heard that one of the residents had a low blood copper level. The man was receiving total parenteral nutritional (TPN) therapy. You wondered if his TPN therapy may be the cause of his low blood copper level (Behan, 2006; Dudek, 2006; Nix, 2005). TPN is a cause for low blood copper levels.

Manganese is associated with metabolic functions and blood clotting. Main sources of manganese are breads, whole grains, legumes, fruits, and vegetables. Deficiencies in manganese are rare (Dudek, 2006; Nix, 2005).

Chromium improves glucose metabolism. Chromium is found in brewer's yeast, grains, and cereal foods. A deficiency in chromium may lead to poor glucose tolerance (Behan, 2006; Dudek, 2006; Nix, 2005). Why would chromium be important in Mrs. Rice's diet?

Molybdenum is essential to many metabolic activities. Molybdenum is found in whole grains, legumes, milk, leafy vegetables, and organ meats. There are few symptoms that indicate lack of or excessive molybdenum in the diet (Behan, 2006; Dudek, 2006).

Fluoride has a role in bone and dental integrity. Fluoride's main source is water, to which it has been added as a supplement.

Osteoporosis may result from a lack of fluoride in the diet. Excess fluoride in the diet may cause nausea, vomiting, diarrhea, and chest pain (Behan, 2006; Dudek, 2006).

The quality of foods containing minerals is related to the soil where the foods are grown. Fruits and vegetables that are grown in soils rich in a particular mineral contain more of that mineral. For example, grains grown in soil rich in selenium contain more selenium. The mineral content of foods is hard to determine because fruits and vegetables are grown in various areas of the world (Dudek, 2006; Nix, 2005).

Water

Fluids are considered an essential component of the older adult's nutrition plan. Water is the most plentiful and easiest dietary means of fluid intake. How much water or fluid the older adult should consume is determined by gender, age, chronic diseases, physical activity, metabolic activity, and heat exposure (Nix, 2005; Dudek, 2006). Older adults are at risk for dehydration because they often neglect drinking adequate fluids during the day. It is important for you to ask the Rices about their fluid intake. Monitoring Mrs. Salvador's fluid intake is part of your nursing assessment.

Water is the main component of the body and has a vital role in maintaining body temperature. It serves as a transport for nutrients and wastes, is a lubricant to body parts, is a solvent for the body's chemical processes, and gives form to the cells and tissues of the body. Water can be found in soft drinks, juices, coffee, tea, milk, and foods containing high contents of water (Dudek, 2006; Nix, 2005). Part of your assessment of the Rices' daily fluids would be to have them report all drinks they consume during the day. Part of being a good LPN is monitoring your patient's fluids during your shift.

Water helps maintain the body's temperature. Heat may be lost from the body by physical activity or an increase in temperature in the environment. The water lost by sweating during an activity or the increase of environmental temperature serves as a coolant to maintain a normal temperature. When fluid is lost through the cooling process, older adults need to increase fluid intake (Nix, 2005).

Blood and other body and tissue secretions are transported or circulate through the body. The circulated fluids carry oxygen, nutrients, and other materials to all body cells. Circulating fluids also carry waste materials from the cells. Fluids provide for smooth joint activity. Fluid also cushions the contact between the organs (Dudek, 2006).

Water is essential for the chemical processes in the body. Water is the necessary solvent the body uses for producing the chemical solutions required for health maintenance. It is vital for the body to maintain a water balance. Older adults are at risk for dehydration because of inadequate fluid intake, not feeling thirsty, medications, perspiration, and chronic diseases. You must remember to assess the older adult for oral fluid intake. Water leaves the body through the skin, lungs, kidneys, and stool. Asking the Rices about their urination is one way to assess for dehydration. You also can assess the skin for dryness and loss of turgor.

Body Electrolytes

As mentioned earlier in the chapter, the particles (minerals) in the body's solutions are made up of electrolytes and plasma proteins (Nix, 2005). The minerals that make up the body's electrolytes are calcium, phosphorus, sodium, magnesium, chloride, and potassium. Each of these minerals carries a chemical charge. Some have a positive charge, and others have a negative charge. You may decide to do a quick review of chemistry to understand better the chemical processes that happen in maintaining an electrolyte balance. For now, you need to be aware that all of the electrolytes must be maintained in a chemical state of neutrality. Any imbalance puts a person at risk for complications. These electrolytes are moved through the body by fluids. Consider fluids and electrolytes lost as a result of vomiting, diarrhea, excessive perspiration, or urination, and then consider the person's potential for electrolyte imbalance.

POINT OF INTEREST

It is best to check skin turgor over the forehead or sternum in older adults. You check the skin turgor by softly pinching the skin and then observing how fast the skin returns to normal. If it is slow to return to normal, the person is dehydrated.

Plasma proteins consist of protein and globulin. They are the major substance in blood circulation and control the water movement in and out of cells. With this understanding, you should realize that blood volume is strongly influenced by plasma proteins. Electrolytes and plasma proteins must be kept in balance to maintain healthy body functions (Nix, 2005). Plasma proteins were discussed earlier in this chapter.

⬤ LABORATORY TESTS AND OTHER ASSESSMENT INFORMATION

Laboratory tests may be performed on either blood or urine. Blood tests measure serum albumin, hemoglobin, hematocrit, electrolytes, nitrogen levels, other minerals, serum lipids, and glucose. Urine tests measure glucose, ketones, protein, nitrogen, and blood (Nix, 2005; Tabloski, 2006). Chapter 21 contains more information on laboratory tests.

Along with the laboratory reports, the physician will need the person's nutritional assessment and a current list of all medications. The physician writes the orders for the older adult's dietary needs. The diet may be modified or changed according to the person's history and laboratory results and your assessment of the person's diet and medication history.

You, the LPN, are in a key position to assess Mrs. Salvador's and the Rices' diets. You will want to assess if they have a variety of fruits and vegetables, meats or other protein-rich foods, and bread and cereals in their daily diets. A poor nutritional intake would put Mrs. Salvador and the Rices at risk for potential health problems. The physician orders laboratory tests if there is a question about their nutritional status.

⬤ DIET PLANS

As the LPN, you need to be aware of the various diet plans that can be used to meet the nutritional needs of the people in your care. You are aware that several of the residents at the Sea Side have different diets.

A regular diet is given to older adults who are healthy, have no special nutritional needs, and are capable of making nutritious food choices. Amounts of foods depend on the person's appetite, and selections of foods are made by personal likes and dislikes. Mrs. Salvador is receiving a regular diet.

A modified diet is given to older adults if they have a prolonged illness and have not eaten or if they have difficulty chewing or swallowing food. Foods in the modified diet range in consistency from clear liquids to soft foods.

Clear-liquid diets are foods that are liquid at room temperature and can be seen through. The physician or dietitian needs to write directions about what foods are to be included in this diet. Clear or strained juices, teas, carbonated drinks, clear broths, and gelatins are some of the choices. Most clear-liquid diets do not provide adequate nutritional requirements (Dudek, 2006). Patients receiving clear-liquid diets are moved to a full-liquid diet as soon as their health condition allows.

Full-liquid diets are composed of the foods included in the clear-liquid diet with the addition of foods that are liquid at room temperature but are not necessarily clear. This includes custards, ice cream, milk, some strained cereals, fruits, and vegetables. The full-liquid diet meets more of the person's dietary requirements but not all nutritional requirements. The dietitian gives you instructions on the food to include in a full-liquid diet.

Foods in the soft diet include those from a regular diet that have been modified for people who have difficulty chewing foods. An example is Ms. Taylor, who has had problems with her dentures. Her dentures should be repaired soon, but she will probably continue to request a soft diet because of sore gums. Foods in this diet are mashed, chopped, or ground.

A therapeutic diet may be ordered for people who need tailored nutritional choices. The person may need more calories or fewer calories in the diet. There may be an order to increase or decrease the amounts of carbohydrates, proteins, or fats in the diet. The person may need dietary restriction on foods containing sodium, potassium, iron, or micronutrients. Examples of therapeutic diets are a diabetic diet or a low-sodium diet for a person with hypertension. Fluid restrictions may be necessary for some patients with chronic kidney disease. Older adults may have food allergies or may be unable to tolerate some foods; such foods should not be included in the diet.

There are health conditions in which a person's GI system can digest food but the person may be unable to consume food. Enteral, or tube, feedings are required for these people. Commercial or blended formulas are used to provide nutritional support by using a feeding tube that can be placed in the nose or directly into the GI tract through the abdomen (Dudek, 2006; Nix, 2005). The physician and dietitian determine types and amounts of formulas to be used.

Older adults with more extensive illnesses or injuries may require TPN or parenteral nutrition (PN). TPN is administered through a percutaneous endoscopic gastrostomy tube. PN is administered intravenously. An RN is responsible for the maintenance and monitoring of both types of feeding tubes (Dudek, 2006; Nix, 2005). The RN instructs you, the LPN, on your responsibility in monitoring a patient receiving TPN or PN. Be sure you are very clear on what the RN wants you to do and not do. If you need specific information on these therapies, be sure to ask. Do not pretend you know what you are doing if the opposite is true.

CONCLUSION

Regardless of the type of diet the older adult you are caring for may be eating, you must remember to provide a pleasant atmosphere to encourage eating. Clear the area where the food will be set. Be unhurried and pleasant, and talk to each person. It may be necessary for you to assist the person in eating the meal. If so, be patient and kind as you perform this aspect of your job. Spending time with the person and sharing a pleasant conversation is a good time for you to educate, support, and assess the older adult's dietary needs.

Not all older adults for whom you will be caring for are in frail health. People are living longer and may have chronic diseases such as arthritis, heart disease, or diabetes. Many older adults consider themselves to be healthy, however, even with these chronic conditions. Under the supervision of the RN, you will have the opportunity to teach older adults about proper nutrition.

You know what nutrients in Mrs. Salvador's diet will aid in healing her fractures and her recent surgery. Nutrition will have an impact on the chronic diseases the Rices are experiencing as well. You know that nutrients affect the immune system, aid in healing, and influence chronic conditions. You must be careful when offering nutritional advice because older adults have issues with food likes and dislikes, economics, and physiological conditions, along with psychosocial issues that they experience.

CRITICALLY EXAMINE THE FOLLOWING:

You are assigned to care for Mrs. Pearson, an 81-year-old woman who has had abdominal pain, nausea, and vomiting. Which type of diet most likely will be ordered for her? Explain why.

Mrs. Pearson's symptoms become much worse. Her skin turgor indicates dehydration. What laboratory tests might the physician order? Which diet is most likely to be ordered by the physician? Think through Mrs. Pearson's health-care needs and come to class prepared to discuss them.

Because you have been thinking about the nutritional needs of Mrs. Salvador and the Rices throughout this chapter, you can consider them as your case study. Write a 1-page summary regarding their health and nutritional needs to submit to the faculty person. Consider each person separately, and then address the following:

1. List their health problems that are related to nutrition.

2. List the nutrients they need and why.
3. List the foods they should eat to have the appropriate nutrients.

Select the best answer to each question.

1. All of the following should be assessed when monitoring an older adult's nutrition *except:*

   a. Does the older adult eat at least two meals each day?

   b. What amount of fluid does the older adult drink each day?

   c. Does the older adult eat with others at least two times each week?

   d. Does the older adult eat foods rich in vitamins?

2. Consider an older adult with bone and soft tissue injuries from a fall. Which diet would be the most effective for this type of person?

   a. High-carbohydrate diet, which would assist in giving the person enough energy for physical therapy.

   b. 1000-calorie diet, which would assist in weight reduction and make ambulation easier.

   c. High-protein, high-carbohydrate diet, which would assist in cellular rebuilding and energy.

   d. TPN, which would provide all nutrients and save energy for the older person.

3. Which of the following diets would be appropriate for an older adult who has problems with blood clotting?

   a. Full-liquid diet

   b. Diet low in potassium

   c. TPN

   d. Diet high in vitamin K

4. All of the following can cause electrolyte imbalances *except:*

   a. Vomiting

   b. Diuretics

   c. Diarrhea

   d. Antibiotics

5. You admit a man who is very lethargic. Through your admission interview, you identify that he is a chronic alcoholic. He is thin and has poor skin turgor. You are concerned about his overall nutrition. He states that he *never* eats green and leafy vegetables. What nutrient do you recognize he needs and is not receiving?

   a. Magnesium

   b. Chloride

   c. Sodium

   d. Phosphorus

8

Culturally Specific Care

Mary Ann Anderson

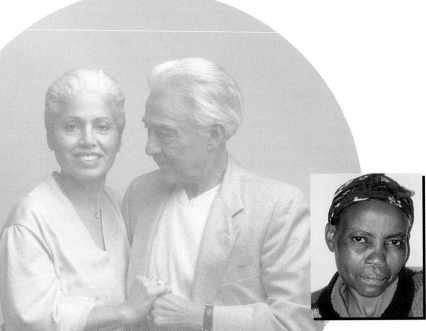

Learning Objectives

After completing this chapter, the student will be able to:

1. Define the differences between culture and ethnicity.
2. Discuss health-care needs of black Americans.
3. Discuss health-care needs of Asian Americans.
4. Discuss health-care needs of Hispanic Americans.
5. Discuss health-care needs of European Americans.
6. Discuss health-care needs of Jewish Americans.
7. Discuss health-care needs of Native Americans.

INTRODUCTION

I was raised in a state where 75% of the population is white, and 75% to 80% is Christian. Utah is a farming state, and I knew many Latinos who traveled through as they worked in the fields, but I didn't see a black person until I was 16. (I saw them on television, but not in person.) Because there are two reservations in Utah, I knew about Native Americans, but I did not actually know any because they lived and went to school on the reservations. My ancestors were Utah pioneers who sacrificed much to live where they had religious freedom. I feel confident in saying that unless you were born and raised in Utah, our cultures are very different.

The concept of culture is complex, but I have a definition that you should find useful. Culture consists of the nonphysical traits we inherit. I am referring to the stories our parents and grandparents tell us (for me it was the pioneer stories of my ancestors) and the traits we learn from simply being in our family or community groups. For me, it was a strong Scandinavian work ethic, family closeness, and a desire to better one's life. My Danish and Swedish emigrant ancestors were very poor, and each generation has worked to provide a higher standard of living for their children. Religion often is considered a significant aspect of one's cultural identity as well.

One common problem with culturally specific care is the tendency for each of us to be ethnocentric. This means that we, as people, think that our "way" is the best way. When one thinks that his or her culture is superior to all others, there is a tendency to dismiss the cultural needs of other people—the thought being that each person should want to be just like you and your culture! This is an act of human nature. For example, when Christian missionaries traveled to the Pacific Islands, they tried to turn the natives into "proper" English men and women. The same thing happened to the Native Americans. Children were taken from their parents during the 9-month school year and were placed in the homes of "proper" white families in an effort to acculturate them. Hitler and others displayed their ethnocentric behavior by killing the "lesser" culture.

As a soon-to-be professional nurse, you need to be aware of any tendencies you have at ethnocentrism and squash them when you are in the clinical setting. As a professional nurse, your objective—your priority—needs to be cultural sensitivity that results in culturally specific care.

Culture is related to ethnicity, but it is not the same thing. Culture is our nonphysical inheritance, whereas ethnicity is the physical inheritance. I have blonde and blue-eyed sisters (you guessed it!); they got those physical characteristics from the Swedes and Danes on my family tree. When you discuss ethnic and cultural aspects of people, you are talking about transcultural nursing. This is a specialized arena of nursing in which cultural awareness is a priority of care. Nurses can earn a master's degree in transcultural nursing; however, you are not expected to know that body of information on such a high level. You simply need to recognize that ethnic and cultural aspects of older adults are an important concept of care.

A basic principle of transcultural nursing is being aware of the need to focus on it to give the best care possible. The other concept reinforced in this chapter is the common sense needed to give transcultural or culturally specific care to others that also addresses ethnic needs. For example, it just does not make sense to assist a Christian out of bed five times a day to face east and pray, just as it does not make sense to require a Muslim to stay in bed when what he wants is to get out of bed, face east, and pray five times a day. You need to be sensitive to the cultural needs of others in all aspects of their lives. Promoting the cultural values of any person assists them in achieving the developmental task of gerotranscendence, which is a concept you should recognize as essential to aging well. In this chapter, your common sense will be enhanced as we discuss ethnicity and culture in several different ways.

▲ PRIORITY SETTING 8.1

The priority for this chapter is clear: for you to give culturally specific care. That requires the skills of holism and caring and the ability to use the nursing process. This chapter gives you a basic background for several different cultural and ethnic groups. You need to focus on the individual, however. Talk to the person; take the time and make a genuine effort to understand the individual's personal needs based on culture and ethnicity as well as the more routine information you need to gather such as health and medication history. What you discover as personal needs for the individual may amaze you. Your responsibility is to meet those needs to promote healing.

ETHNICITY AND CULTURE AS CARING BEHAVIORS

There are multiple aspects to ethnicity and culture. Following is a story from an experienced nurse that addresses ethnicity and culture:

When I was younger and unmarried, I wanted to travel and still use my nursing skills. My ancestors were from Denmark, so that was a place I wanted to spend some time. I finally found a hospital that was eager to take me even though I did not speak Danish. I got my passport and traveled to the land of my ancestors. It all was very exciting. When I reported to work the first day, I realized I had entered a world totally unknown to me as an American citizen. The name of the hospital was exotic and quite beautiful when it was written in Danish. However, the translation to English was something like "The Torture Victims' Hospital." I was confident in my nursing skills before leaving for Denmark. I had worked for 3 years in a high-level intensive care unit (ICU) and knew my way around the system of health care. However, nothing had prepared me for my new job.

Torture victims? There was nothing like that in the United States! I was stunned when the nurse orienting me toured me through the building. The lights were turned low, and everyone walked quietly and spoke in semi-whispers. There was not an overhead public address system, nor were there visitors milling around. It was a building filled with men and health-care providers who moved about in the semi-darkness in a quiet and surreal manner.

I learned that the men, mostly former soldiers and spies from across Europe, were victims of torture from the Communist regimes of Eastern Europe. These were men who had fought or spied in places with danger that was absolutely unknown to me. My entire life changed because of the 6 months I was there. I learned much more than simply discovering the land of my ancestors. The men there often could not be touched because it brought back memories and/or fears of their torture. It took months for a patient to develop trust with any of the hospital employees. They didn't even trust each other because so many of them had been spies and felt that others were spying on them. It was a place of no laughter. The low lighting and diminished sound were to avoid startling the men, as they had the basic "fight" reaction to being startled. They were, after all, soldiers.

Because most of the men had been spies, they spoke English, as do most Danish citizens, so the language was not a problem for me. I spent my 6 months there quietly serving those men in any way I could. In addition, I learned a harsh reality concerning the price of freedom.

The ethnicity of the patients in this story would indicate that they inherited high IQs; healthy, strong bodies without chronic diseases; and strong will or self-concept that allowed them to survive torture without mental illness. The cultural aspects of the men indicated that they were patriotic and loyal, self-disciplined, and tenacious (they didn't give up).

The ethnicity (physical changes) of the United States is ever changing. The 2000 Census (2001) indicated that 74% of the U.S. population was white. The prediction is that in 2050 that number will decrease to 53%. The prediction also indicates that the Hispanic population will grow from 10.2% to 24.5%; Asian, from 3.3% to 8.2%; and black, from 12% to 13.6%. I realize that 2050 is a long way into the future; however, these numbers relate an ethnic trend. As you work in health care, the number of older people will increase, and the cultural diversity of those older adults will become even more diverse. The challenge is to be able to give culturally competent care to a greater number of older adults who are more and more diverse. To do so requires learning about different cultures and paying attention to people and their cultural needs as you give them care. Culturally competent care is a basic concept of administering holistic care to others. It is impossible to do this unless you understand and respect the ethnic and cultural core of each person in your care.

One of my nephews was 20 when he left his small rural community to visit other countries. His first real experience was in Latvia, a small country between the Baltic Sea and Russia. He flew into the capital city, Riga, and stayed there for a year. He spoke the native language (he studied it before going to Latvia) and took the time to meet individuals and families.

He was a teacher and spent a great deal of time with people outside of class as well. While in Latvia, he learned about the cultural and ethnic traits of the society. It was fascinating!

This chapter contains a brief overview of the ethnic and cultural traits of several different groups found in the United States. You may be familiar with many of these groups already, but if you aren't, this is a good time to sit down and be "fascinated" by what you are learning. An example of what I mean is in the following story:

I remember one occasion when the daughter of one of the families in Latvia had a bad cold. Her mother called me and asked me to go to the hospital to visit her. I was amazed that her daughter had gone to the hospital and was admitted for a cold. The young lady was in the hospital for 4 days! I also met people (more than one) who took the standard 3 weeks off from work for the flu. I know I wouldn't have a job if I took 3 weeks off for the flu in the United States. The Latvian people look at sickness in a very different way from most Americans. From my personal experience of having a cold, I can say that all I got was cough syrup and my Dad telling me to buck up and get to school. The people of Latvia were responding to their illnesses in the way that was standard for their cultural norm.

BLACK AMERICANS

I will be referring to people whose ancestors came from Africa as blacks or black people. This phrase refers to people who have origins in any of the black racial groups of Africa predominately, but it also includes people from other nationalities with skin that is black in color. Most members of black communities in the United States descend from people who were brought here as slaves from the west coast of Africa. The largest importation of slaves occurred in the 17th and 18th centuries, which means that black people have been living in the United States for several generations. In modern times, numerous black people have immigrated to the United States voluntarily and have traveled from Africa, the West Indian Islands, the Dominican Republic, Haiti, and Jamaica.

Blacks live in all regions of the United States and are represented in every socioeconomic group. They are disproportionately poor, however,

CRITICALLY EXAMINE THE FOLLOWING

Imagine that you are in a part of the United States where you never have been previously. While there, you encounter the ethnic groups listed in this chapter. Read about the people, and then think about the information. See if you agree with what is written, as I know you have your own experiences with different ethnic and cultural groups. Consider the health-care implications of what you read. Always keep in mind that the information is not designed to stereotype people but to give a general background to different groups of people. Do your best thinking and come to class prepared to discuss your insights and ideas for this chapter.

with 22.1% of all black people living in poverty. In addition, greater than 50% of black people live in urban areas surrounded by the symptoms of poverty—crowded and inadequate housing, poor-quality schools, and high crime rates. The living conditions and poverty of many older black adults are considered major contributors to the fact that black men and women die at a significantly younger age than white men and women (Table 8.1).

Black people hold older members of their communities in high esteem because they value the wisdom and knowledge that comes with aging. This valuing results in fewer black older adults in nursing homes than white older adults. It is unknown if difficulty accessing the health-care system also contributes to this fact.

Older black people often embrace the customs and traditions of their ancestors. The core of their health-care beliefs is often based on harmony with nature. They also consider the body, mind, and spirit as interconnected. When you give care to older black adults, take the time to determine how you can support the person's

TABLE 8.1 Life Expectancy of Older Whites and Blacks in the United States

Group	Life Expectancy (Years)
White men	73.8
White women	79.6
Black men	66.1
Black women	74.2

Source: Stolberg, S. G. (2002). U.S. life expectancy hits new high. New York Times, Sept. 12.

Poverty is defined as a family of four with an income of $18,000 or less per annum

Government Assistance

Public housing

Government loans for school

Medicaid

Aid to families with dependent children (AFDC)

Food stamps

Head Start programs

Free school lunch

Note: The 2000 Census notes that people over the age of 65 are at their lowest income level since the census has been taken.

Living Conditions

Overcrowded housing

Poor sanitation

Homelessness

Poor nutrition

Higher crime rates

Crowded schools

Impact on Health

Tuberculosis

Spread of infectious diseases

Diminished personal space

Diseases of the GI system

Emotional detachment from society

Nonproductive life

Malnutrition

Obesity

Diabetes mellitus

Frequent homicide and suicide

Violence in the streets

Lack of personal safety

Poor education with less opportunity for achievement

---

health beliefs. That can involve a religious practitioner, the need for plants (nature) in the room, or a traditional healer.

Many members of the black community are Muslims. Some are descendents of Muslims who were brought here as slaves, and others have chosen to convert to Islam. Religious beliefs are an important part of the Muslim lifestyle, and as a health-care provider, you need to be familiar with them. Practicing Muslims eat a Halal diet, which means they do not eat pork or any pork products. You should work with the dietitian to ensure that the food of a Muslim patient is not "contaminated" with pork. There is a potentially serious problem with diabetic Muslims as well. Because most insulin is made from pork pancreas, a practicing Muslim will refuse to take it. Consult with the pharmacy to obtain nonpork insulin, and then assure the patient that the insulin is *not* made from parts of a pig so that there will be compliance in taking this critical medication.

Sickle cell anemia is a disease that affects only black people. It is genetically inherited, and scientists have concluded that it originally was an adaptation to fight the disease malaria. Sickle cells result in hemolysis and thrombosis of the red blood cells because the deformed cells do not flow properly through the blood vessels.

The symptoms of sickle cell anemia include hemolysis, anemia, and severe pain in the areas of the body where the thrombosed red blood cells are located. Statistics indicate that only 50% of children with sickle cell anemia live to adulthood. Some children develop complications that exist for the duration of their lives. The only way to prevent sickle cell anemia is to provide genetic testing and counseling to adults before they have children. This often does not happen because of the prohibitive cost of genetic testing.

The leading causes of death are the same for black and white populations; however, black mortality rates are higher. Blacks die from strokes at almost twice the rate of whites. Coronary heart disease death rates are higher; black men experience a higher risk of cancer of the prostate; homicide is the most frequent cause of death for black men 15 to 34 years old (although these are not elderly men, older men do live in the communities with high homicide rates); and the rate of AIDS is higher for black men than it is for white men (Spector, 2004).

There are many conclusions you can draw from the information you have just read that will assist you in understanding the needs of older black adults in your care. My purpose is to

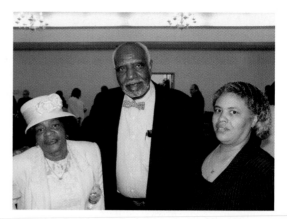

These black older adults have a strong religious background that assists them in the quality of their lives. Would their religion be considered ethnicity or culture?

inform you so that you can apply the information to your nursing practice. Your purpose is to learn the information and then determine ways, based on the needs of each individual, to increase your sensitivity to the person's personal health-care needs.

NATIVE AMERICANS

American Indians, Alaskan Natives (Eskimos), and Aleuts (who also live predominately in Alaska) are included in the category of Native Americans. In this chapter, *Native American* is the inclusive term used because the aforementioned ethnic groups all were on this continent long before any other people. They were well established before the Europeans came here. In A.D. 1010, they repulsed the Vikings. The Vikings were here for a decade and then left in frustration. As more and more people came to the Eastern shores, the natives of this country were pushed by force west into the wilderness. They died because of exposure to disease brought by the Europeans, which their bodies did not have antibodies to fight, and they died in war trying to defend their homeland.

As Native Americans migrated westward against their will, they carried with them fragments of their culture. Their lives were disrupted, their lands were lost, and many of their leaders and teachers were killed. Yet much of their history and culture remain. Native Americans essentially live in 26 states, including Alaska, with most of them living in the Western states. Although many Native Americans live on reservations, others live in rural and urban areas.

The Indian Health Service recognizes 560 tribes of Native Americans in the United States. Each tribe has its own culture, folklore, and folk medicine. To tell you about 1 tribe is to leave out the specifics of 559 other tribes. All tribes have traditional beliefs in Mother Earth and the necessity of having harmony with nature, however. If a person is ill, it is thought to hurt Mother Earth, just as when Mother Earth is hurt by disrespectful behavior (such as pollution and litter), it hurts people. Many traditional Native Americans believe there is a reason for every sickness and pain that relates to their behavior. They often believe that illness is the price to be paid for something they have done in the past or something they are going to do in the future. Often, traditional Native Americans who are ill believe that the illness is the best possible price they can pay for what they have done or will do. Native Americans believe in treating illness despite the person's behavior having been the cause.

Traditional tribes have a medicine man or woman. For some tribes, this person is referred to as a shaman. The shaman is someone who should be welcomed into the room of the person who is ill. There may be dancing and chanting; family members may gather in the room and perform a healing "sing" with the shaman; or there could be incense or healing sand paintings. All of these traditional healing methods need to be respected. It is important for you to provide privacy to the people who come to participate, treat them and what they are doing with respect, and obtain any items they request. Working with a person in this manner is truly practicing holistic health care.

Native Americans often are caught in limbo in terms of modern health care. They are caught between their traditions and modern treatment— the shaman and the physician. Finally, they often are "lost" between the Indian Health Care Services (free access to care for people who live on reservations) and services in the community. At least one-third of all Native Americans live in abject poverty. With such destitution comes poor living conditions and the problems that follow such situations. Native Americans have the diseases of the poor, such as malnutrition, tuberculosis, and high maternal and infant death rates. They also have a greater incidence of diabetes mellitus: one in five have the disease. In other ethnic groups, the incidence is 1 in 10. At the beginning of the 20th century, diabetes was very rare in Native Americans. Why the change in a manageable disease? Some say diet and exercise changes from the traditional lifestyle were the causative factors. I was surprised to learn that the cancer survival rate among Native Americans is the lowest of any group in the United States. Scientists do not give an explanation for this occurrence. Now that you know this fact, you have an obligation to take extra time to promote health screening and to perform health education related to cancer to assist older Native Americans in reducing their risks and identifying health problems early.

CRITICALLY EXAMINE THE FOLLOWING

What are the first five causes of death in your cultural or ethnic group? If you don't know, make an intelligent guess and prepare a list. Is suicide, homicide, or alcoholism on the list? What does it mean to a society when deaths of that nature are on the list of the most common causes of death? What does it mean to have so many people dying from tuberculosis and diabetes? Do you know any Native Americans? If so, perhaps you could talk with one of the elders in the family and ask them what they think of modern health care. You also should learn about traditional healing methods from them. I am sure you will find it very interesting!

Prepare a paper of no longer than two pages to discuss the aforementioned questions and any others you would like to have answered about health care for older Native Americans and their culture. Be prepared to submit your paper to the faculty person. If you cannot locate someone to interview, do a thorough discussion on the questions that relate to your cultural group.

The seven leading causes of death, in order of frequency, among Native Americans are:

1. Alcoholism
2. Tuberculosis
3. Diabetes mellitus
4. Accidents
5. Suicide
6. Pneumonia and influenza
7. Homicide

Close family bonds are typical in Native American groups, with elderly persons being treated as people with wisdom who are to be respected. It is becoming common for younger people to feel that the advice of their elders is no longer relevant to their modern lives, and they tend to ignore older adults.

Many traditional Native Americans may find the questions asked during an assessment or history taking offensive. Asking personal questions can be seen as probing and being disrespectful. You may find it necessary to develop a relationship with the older person before asking the questions you need answered. It would be wise to ask younger family members (adult children) for much of the history, so that you will be seen as less intrusive by the older person. Be sensitive to the nonverbal reactions of the person, and use your common sense based on your knowledge of the culture, communication, and the disease process.

● ASIAN AMERICANS

There are nearly 12 million Asian Americans in the United States; they constitute the third largest minority group (Spector, 2004). Asian Americans come from many different countries. The category of Asians includes people from China, Japan, Korea, Cambodia, India, Malaysia, Pakistan, and the Philippine Islands. The term *Asian* refers to people with origins in the Far East, Southeast Asia, and the continent of India.

The different groups of Asians came to this country for various reasons. The Chinese migration began in the mid-1800s because of a severe drought in China. The Chinese workers were hired for cheap wages to assist in the gold rush and to build the transcontinental railroad. They were victimized and generally treated poorly by Americans who were concerned about them taking their jobs. Many Chinese lived in Chinatowns, which were neighborhoods within larger cities where they went as a place of refuge from the abuse they received from others.

Japanese immigrants started to arrive at about the same time as the Chinese. Similar to the Chinese, they took any job offered to them so that they could support their families. This resulted in a strong prejudice from men who also were afraid of losing their jobs. Restrictive laws were passed that limited immigration and did not allow a person from Japanese descent to marry native-born Americans. The greatest indignity occurred during World War II, when 70,000 American-born Japanese were confined to relocation camps. Immigration laws also restricted Japanese people from coming to the United States at that time.

Filipinos began to immigrate in the 1900s and were employed as farm workers. Koreans began to immigrate in the early 1900s to work on plantations, predominately in Hawaii. Another group of Koreans came to the United States with their husbands, American servicemen, after the Korean War. After the Vietnam War, there was an influx of Vietnamese and Cambodians seeking political refuge.

Asian Americans have the highest median income of any foreign-born group; only 13% were poor in 1999; 39% are employed as managers or have professional job specialties; and 53% have employment-based health-care insurance (U.S. Census Bureau, 2008). All of these factors assist them in being healthier people. Yet they are from a variety of cultures, each with definite concepts and opinions.

The following story from an experienced nurse may help you to understand the involvement of traditional elders in many Asian cultures:

The nurse was working on the pediatric intensive care unit (PICU) and was the primary nurse for a 6-year-old boy who had been hit by a car. He and his parents were of Japanese descent and were American citizens. He had severe injuries and faced a prolonged treatment and rehabilitation regimen. Every day there were new decisions that needed to be made regarding his treatment plan. It was the nurse's responsibility to talk to the parents and explain all options to them for every decision. On the very first day, the nurse became concerned about the parents' inability to make decisions regarding their son's care. The nurse, Roger, needed answers and had concerns that could not wait until the next day as the parents requested. Roger wondered if language was a problem but learned that the parents were born in the United States and had university educations. The nurse shared his experience with the doctor, who also became concerned about the management of the little boy and his multiple problems. Delays were not a good idea based on the criticality of the boy's condition.

It was 2:00 p.m. before the parents came to Roger with a decision. With them were the father's parents. They were immigrants to the United States and were dressed in traditional Japanese clothing. The son was quite formal when he introduced Roger to his father and mother. Something in the way he did the introductions indicated to Roger that it was more than a simple courtesy. Roger invited the four of them to the unit's counseling room for privacy and sat down with them. What he learned in the next few minutes was of priority importance to the care of his young patient. In the traditional culture of this family, the oldest male made all important decisions for family members. If the grandfather was deceased, the grandmother would make the decisions for everyone. This process is based on the traditional Asian respect for the wisdom of older people. The parents wouldn't make decisions that they believed should be made by their parents.

Roger obtained the necessary contact information for the grandfather, introduced the grandparents to the physician and other nursing staff, and felt relief over the management of the care for the little boy. It was clear on the care plan to contact the grandfather for all decision making, and the process worked well. The grandparents always notified the parents about what had or was going to happen, and the family structure was kept intact. Most important, the little boy received the best care that could be given, and there was no communication frustration or distress.

The previous story indicates how most Asian people feel about their elders. Similar to the black and Native American cultures, there is a great deal of respect for older people and their wisdom. As you give care to people from these cultures, *be sure* you address the older person with his or her formal name, such as Mr. Fudano or Mrs. Begay. Do not assume a

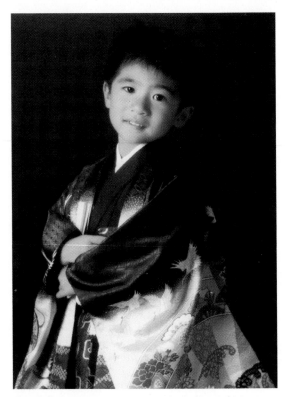

This little boy's name is Youta. He is dressed in traditional Japanese clothing in honor of his grandfather's birthday.

casual relationship with any older adult. I believe that older people from all cultures deserve the highest level of respect they can be given. This includes how you speak to them, preserve their modesty, and listen to them because it is their wisdom that is so highly valued. You should never give a command to an Asian older adult because it is a definite insult.

In traditional Asian families, older family members are cared for at home. This decision is based on the value the family members place on someone older. Another story that emphasizes this concept happened to a doctorally prepared nurse who was visiting the People's Republic of China in an official capacity:

> One evening she had dinner with Madame Chou, the President of the Chinese Nurses Association. This is a very powerful position and one that is appointed by the government. Madame Chou was in her early 60s, and the conversation was done through a Chinese interpreter. Madame Chou asked the American nurse what type of nursing she did in the United States.

The nurse, who loved old people and her work in nursing homes, explained with excitement where she did her clinical practice in nursing homes. Madame Chou visibly reacted negatively to what was being said. She even pulled back from the table. The nurse quit talking and apologized for anything she said that had been offensive. Madame Chou responded that she was concerned that the nurse was so happy to be cruel to the older people in her country. The dinner did not end on a pleasant note. The next morning the two women were to have breakfast together and then part, as the American nurse was moving on to another part of China. At breakfast, the American nurse apologized again and asked Madame Chou about nursing homes in China. Madame Chou thought for a few seconds and then said there are five. Keep in mind that this is a country with one-fifth of the world's population, and there were five nursing homes! She said they existed for those older people who did not want to be around little children or who had no family with whom they could live when they needed help. Then she made arrangements for the nurse to visit a rural nursing home.

I tell this story to emphasize that you must always be sensitive to the older person in your care; this is a time to develop good common sense based on information about older adults.

Asian Americans born in the United States have the same general good health and similar health problems as other citizens. People from most Asian cultures are comfortable with a physician being in charge of their health management for acute conditions. It is common, however, to use traditional remedies for chronic illnesses. These remedies may include herbs, acupuncture and acupressure, cupping, and spirituality. Allow and support their personal remedies and assist in any way that is appropriate. Always inform the registered nurse (RN) about what is taking place.

● EUROPEAN AMERICANS

Most European Americans have white skin and are easily mistaken for someone who has lived in the United States throughout his or her life. Many of them speak English, and, depending on how long the European has spoken English, there may

or may not be an accent of the person's country of origin. European immigration started with the Pilgrims and has continued since that time.

Each European country, similar to each Native American tribe, has its own individual culture from its region of the world. European Americans are as diverse as the people of the United States because all European countries have experienced constant immigration. The following story makes a point about the need for your sensitivity and thoroughness in giving nursing care to Europeans:

I remember being assigned an older white man who was admitted to the surgical preoperative area. The man was there for abdominal surgery that day; his wife accompanied him. The couple was well dressed and knowledgeable about the surgery. All went well until I came back on duty early the next morning and noted that Mr. Swensen had not received any pain medication since his late return from the recovery room. Being a firm believer in the concept that pain must be managed for optimum healing to take place, I went to his room immediately. He was pale; however, his dressing was secure and without drainage, his vital signs were within normal limits, and when asked if he wanted anything for pain, he simply stated, "No, thank you."

I felt concern for this man but also believed in the adage that "what a patient states is his pain level is his pain level." Within an hour, his wife came to visit him and then rushed to the nurse's station screaming with frustration. When I listened to her (I mean really listened without thinking of how to defend myself, just like I was taught in the communication chapter), I learned a valuable lesson. She was very upset because her husband had not received any pain medication since his surgery. According to her, he had severe pain, and she couldn't bear to see him so uncomfortable! I gently took her with me to a quiet place to talk after I asked another nurse to give Mr. Swensen the appropriate pain medication. Mrs. Swensen, an American citizen, had only recently married Mr. Swensen, a native of Sweden. In the Swedish culture, it is considered rude for a person to accept something the first time it is offered. Mr. Swensen was a very proper gentleman who was waiting for the nurse to make the, to him, mandatory second *offer of the pain medication. When she did not, his upbringing required him to endure the pain unnecessarily. This very unfortunate situation would not have happened if I had known more about his culture, talked with him in more depth about his pain, or talked with his wife. I feel that I missed this critical aspect of Mr. Swensen's health care because I did not use the principles of holistic nursing care.*

One of the major differences in health-care delivery between most European countries and the United States is the understanding each has about the responsibility and delivery of health care. Because many European countries have national health-care plans with socialized medicine, there is an expectation that the federal government is responsible for each person's health care. This is in sharp contrast to the United States, which is more individualistic in terms of health care. Health care in the United States is seen as being reliant on family or extended family groups. This change is often a challenging one for older European adults to accept. It definitely makes working within the health-care system challenging. As the nurse, you need to be aware of this potential problem and refer the person or the family to a social worker for more information. Assist the individual by making an appointment with the social worker if necessary.

HISPANIC AMERICANS

The second largest emerging minority group, soon to be the largest, in the United States is the Latino and Hispanic populations. The terms *Hispanic* and *Latino* are used interchangeably throughout this section because they are the terms recognized by the U.S. government. These terms refer to people, or their predecessors, who immigrated from Mexico, Puerto Rico, Cuba, Central and South America, Spain, and other Spanish-speaking communities to the United States. Hispanics are the fastest growing ethnic group in the United States, and with a mean age of 25.8 years, they are the youngest group as well (Spector, 2004). This young group also has the following characteristics:

1. Hispanics live in family households that are larger than those of non-Hispanic whites.
2. More than two in five Hispanics have not graduated from high school, and there is a variation in educational attainment: 73% of

the Cuban population has completed high school compared with 51% of the Mexican population.
3. Hispanics are much more likely to be unemployed than non-Hispanic whites.
4. Hispanic workers earn less than non-Hispanic workers.
5. Hispanics are more likely than non-Hispanic whites to live in poverty (Therrien & Ramirez, 2001).

The previous facts allow us to make several general assumptions. First, the mean (average) age of 25.8 years for this group indicates that there are not as many older people in the Hispanic population. Many of them live in multigenerational homes, which is a positive thing. They probably are poor and do not have a high school education. There are people who are the opposite of this generalized picture, however. As with all ethnic and cultural groups, you need to avoid stereotyping people while still meeting their needs. It is a challenge.

For older Hispanics, traditional beliefs concerning health do not readily work well with modern health-care treatments. Some traditional Hispanics think that good health is "good luck." When their health is not good, that is simply a mechanism of the "bad luck" they are experiencing. Other traditional Hispanics believe that good

---

CRITICALLY EXAMINE THE FOLLOWING

Read the following story and ponder what it means in terms of recognizing individual rights of people regarding their ethnicity or culture. What is the Nigerian woman really asking for from the class? Does the same need exist in the culturally diverse people to whom you give care? If so, how can you meet that need? *Hint*: The need is to be recognized as an individual.

Do your best thinking and come to class prepared to discuss the following incident.

I was in a class where one of the nursing students, a woman from Nigeria, was loudly protesting that she was not an African American, but that she was a Nigerian American. She was very upset because no one in the class commented on something that obviously was very important to her. I finally spoke up and said, "Neta, I will recognize you as a Nigerian American when people start recognizing me as a Danish American." My point was that it just won't happen!

health is a gift from God, and as such, it is something not to take for granted. People with this philosophy are expected to maintain their own good health by eating nutritious food, exercising, and getting enough rest. It is the person's responsibility to maintain his or her balance in the universe. Illness is seen as a punishment for wrongdoings. It is combated through prayer and the use of amulets (small figures made of clay or metal), herbs, and spices (Spector, 2004).

Overall, Hispanic cultures assume the responsibility of caring for elderly persons. There are so few older adults that those who live to be older are treated with respect and love. Hispanic people generally do not admit an elderly person to a nursing home; they try to avoid hospital admissions as well. They keenly feel the responsibility to care for older adults in the home surrounded with family. As a culturally aware care provider, you need to assume the role of patient advocate and inform the nurse and appropriate others of the desire for the older person to be cared for in the home, if that is true. In many situations, a hospital admission can be avoided with a strong home health-care plan. This approach requires effective teaching for the family members who are assuming responsibility for the care, and teaching can be a challenge when English is the second language for the people you are teaching. Read the following story from an experienced nurse, and consider how you will teach people with minimal English skills:

I always have been a coronary care nurse and enjoyed the challenge of family and patient teaching very much. There was one situation where I did not feel successful until I did something drastic. Mr. Lopez, a 73-year-old Hispanic man, was admitted to the unit with a massive coronary (heart attack). He had a charming wife and three adult children. None of them spoke English well, and I did not speak any Spanish. Because of the language problem, I felt I was not being successful with the teaching. This man had a strict medication regimen, was scheduled for cardiac rehabilitation (a supervised rehabilitation program at the hospital) three times a week and for an echocardiogram (ultrasound examination of the heart), and had critical follow-up appointments with the physician. I had pictures of the medications with their time and dosage, a picture of the supervisor for cardiac rehab (I had the supervisor meet Mr. Lopez earlier in the week) with times and dates, and the appointments written down with directions on how to get to them.

➤ POINT OF INTEREST

Envidia, or envy, is considered to be a cause of illness and bad luck. Many traditional Hispanic people think that to succeed actually is a failure. This is based on the idea that people envy a successful person. When friends, family, and neighbors envy a person in the community who has achieved success, that person will blame the envy for any illnesses. Several social scientists have determined that the low economic and success rates of some Hispanic groups can be attributed to belief in Envidia.

I went over the information for the last time on the day the man was to be discharged. In his broken English, he kept saying, "You have fixed me." I would respond, "No" and would explain again the regimen he needed to follow. He seemed to think that because he was feeling so much better, he was healthy again. I sensed that he would not be following his discharge instructions and was very concerned. This went on for several minutes until I stopped and drew another picture. It was a stick figure of his family. He recognized who they were and was smiling. Then I took a marker and "Xed" out the figure of him and nearly shouted, "You will be dead!" He was taken back by what I said. Then he looked at the picture of his family and the teaching pictures and information I had made for him. He turned toward me and said, "I understand." For the first time, I felt that he did. With his new understanding, I went over the teaching plan again, and he really listened. He took out his pocket calendar and wrote things on it in Spanish. He spoke to his wife in his own language and explained things to her. I felt like there was a future for this man and his family.

I don't know if shouting "You will die!" at someone is the best teaching approach. In this situation, it was effective, although unconventional. For you to be good at teaching people who speak English as a second language, you need to focus on your skills and awareness. If you do not speak a second language that is useful, you or your facility need to have a list of people with language skills who can be called in such situations.

Another concern to address when caring for older Hispanic people is the weather, especially if this is the first year they are in the United States and your winter climate gets cold. Many Spanish-speaking countries have warm climates, and cold weather is nonexistent. These people need to be taught about Pneumovax and the annual flu shot. You also should check to be sure they have or can afford fuel for warming their homes. The federal government has assistance programs for household heat. You should refer a person in need to a social worker for information.

Another barrier to health care that many Hispanic people encounter is poverty. Similar to so many others we have discussed in this chapter, Hispanic people tend to be poor. Along with

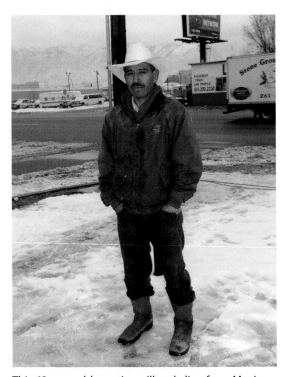

This 63-year-old man is an illegal alien from Mexico. He does not have health-care insurance or a steady job. He stands, sometimes for hours, on a specific street corner where people who want day help come to hire him and others like him. His objective for each day is to make enough money to buy food for him and his wife. If there is any left over, it goes toward the money they need each month for rent and utilities. As he ages, how will his lifestyle affect his overall health? Consider that he has no insurance, no guaranteed income, and minimal finances for essentials and that he stands on a cold (or hot) street corner each day hoping for work.

poverty are the diseases of poverty, including malnutrition, tuberculosis, and homicide. Knowing this should cause you to check each older Hispanic person for tuberculosis on a yearly schedule. You also should check the person's laboratory work to determine if malnutrition is a problem.

It is important to ask older Hispanic adults if they feel safe in their neighborhood. Do they go out for walks? Do they visit a local recreation center? Do they visit with their neighbors? If they do not feel safe doing these things, they may be staying in the house for prolonged periods and should be assessed for depression, muscle disuse, and loneliness. Be creative and use your common sense based on knowledge to assist in resolving such problems. Could a group of elders go for a walk together and, perhaps, be safer? Does the senior center have a bus that could pick the older person up routinely? Including the older adult and the extended family in a discussion of such problems may result in creative solutions.

A serious barrier to receiving modern health care is time orientation. To most Hispanics, time is a relative event because minimal attention is given to the exact time of day. This attitude toward time becomes a problem when the Hispanic person leaves the folk healer and goes to see a physician because of worsening health. The folk healer comes to the patient's home 24 hours a day, 7 days a week. The physician can be seen only if the older adult goes to the office and waits a long time to be seen. It is ironic to these older adults that they cannot be late (which they often are), but the physician can be very late without criticism. Older Hispanic adults often are slow in coming into the health-care system; by that, I mean that their disease is well developed by the time they get there. This often is because they have gone through all of the folk healers and their suggestions in their local community before coming to a physician. It is important to understand this behavior rather than criticize it.

Traditional Hispanic people, especially older people, have a belief system based on treating "hot" diseases with "cold" remedies or vice versa. An example is that penicillin, a "hot" prescription, may not be taken for diarrhea, constipation, or a rash because they also are "hot" diseases. The only way you will know what is "hot" and "cold" is to ask. Write down the pertinent items and add them to the care plan. You also should tell the nurse or team leader verbally so that the information can be shared with the members of other shifts. Another example relates to the use of diuretics. When a diuretic is prescribed, along with encouragement to eat more bananas and raisins for potassium replacement, the bananas and raisins may not be eaten. They are considered "cold" foods and cannot be eaten with a "cold" disease. The resolution to this problem is to determine what the "hot" and "cold" diseases are and decide if there is a way to word the current illness so that it is a "hot" disease (never lie, however). The purpose of mixing "hot" and "cold" diseases and treatments is to find and maintain the individual's personal balance.

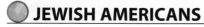

JEWISH AMERICANS

The strength of the Jewish religion binds Jewish people together. Jews from many parts of the world have immigrated to the United States. It is estimated that 50% of all Jews live in the United States, which is approximately 6 million. There were several waves of immigration, most of them resulting from the horrors of prejudicial behavior from dominant societies. The most significant example of this behavior is the death of 6 million Jews during Hitler's "ethnic cleansing" of Germany. I recall doing an evaluative visit to a large Jewish nursing home on the East coast. While there, I met several survivors of the Holocaust. I listened to their stories and touched their tattoos (numbers tattooed on the wrists of all prisoners as a form of identification), and my life was changed forever. I suppose most of them are dead now, but they did live to a wonderful old age.

When Jewish immigrants arrived, they were forced to work in factories and live in tenement housing, while experiencing prejudice from many people. Yet, they have shown excellent leadership in business, arts, and sciences and have made major contributions to American society. Eighty percent of all Jewish Americans have a college education. When you have an older Jewish adult as a patient, you need to recognize their personal strength and motivation and that they may have more education than you do. Although Yiddish is a traditional language for Jewish people to use with each other, essentially everyone speaks English as well.

Traditional Jews recognize two aspects of health: the spirit and the body. Maintaining good health is an expectation. The use of modern medicine is encouraged; however, a rabbi (religious leader) may be consulted when transplantation or life-and-death issues need to be decided. Prayer is used to ask God for improvement of a condition or healing of one's body. The Torah (the holy book of the Jews) teaches Jewish people to visit and assist the sick. Most elderly Jews have a strong family and community support system.

Traditional Jewish people follow a kosher diet; they avoid mixing meat and dairy products, and eating shellfish and pork are forbidden. The Jewish culture has many holy days that are observed in a formal manner. You are responsible for assisting older Jewish adults to maintain their healing process as well as meet their need to observe any holy day that may occur while they are in your care.

The following story happened to an experienced nurse who successfully managed what could have been a very negative situation:

One day I was assigned an older woman who was recovering from surgery for a ruptured appendix. She was doing well considering what had happened. I had not been assigned to her before, but I noticed that on the previous day she was bright and pleasant. I was excited to spend time with her. You can imagine my surprise when I went into her room and found her arguing with the certified nursing assistant (CNA). I invited the CNA out of the room and asked her what had happened. After I listened to her identify the problem, I explained to her that she must never argue with the patients and that she should bring all problems that might cause an argument to me, as the licensed nurse. Then I went in the room to talk to the patient, Mrs. Goldstein.

The argument was based on the fact that Mrs. Goldstein would not eat or drink anything. She asked the CNA to remove her water pitcher and her breakfast tray, as well as cancel her meals for the rest of the day. Then she asked the CNA to see to it that she not be disturbed throughout the day. You can see the problem with these requests. Mrs. Goldstein was recovering from a very serious peritonitis caused by the ruptured appendix. She should not be NPO (nothing by mouth), and the staff would need to check on her and assist her with ambulation, administer pain medication, and check her vital signs and dressing. Also, when the body is recovering from something serious, it does need nutrients. I had a problem, and it was critical that I resolve it well.

I went into the room and sat down by Mrs. Goldstein. I asked her to tell me what the problem was. I felt it was essential that I get her version of what had happened. I reached out and touched her hand and made sure I was close to the bed so we both could see and hear each other. Mrs. Goldstein simply and clearly told me that she was Jewish and that it was Yom Kippur, the Day of Atonement. She went on to explain that Yom Kippur was the High Holy Day of the Holy Days for her religion. It was sacred to her. Yom Kippur was a day of repentance. No one drives; therefore, her family would not be visiting. And she needed to fast, so she would not be eating or drinking during the day. She felt that this would allow her to be cleansed spiritually and enable her to repent of her sins. I was very concerned.

It was obvious Mrs. Goldstein was a devout Jew and that the sacredness and traditions of Yom Kippur were deeply embedded within her. How could I meet her needs within the framework of respecting her body, mind, and spirit? I talked to her and listened, and then we made a plan.

Mrs. Goldstein agreed that God would understand if she did not observe Yom Kippur in the manner she usually did after I explained the importance of fluids to her healing body. As a result, she agreed to drink water only. Then we talked about nutrition and the work her body cells were doing to heal her. She agreed they needed fuel and said light meals would be satisfactory. I promised her that the staff would come in only for essential activities so she would have time to meditate and ask forgiveness of her sins. She seemed happy with our decisions.

I spent nearly an hour with this wonderful older woman working out a satisfactory solution that would meet her needs holistically. Then it took another 30 minutes to make the necessary arrangements for the day. Fortunately, I work with a team of nurses who "covered" my other patients while I worked with Mrs. Goldstein. I called dietary and organized her meals, including another breakfast. I put a note on her door that said she was not to be disturbed without consulting me. Then I asked the CNA to take the water pitcher back into her room and coached her on a way to apologize for her aggressive behavior and express understanding for the sacredness of the day for Mrs. Goldstein. Fortunately, the CNA was willing to do as I suggested, as she felt badly about her previous interaction.

It was a hectic but satisfying day. Mrs. Goldstein's needs were met on every level without endangering her body. She had a wonderful day and expressed her gratitude to everyone she saw on the following day. I was appreciative to the staff for understanding her needs and assisting me to meet them; it really took a team effort.

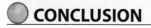

CONCLUSION

Giving culturally competent care in a caring and holistic manner requires a great deal of attention, sensitivity, and knowledge. This chapter gives you a basic background about common minority groups in the United States. Ethnic and cultural aspects of care were discussed. As the number of aging people in the United States increases and their diversity expands, it is crucial that you become familiar with the needs of older adults from all backgrounds. When you learn to do this, you will be giving culturally competent care, which is the goal.

Ask questions of older adults and partake of their wisdom as you learn about them and their lives. Advocate for them as they live their culture and religion. Provide them with the items they need to practice their health beliefs. Respect them for the lives they have lived and the reasons they have lived them.

During the genetic cleansing that took place in the former Yugoslavia, numerous refugees came to your community to live. Many of them had watched their family members be raped, tortured, and killed. They had nothing of material value and often no family.

You were assigned, as a volunteer, to work with one family. That was amazing in itself because it was an entire family! You met them at the airport and took them to their roomy and fully furnished apartment. You showed them how the bathroom worked and the shiny new oven and refrigerator and were pleased that there were enough bedrooms for them to sleep comfortably. Supper had been brought in by a local church group, so you left them in their new home and confirmed that you would be back in the morning to assist them in any way you could. It all felt good to you.

The next morning you were at their home bright and early because you were excited about what you would do with them that day. After knocking several times, you let yourself in and were shocked by what you found. No one slept in the beds, no one used the new sheets and blankets, and it appeared that no one used the toilet or shower (the new towels were unused on the racks). You found the family in the living room all sleeping together in a big knot of people. Also, there was a stack of small pieces of wood by the oven. You knew by what you saw that you had missed something major when you oriented these people to their new surroundings. After finding the family in the situation described, what are you going to do?

Solution

First, you would control your surprise and that bit of criticism that some people may feel. Then you would think about what you know about the culture of these people because the problem seems to be one of cultural differences. The following is what I would have done. You may have other ideas that also would work. Remember that my thoughts are not the only answer, or even the best answer. Value your own thinking.

I hope I would have thought to bring breakfast. I would have had the family gather around the table and eat. Because I wouldn't have known their religion or preferences regarding blessing the food, I would have asked them what would be appropriate. While we were eating, I would have listened to what happened after I left them. Remember, they were refugees from a war-torn country where the military government had tried to kill everyone of their ethnic background. They would have told me stories of how they had to live to survive. They were poor and oppressed people to begin with and had been homeless for several months; they were accustomed to living off the streets or stealing to eat. They were from a very poor country and did not know what the oven and refrigerator were designed to do. The children had gathered the stack of sticks so they could be put into the oven to cook. The bathroom was another complete

mystery to them. (They had gone outside to take care of their elimination needs.) They thought the towels and sheets were too pretty to use! Why were they sleeping on the floor? That was how they slept to keep warm and to be together if soldiers came.

By listening to these people, really taking the time to listen, I would have learned where to begin to acculturate them to modern Western society. I would have patiently explained the details of the items in their apartment, and then I would have demonstrated how things worked and let them do what they emotionally could. My only rule would have been that they could not build a fire inside the oven! It might have taken weeks before they could sleep in beds and even longer before they could sleep in separate beds.

With support and respect, this family could make a successful transition to their new lives. It might take more time than I originally planned, but it all would be very rewarding. I would have continued to work with them until the father got a job and the mother learned to shop and cook in her new country. English-as-a-second-language classes would have been a priority for everyone, and when the children seemed adjusted to the new culture, I would have assisted the family in getting them into school.

Select the best answer to each question.

1. Compared with white Americans, black Americans have a life expectancy that:

   a. Is longer by 3.2 years

   b. Is longer for black women and shorter for white men

   c. Is generally equal because they all are Americans

   d. Is shorter for women and men

2. The leading cause of death for Native Americans is:

   a. Homicide

   b. Alcoholism

   c. Diabetes mellitus

   d. Tuberculosis

3. The median income of Asian Americans is:

   a. Comparable with that of white Americans

   b. One of the lowest of the minority groups

   c. The highest of the minority groups

   d. At a level that keeps them in abject poverty

4. Among the Hispanic cultures, the Cuban population has:

   a. The highest level of illegal aliens

   b. The highest level of high school graduates

   c. The highest level of tuberculosis

   d. The highest level of older people

5. The kosher diet of traditional Jews must strictly follow which basic rule?

   a. No pork, shellfish, or white flour products

   b. No dairy products served with meat, and no beef or shellfish

   c. No white flour products, pork, or dairy products

   d. No dairy products served with meat, and no pork or shellfish

9 Activity, Rest, and Sleep as Criteria for Health

Mary Ann Anderson

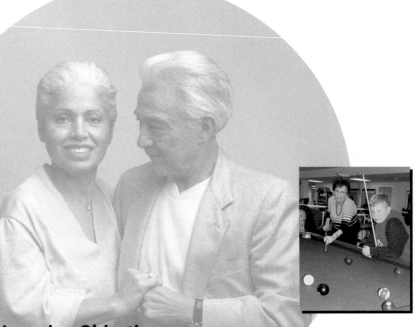

Learning Objectives

After completing this chapter, the student will be able to:

1. Express an understanding of the importance of activity for all older adults, including the most disabled.
2. Discuss the significance of activity for people with and without chronic diseases.
3. Describe normal rest and sleep patterns for older adults.
4. Identify older adults who are most at risk for developing rest and sleep disturbances.
5. Apply nursing interventions to older adults who are experiencing problems with activity, rest, or sleep.

INTRODUCTION

At age 59, I finally got to be a grandma! My darling, whose name is Kedzie, moves constantly. She is only 7 months old, but her arms are flinging, her legs are in constant motion, and her physical flexibility allows her to suck her great toe—if her mother isn't looking! Then when she is tired, she simply goes to sleep. She naps several times a day and sleeps for 8 to 9 hours a night. It is the perfect life.

This chapter discusses activities similar to Kedzie's in older adults. Activity, rest, and sleep are not nearly as simple for older adults as they are for children. That is why it is important to discuss them here.

Activity promotes life physically and psychologically. Even minimal activity can help prevent or manage diabetes mellitus, osteoporosis, heart disease, arthritis, and most pulmonary conditions. The psychological benefits include the sense of well-being that comes with having the freedom to move from one place to the other and to take care of oneself, even if that care is minimal. Rest is a luxury that I assume you do not get to experience a great deal because you are a student who probably also is working and taking care of a family. The peaceful feeling that comes from an afternoon nap is a wonderful thing. Kedzie and other babies simply fall asleep if they are tired. If you tried that, you would have trouble staying in school or managing your job.

▲ PRIORITY SETTING 9.1

The priority for this chapter is for you to allow all older adults to do as much for themselves as possible. It is that simple. The challenge is that the person may not want to do all he or she can do. Perhaps the person's family members have pampered and waited on him or her more than is healthy for the older person. Perhaps he or she needs good pain management so that moving is not so painful. Whatever the challenge, you need to use the information in this chapter to determine what is keeping the person from doing everything possible as independently as possible. Be clever, be smart, be caring, and be holistic. But you must get the job done!

Adults have to work at getting enough rest, which leads us to sleep. I feel confident that there are days, perhaps even right now, when you feel sleep deprived. It is a difficult way to go through your life, isn't it? I am hopeful that this will not be a permanent condition for you. There should be a time, when you are through with school, when you will be able to get more sleep. I want you to consider, however, what it would be like to be an older adult whose sleep patterns have changed from what they always have been and whose sleep definitely has diminished in quality and quantity. Sleep deprivation in older persons can be a very serious consideration when planning nursing care. The importance of managing activity, rest, and sleep is critical in giving care to older people.

ACTIVITY

Activity for people in the United States has changed dramatically over the years. As society has moved from an agrarian (farming) society to an industrial one, the natural activities that dominated society have changed as well. No longer do teens get up at 4:00 a.m. to milk cows, thin sugar beets in the cool of the day, or "buck" (lift and move) bales of hay. Many of those activities are now automated, and there are fewer and fewer farms.

Instead of cutting trees, building houses, and having "barn raisings" along with the farming (I know this is dated, but think of what great exercise it was!), people now go to gyms or join organized community sports groups to get enough exercise to be healthy. Others participate in sports as a spectator only and spend a great percentage of their free time watching television or sitting with a computer. It is as if exercise is now a luxury instead of a necessity for good health. With the growing obesity problem in the United States, the lack of exercise as a normal part of one's day should be a serious concern for you as a health-care provider.

It is a delight to me to see older persons golfing, mowing their lawns, or walking their dogs. In my mind, I simply say "yea!" What I see are people who are using the health they have and are working to maintain it. I even get excited when I see someone with a cane and oxygen zooming around the grocery store in an electric cart. Even though they are not walking, I appreciate the effort it took for them to get to the store. They had to get up, eat, dress, and manage getting to their car and then the store. They are interacting with an environment different from their home and have to stretch and move to get the items they need from the shelves. It is wonderful to see people moving at whatever their physical activity level is. The idea of exercise, for all of us, is if we keep moving, we *will* keep moving!

Advantages and Disadvantages of Exercise

As a nurse giving care to older adults, you have several complex concerns to manage in terms of activity and exercise for older adults. The number one problem often is managing an older person's chronic diseases (Box 9.1). Degenerative arthritis makes it difficult to walk; pulmonary disease makes it challenging to move at all. With the aging of society, many old-old people use canes, walkers, wheelchairs, and oxygen that add to the need for planning when exercising. Nevertheless, elderly people need to exercise.

When people exercise, they are assisting all of their major systems. Exercise improves the

BOX 9.1 **Ten Most Common Chronic Diseases in People Older Than Age 65 in the United States**

1. Arthritis
2. Hypertension
3. Problems hearing
4. Heart conditions
5. Visual impairment
6. Deformities or orthopedic disability
7. Diabetes
8. Chronic sinusitis
9. Hay fever and allergic rhinitis
10. Varicose veins

Bureau of National Health Statistics (2007).

functioning of the heart and lungs, the musculoskeletal system, and the digestive and excretory systems, and it provides feelings of self-satisfaction. Setting goals and having meaningful things to do, all of which require some activity, combats depression, insomnia, and boredom.

When older people do not exercise, they are subject to osteoporosis; joint immobility; indigestion; constipation; pneumonia; weakened cardiac and other muscles; pressure ulcers; and the depression, insomnia, and boredom mentioned. The aging process is a challenge to maintaining a healthy lifestyle. The instrument for avoiding the pitfalls of inactivity in older adults is the care given by you, as a licensed practical nurse (LPN), and the members of the family, who you are responsible to teach.

How to Keep Older Adults Active

The first rule when working with older persons and their exercise needs is to allow them to do as much for themselves as possible. This sounds very simple; however, in the real world of your clinical practice, it is not. There is pressure to get everyone to the lunch room in a nursing home in a timely manner, and walking residents to meals is more time-consuming than putting them in wheelchairs to transport them. Yet, walking residents to the lunch room is an excellent way to give them some exercise despite the time crunch. This could become problematic for you as you organize your time. It is critical that you and the people you manage (the nursing assistants) organize yourselves so that everyone can be assisted in walking to their meals, if possible. Once there, the residents can use their time to visit with each other, discuss the day's events, and compliment or complain about the

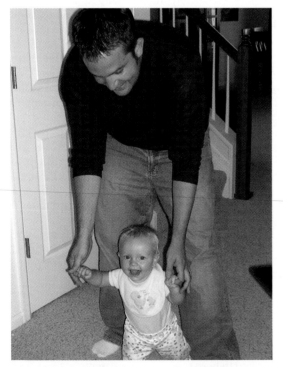

When Kedzie was learning to walk, she needed assistance from her parents. She would walk and walk and walk until she learned to do it independently. Can you draw an analogy from Kedzie to an older adult who has experienced an injury that limits mobility?

food. The difference between getting them to lunch at your convenience and ambulating them to lunch with time for socialization is one of quality of care and caring.

In the hospital, you may need to assist an older adult to a chair so that meals can be eaten while sitting upright (better digestion, less acid reflux). Assisting someone to the toileting room, without the use of a wheelchair, promotes bowel elimination, and the walking is important for muscle strengthening (including the heart) and the avoidance of increased osteoporosis.

The "allowing people to do as much for themselves as possible" rule extends to all of the care you render to people in a nursing home, hospital, or home. Allow individuals to brush their own teeth, comb their own hair, and dress themselves as much as possible. All of these actions take time but are excellent for range of motion and self-esteem building. Teaching this principle to family and friends further enhances the quality of life of older adults. Tell them what you are doing and explain the "why." You need to role-model safe and caring ways for assisting the person in your care. During the time you are assisting older persons, talk to them, listen to what they have to say, and value their wisdom and experience. This valuing behavior helps build self-esteem, and it is a caring and wise way to use the time you are spending in activity with your clients.

While planning exercise for specific older adults in your care, be aware of their physical ability. It is not helpful to put persons in a situation that makes major demands on their bodies that could be unsafe. For some people, sitting in a circle and throwing a ball from one to another is good use of their upper body and is fun. For other persons, it could be boring and beneath their physical abilities. Begin with a conservative plan, and increase it if it does not physically stress the person.

● REST

Rest is something most people want to experience more than they generally do. I am sure you would like some time off to do nothing but rest; I do find that to be common among busy students. When dealing with older adults, you have a specialized group of people who have specialized rest needs.

Because of the number of chronic diseases older people tend to have, they may be unable to rest owing to pain or stress over their diseases. In another scenario, the person may feel that all he or she does is rest! The key to managing the rest needs of older people is to identify what their needs are.

Pain

A common reason people cannot rest is because they have pain that keeps them awake. Pain needs to be identified and managed. It not only interferes with rest and sleep, but it also decreases

---

FOCUSED LEARNING CHART

Advantages of exercise

Assist to Prevent	Assist to Manage	Can Improve
Osteoporosis	Pressure ulcers	Joint immobility
Diabetes mellitus	Arthritis	Most pulmonary conditions
Heart disease	Depression	Insomnia
Boredom	Obesity	Indigestion
	Psychosocial health	Constipation

activity. It is your responsibility, as the LPN, to identify the pain and share that information with the registered nurse (RN) or physician. It is the responsibility of the RN or physician to do a comprehensive assessment to determine the causative factors related to the pain. Your responsibility, besides reporting the pain and its impact on the resident or patient, is to check for more common possible causes of the pain. Is the individual positioned properly? Are position changes made often enough to prevent pressure ulcers from starting? Have you checked the medications to see if there is a drug reaction or interaction? Listen to the person experiencing the pain and carefully describe it when you chart. You also should consider having the older person self-evaluate the pain by using a scale (e.g., 1–10). When using the 1-to-10 scale, you ask the person to pick a number that describes the pain on a scale of 1 to 10, with 10 being the worst pain imaginable. When you regularly chart this self-evaluation, it could give the RN or physician valuable information that would assist in pain management.

Stress

Every person has his or her own personal ability to manage stress. This is very important because stress is a normal part of life. Think of the stress in your own life. Without deadlines, you would

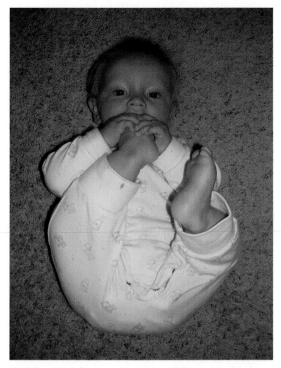

Kedzie enjoys just resting. She will lie on her back and talk to her mother or herself or play with her toys. This generally is the time she will demonstrate her flexibility and suck her toe when her mom isn't looking! Older adults also need their rest. Short naps during the day help them to have more energy for their daily activities.

not be stressed enough to get your school papers or care plans written and prepare for your tests. Every day people manage the stress of weather changes, worldwide events (war, hurricanes, floods), interactions with others, time constraints (such as your school assignments), and other physical and emotional stressors. For some people, getting up and getting dressed in the morning are major stress points. Stress is part of everyone's life, and it will not go away. The key to stress is not elimination; it is management.

Life is a series of stressful events. Much of the stress actually enhances our lives (getting up in the morning and getting dressed). Some stress assists us in achieving our goals (school assignments), and other stress simply makes us feel alive and assists us in avoiding boredom. The problem with stress is that there can be too much of it; this is called "distress" and can be damaging to our lives physically and emotionally. The potential for the negative effects of distress is why stress management is crucial to understand. The informative section in the chapter on promoting wellness (Chapter 6) would be valuable for you to reread. The content supports the principles of achieving rest by managing stress. Refer back to Chapter 6 and apply the information to the concept of appropriate rest for older adults.

"All I Do Is Rest!"

If you hear this or similar comments from your elderly clients, you need to assist them and their family members to understand the information in the activity section of this chapter. All people need to move to the extent of their ability. The movement works their muscles, and that encourages the body to rest. One of the main considerations when planning activity and rest is to assist the older person to alternate them throughout the day. Many older people have worked for most of their lives and consider daytime the right time to "do their work" or activities, and they rest in the evening.

As most of us age, we have less stamina for prolonged activities, such as working for 8 consecutive hours. It is important to teach older people and their families that the individual really is retired and need not work for so many hours at a time. A combination of activity and then rest, activity and then rest again is generally the best way to stay healthy and happy as an aging person. The older one becomes, the more common this tends to be. I personally think that naps are the second greatest thing ever invented! (The first, of course, is being a grandma.) It is common for older people to take two or three naps a day. Napping is perfectly natural because of the aging body. Encourage naps that are intermingled with episodes of activity throughout the day. You need to be aware of the possibility of oversleeping because of boredom or depression, however.

Take a moment to consider if the person is bored. Should the individual be going to the senior citizen center two to three times a week for lunch and socialization? Most senior centers also have classes and crafts that help maintain a person's interest in life and living. Should a craft be brought into the home or nursing home for the individual to do? Do the neighbors need to know that their visits are very welcome, or is there an adopt-a-grandparent program at the local high school? An adopt-a-grandparent program is where teens volunteer to be with one particular older person. Generally, this arrangement results in a very satisfying relationship for both individuals.

Because it is so important, I again mention the need for you to take time to talk to the older adults to whom you give care. Learn about their lives and the courage and creativity it has taken older people to survive two world wars, the Great Depression, and living in a predominately ageist society. Old people are strong, they are interesting, and they are wise. You need to learn the truth of what I have just said for yourself by talking to them and learning to value them.

 SLEEP

Sleep is the most significant activity people can participate in for quality health. Every person, at whatever age, needs sleep to function normally. During sleep, the body physically repairs body tissues and emotionally resolves the issues of the day. Some people need only 6 hours of sleep, whereas many need the traditional 8 hours. Generally when people age, they feel less rested, and many need more sleep than they get.

What Is Sleep?

The central nervous system controls sleep-wake patterns. There are two types of sleep: rapid eye movement (REM) and nonrapid eye movement (NREM). Every individual of every age needs to experience both types of sleep every night. The sleep cycle has four stages of NREM and one stage of REM. The NREM stages go from relaxation to deeper and deeper sleep. The REM stage is the deepest sleep and is essential for a good night's

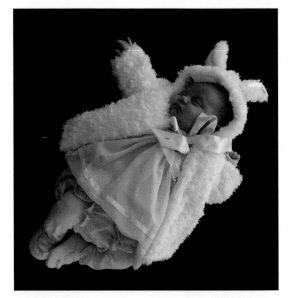

When Kedzie is tired, she falls asleep; it does not matter where she is or what she is doing. I have observed older people who nod off or stay home from a shopping trip because of their fatigue. Everyone needs enough sleep to be at the optimal level of alertness and health. Devise strategies for the people to whom you give care that will allow them the sleep they need.

rest. People often go through this sleep cycle four times a night, with each cycle allowing for deeper and more restful REM sleep. If the person's sleep is interrupted, the cycle starts over again from the beginning, and much of the deep sleep needed for optimal health is lost. This deep sleep is the healing sleep. When you wake up from a night's sleep and feel really great, you have, in all probability, had uninterrupted cycles of sleep.

Another aspect of individual sleep patterns is the person's circadian rhythm. This is the body's response to the day-night cycle of the sun. Within this cycle, people develop personal responses to their sleep needs. A common problem is that as people age, they wake up earlier. As a result, they get tired during the day and need one or more naps. The daytime fatigue comes from normal physiological changes in the person's circadian rhythm. Research indicates that circadian rhythms change over time, resulting in younger people sleeping late in the morning (think of your own teen years) and older people awaking earlier. This normal physiological change causes many older people to want to stay up late so that they do not wake up at 4:00 or 5:00 in the morning. Getting up early also reinforces the need for naps throughout the daytime hours.

Sleep Disorders

There are various sleep disorders diagnosed, but the end result tends to be the same. Older adults often have trouble falling asleep and staying asleep, and they awaken fatigued, which can last throughout the day. As you probably know from personal experience, people who do not get enough sleep are often irritable, and in older adults, that can lead to confusion. The management of sleep disorders is an important aspect of the care you need to be giving to elders.

A common sleep disorder is insomnia. Insomnia occurs when people have difficulty getting to sleep or remaining asleep, or they simply feel that they do not get enough sleep. Insomnia is not a disease, but rather it is the result of some other condition. Imagine the pain from arthritis without effective pain management. You may be too young to know how devastating arthritic pain can be, but it definitely is enough to keep a person awake. One of my sisters has insomnia every time a storm "blows in." She complains of her lack of sleep until I remind her that the cause is her pain. Then she takes a long-lasting analgesic before going to bed, and this works for her.

Another common cause of insomnia is sleep apnea. Sleep apnea occurs when a person's airway is partially obstructed during sleep. The classic symptom is fatigue on awakening and throughout the day. People with sleep apnea are very tired *all* of the time. They often snore throughout the night, which can result in insomnia for their sleep partner. People with sleep apnea are frequently obese.

Sleep apnea is treated with continuous positive airway pressure (CPAP) while sleeping. The CPAP machine eliminates the airway obstruction by forcing air into the trachea throughout the sleep period. This is done through a mask that is strapped to the person's nose. Untreated sleep apnea can lead to right-sided heart failure and eventually pulmonary hypertension. You need to pay attention to people who complain of constant fatigue. It is your responsibility to report such complaints to the RN or physician rather than dismiss the complaint.

Other common reasons for insomnia include frequent urination, acid reflux, chronic obstructive pulmonary disease (COPD), and congestive heart failure (CHF). These medical conditions should be treated by the physician. It is your responsibility, as the LPN, to report symptoms related to these diseases and their management to the RN or physician. Then, as the excellent nurse you are or will become, go a step further by applying nursing interventions where applicable. People with COPD and CHF sleep better if the head of the bed is raised. The same is true of someone with acid reflux. Also, a person with acid reflux should never take medications on an empty stomach.

Nocturnal movement is another physiological condition that causes insomnia. There are two common types of nocturnal movement. The most common is restless legs syndrome (RLS), which is an irresistible urge to move one's legs. This can happen several times a night, and each episode is capable of awakening the person experiencing the situation. RLS can be managed with medication. For some people, heat application also helps the legs to relax. Be sure to report this disruptive complaint to the RN or physician so that it can be effectively treated.

Another disruption to sleep is nocturnal myoclonus, which is sudden moving or kicking movements of the lower extremities. This happens without warning and is very disruptive to sleep. Again, report it rather than ignore it as "just another complaint" because medications can assist in managing the disorder. These problems are legitimate concerns when considering sleep patterns and, subsequently, the overall health of the people to whom you give care.

Dementia is a deterrent to effective sleep for the person with dementia and his or her sleep partner. Sleep patterns are altered in someone who is demented, which often results in being awake and wandering at night. This is very disruptive for the caregiver, who most often is the spouse of the demented individual. The result is two people who are sleep deprived and having difficulty because of fatigue. This is one reason that many communities have respite programs for caregivers of persons with dementia. The person with dementia is taken to the respite center for constant care, and the caregiver has a few hours or a weekend to rest, visit relatives, or engage in other activities important to a quality of life.

Psychological conditions often are detrimental to effective sleep patterns. People who are depressed often awake early and have hypersomnia, which is sleeping during the time people

---

CRITICALLY EXAMINE THE FOLLOWING

Nursing interventions often bring the needed information and comfort to patients and residents experiencing insomnia. Take the situation of frequent urination as a causative factor for insomnia. There are nursing actions that theoretically can improve this situation. Make a list of things you can do and the reasons why. Focus on nursing knowledge and not medical knowledge, such as medications. I will write one action and rationale for you as an example; then you need to complete the list. Be prepared to submit your plan to the faculty person.

1. ACTION: If possible, terminate drinking fluids at 6:00 p.m. This is a challenge for anyone accustomed to drinking throughout the evening, but a worthwhile behavior. The nurse will need to give sips of fluids with medications at bedtime. Be pleasant and supportive to the person giving up the fluids. It is hard!

   RATIONALE: It is simple. If the kidneys do not have fluid to process, there is minimal urine. Remember how important it is that any person sleeping has continuous sleep? If not, then refer back to the previous section. This action may be all that is necessary to stop nightly urination. You should write three more nursing actions that can assist this type of patient.

normally are awake. Anxiety often is related to difficulty falling asleep and frequent awake periods during the night. Psychiatric disorders can be treated with medication and therapy. Several disorders interfere with sleep and other life issues. Be diligent in your awareness of what is going on with the people to whom you give care. Talk to family members to gather information and an accurate past history. Share what you learn with the RN and physician so that a psychiatric assessment can be made and treatment can be started. The benefits will be much more than a good night's sleep.

As you evaluate and teach the patient and the family about healthy sleep, keep the following deterrents to good sleep in mind as part of your teaching plan. The following contribute to poor quality sleep: sedentary lifestyle, alcohol, tobacco, caffeine in the evening, disrupted sleep patterns, noise, and light in the sleeping environment. It is your responsibility to make the environment conducive to sleep, to teach the patient and family members about what disrupts sleep, and to report any medical conditions appropriately so that they can be treated. Carefully examine and talk to any person in your care who seems fatigued. Fatigue is *not* a normal outcome of aging; it is a problem.

CONCLUSION

The care of older adults requires a special sensitivity to their health needs. Their health is the main factor in determining their quality of life. To have maximum health, all people need activity that fits their physiology, rest that accommodates their lifestyle, and sleep that allows them the ability to function without fatigue. You, the nurse, are the key to these things happening for older adults. The ageist stereotype that the United States has for older adults leads many people to believe that lack of activity, taking several naps a day, and complaining of fatigue are simply factors that accompany aging. You now know that when these problems are recognized and documented, they can be managed through an interdisciplinary team approach (you, the RN, the physician, and the family). Many of the problems can be resolved through good nursing care approaches and family involvement. It is your responsibility to facilitate this type of care.

Mrs. McDonald is an 86-year-old woman who lives with her eldest son and his active family of five children. Mr. McDonald died the previous year of heart disease. After his death, Mrs. McDonald became less and less able to care for herself. She cried a great deal and refused to walk to the kitchen to prepare food. She said it was "too much work." She complained of not being able to sleep, yet whenever her son, Sean, came over to see her, she was sleeping in her chair. Being concerned about his mother, Sean moved her into his home with his wife and five children.

Mrs. McDonald had her own room but had to walk a short distance to the bathroom. She often was incontinent because it was "too hard" to get to the toilet. She always was tired and napped four to five times a day. Sean had two teenagers who often had friends over to the house. They were noisy and tended to stay until 9:00 or 10:00 in the evening on the weekends.

There also was a 5-month-old baby who woke up crying twice a night. All of the bedrooms were on the same floor, so each noisy incident awakened Mrs. McDonald.

Sean's wife, Mary, began to complain of having to wait on the children (baby, toddler, 5-year-old, and the teens) and Mrs. McDonald. "She won't get out of her chair or do anything for herself. I can't stand the incontinence; my house smells," Mary told Sean one day as she was crying. Sean felt caught between the needs of his mother and the needs of his wife and children. He was committed to not putting his mother in a nursing home because she was adamant about not going to "live in the county poorhouse." Sean called a local home-care agency to see if they could help him with his problem. You are the nurse assigned to Mrs. McDonald. What are you going to do? This is a holistic problem because the entire family is involved, so approach your solution with that in mind.

Solution

Gathering Information

You ask the admitting RN if you can accompany him on his first visit. He agrees that you should be there. While the RN does the admission, you ask Mary to show you Mrs. McDonald's room and the bathroom. While you are walking down the hallway, you talk to Mary about the problems she is having. It is obvious the entire family needs help if you are going to assist Mrs. McDonald. The following items need your attention.

Depression

Mrs. McDonald's behavior indicates that she could be depressed and has been since the death of her husband. You use the Beck Depression Scale as an assessment tool on Mrs. McDonald; the results indicate that she is clinically depressed. You talk to her and observe her to see if what you hear and see support the results of the test. Your observations lead you to talk to the case manager, who contacts the physician. After talking to Sean, the physician orders a mild antidepressant for Mrs. McDonald. You will observe her closely for the next 3 weeks to determine if there has been a change. If the medication does not relieve the depression symptoms, you may need to suggest some

psychological therapy sessions to assist her in managing her feelings regarding the death of her husband. You know that if the depression is managed, Mrs. McDonald will sleep better and be better able to care for herself during the day.

Strengthening

Mrs. McDonald needs more activity to become stronger. You arrange your first visit to be when the entire family is at home. Mrs. McDonald also is present at this family meeting. You explain the "first rule" of activity for older adults: It is for the person to do all activities possible for himself or herself. Mrs. McDonald is not doing that because she has the 5-year-old and the toddler running errands for her frequently during the day. She refuses to go to the bathroom—hence her incontinence—and she seldom leaves her room "because she is so tired."

Mrs. McDonald likes the idea of being more independent, so she agrees to listen to your plan, which follows. You also explain to everyone that the more activity Mrs. McDonald has, the better she will sleep.

1. She will come to the dining room for all meals. (Mary has been feeding her in her room, which contributes to Mrs. McDonald's

depression.) Mary agrees to walk her to the dining room for breakfast and lunch in time to enjoy eating with the family. The teens agree to take turns walking their grandma to the dining room for dinner.

2. The 5-year-old volunteers to "work out" with grandma while she does arm exercises with a soup can in each hand twice a day. You need to evaluate how many lifts she can do with her current muscle strength. You will reevaluate this frequently.

3. The teenagers agree to take turns taking grandma for a walk each day. You demonstrate how to get her out of the chair and how to use a walking belt (you brought one from the agency that will be left at the home) and emphasize that "a walk" initially will be a short trip in the hallway. You will monitor Mrs. McDonald's strength and add to the distance traveled as is appropriate.

Incontinence

This is a major problem that often is the reason families place their older family member in a nursing home. It is unpleasant for the caregiver and the person experiencing the incontinence. The smell tends to bother the entire family. You see this as an urgent matter. You explain to the family that the exercise will assist Mrs. McDonald in becoming strong enough eventually to ambulate to the bathroom. In the meantime, something must be done to make the situation manageable.

You talk to Mary and Mrs. McDonald privately and suggest adult briefs. Mrs. McDonald is able to change them herself, and their use would diminish the smell in the house and stains on the furniture and floor. You suggest a tight-lidded container as the place to dispose of the briefs. This will help control the smell as well. The container needs to be emptied every day. Mrs. McDonald is excited to have this type of autonomy, and Mary is visibly relieved.

You should advise other methods of bladder control, but because they are not the focus of this case study, they are not discussed here.

Sleep and Rest

Mrs. McDonald naps four to five times a day and still feels exhausted. You should ask her to keep a log (with Sean's help, if necessary) about her sleep. What time does she go to bed? What time does she wake up? How many times a night does she get up or become fully awake? What causes her to awaken? This information should be shared with the RN or the physician so that decisions can be made about sleep apnea tests, medication for RLS, or other medical interventions for Mrs. McDonald's fatigue.

In the meantime, you can get to work on basic nursing interventions. Is the room quiet at night without disruptive lighting? Does Mrs. McDonald avoid alcohol, smoking, and caffeine, as they are things that can disrupt her sleep? Is the room warm enough, and is the bed comfortable for her? Does she need more pillows or a bed that is elevated because of COPD or CHF? Does she need a new nighttime ritual, such as reading a large-print book with a 100-watt lamp? Would she like the family to come into her room and have family prayer at bedtime? There are several interventions you can investigate.

It would be an effective idea for Mrs. McDonald to try to have only two naps a day. She needs to be tired when she goes to bed. Staying awake, if it is reasonable, along with her new strengthening program will help her sleep.

There are other plans you could work out for Mrs. McDonald and her family. Consider at least two more and write them as part of this case study solution.

Select the best answer to each question.

1. When considering activity for older adults, the greatest challenge is:

   a. Getting them up and about without hurting your back.

   b. Keeping their weight within normal limits so that it is easier to move them.

   c. Managing their chronic diseases.

   d. Doing as much for them as possible as a pain management intervention.

2. The normal sleep cycle for older adults:

   a. Has four NREM cycles and an extra REM cycle. This occurs approximately four times a night

   b. Is not affected by the interruption of the NREM/REM cycles.

   c. Has a built-in mechanism, which develops as people age, that makes awakening more difficult.

   d. Does not change or adapt as people age.

3. The normal circadian rhythm:

   a. Changes as people age.

   b. Does *not* change as people age.

   c. Protects older adults from sleepless nights.

   d. Causes significant disruptions in normal sleep patterns in older adults.

4. Older adults who are most at risk for rest/sleep disturbances include all but the following:

   a. Older adults with sleep apnea and obesity

   b. Older adults with depression or dementia

   c. Older adults with RLS or myoclonus

   d. Older adults who are underweight and confused

5. Many sleep/rest problems can be managed with effective nursing interventions. Choose from the following list the activity that is not based on nursing knowledge:

   a. Sleep apnea testing

   b. Appropriate toileting pattern

   c. Strengthening program

   d. Administering the Beck Depression Scale

10

End-of-Life Issues in Older Adults

Emily Ravsten

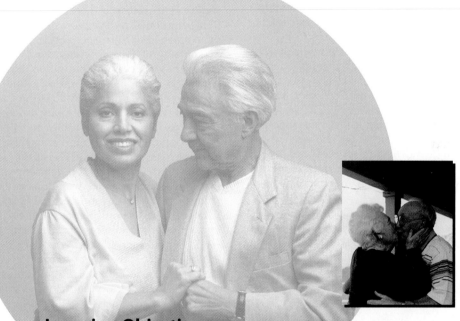

Learning Objectives

After completing this chapter, the student will be able to:

1. Define the essential characteristics of a hospice organization.
2. Identify the five stages of grief as outlined by Kübler-Ross.
3. List the qualities necessary for a nurse to give end-of-life care.
4. Express an opinion on assisted suicide.
5. List the eight signs of imminent death.

⬤ INTRODUCTION

My only living grandparent is Margrette Romer, an 83-year-old woman who keeps on kicking! She gave birth to six daughters, is the grandmother of 16 children, and is the great-grandmother of nine children, with one on the way. She lived her entire life on a farm in rural northern Utah, until 1998, when she fell and broke her hip and femur. She now lives with one of my aunts, who is her caregiver.

Grandma celebrated her 80th birthday with her friends and family and returned to the hospital that evening because of her fractures. Months before, my mom had sat down with Grandma and filled out a living will, which is a document that expressed my Grandma's desires to live or die if she were in a hospital. This preparation was helpful to my Grandma and to her daughters. At the time of her hospitalization, the family realized that she might not live. Her health gradually improved, however. When she was asked why she was fighting to live, she seriously stated that she still had quilts she needed to finish for her grandchildren! Three years later, Grandma is quilting and living a peaceful and pleasant life with her children and grandchildren all around.

I have a deep love for older people. My mom, who is the author of this book, practically raised me in nursing homes as she traveled from one nursing home to another evaluating the facilities and teaching the staff. Through such experiences, I learned that older adults are very wise and experienced. In addition, as they approach the end of their lives, they have the courage to face the multiple, serious decisions that need to be made. The focus of this chapter is to explore how to assist older adults to die well through the excellent care and support you provide them as they approach the end of their lives. Some terms related to end-of-life (EOL) care include the following:

- *EOL issues* are vital issues in health care throughout the United States. Americans want to experience a "good death" without being burdened by symptoms or technology. Nurses have an essential role in maximizing EOL care by improving symptom management; communication; and education about choices, referrals, and psychosocial treatments. You, as the care provider, have the responsibility to explain to older adults and their family members all of the options, referrals, and resources available. As you review some of the options in this chapter, it is very important that you examine your own attitudes, values, and beliefs. You need to consider what happens if your personal beliefs conflict with the choices and decisions made by an older adult in your care.

- *Palliative care* is the term used to describe care that is no longer aimed at a cure or active treatment of a certain medical condition. Instead, the goals of palliative care are to provide older adults with comfort and to manage their symptoms. This type of care is the art and science of quality EOL care. It is your opportunity, as a licensed practical nurse (LPN), to take the initiative in providing palliative care that ensures comprehensive, holistic EOL care for all older adults who are experiencing life-threatening, progressive illness. It is the opportunity to be sensitive and respectful to the older person's values, religious beliefs, family traditions, individual cultures, and beliefs. It is a tremendous amount of responsibility.

- *Terminal restlessness (TR)* is another term for agitated delirium. This is a common occurrence for individuals nearing the end of their lives. It may appear as involuntary muscle twitching or jerks, thrashing or agitation, tossing and turning, or yelling and moaning. These symptoms may not seem to be that

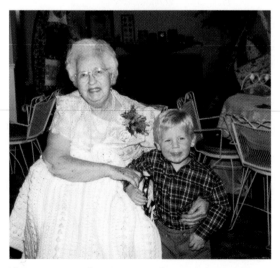

This is my Grandma Romer on her 80th birthday. With her is her youngest great-grandson. Grandma had a fractured hip and femur, but she wasn't going to miss her party! The ambulance was on standby, and as soon as the party was through, it took her to the hospital 50 miles away.

different from the symptoms experienced by residents in long-term care situations. Delirium at the end of one's life is usually multifactorial, however, and intensified by the progressive shutdown of numerous body systems.

- *Hospice* comes from the term *hospitality* and can be traced back to medieval times, when there was a need to find a place of rest for weary and ill travelers. Today, hospice organizations are located all over the United States. A large hospice organization attracts hundreds of people each year with diverse services (Box 10.1). More than 50% of all other hospices report being underused, however. This is poor use of a potentially tremendous service.

Often, referrals to a hospice come "too little, too late" to be most effective. An example of providing successful care is that of patients with Alzheimer's disease (AD). Providing them with palliative care may be the primary long-term mode of care. When death is imminent, generally around the last 6 months of life, a hospice team should be called on to provide their specialized knowledge to the palliation plan of care for the transition from dying to death.

BOX 10.1 Essential Components of Hospice Programs

The following qualities can be found in an excellent hospice program:
- Serves patients, families, and the community with sensitivity to different cultures, values, and beliefs
- Provides interdisciplinary teams of palliative care experts educated to give competent, compassionate, highly skilled, state-of-the-art care to dying people
- Has a small patient-to-worker ratio
- Is responsive 24 hours per day, 7 days per week
- Elicits and responds to patient and family needs and wants and encourages involvement of patient's own physician
- Produces accurate, reliable data about care, outcomes, and costs
- Earns community support

Adapted from St. Christopher's Hospice. (2001). http://www.stchristophers.org.uk/.

THE MYSTERY OF DEATH

More than 70% of annual deaths normally occur in people age 65 and older. By 2020, 2.5 million individuals older than age 65 will die annually in the United States. Dying is an unpredictable event. The exact moment or situation in which someone will die is never known. As the caregiver to older adults, you need to be prepared to be a positive influence for appropriate EOL issues. First, you need to be educated in EOL issues and learn to communicate them. Then, you need to provide the older adults in your care with a high quality of life and a good death. You need skills in working as a team with other caring professionals, families, and the dying person, understanding and applying the guiding principles of gerotranscendence for yourself and your patients. Finally, you need to maintain a positive work environment. Without skills in these areas, the quality of EOL care for older adults is diminished.

PRIORITY SETTING 10.1

This chapter describes the role of an EOL nurse. It talks about what you need to learn and explains many things you should work to understand. In my experience, I have found that people cannot apply information regarding EOL in an effective way unless they have come to an understanding within themselves about death. That is your priority for this chapter. Take the content you read and internalize it. Think about people who have died who were important to you. How did you feel, react, and grieve? If you are confused or uncomfortable with death experiences, where can you go to get more information? Who can you talk to about the death of someone who was close to you? Do you have religious beliefs that comfort you or friends who can assist you to accept the death? Do you understand gerotranscendence, through which individuals plan for their own good death and accept it? Do you apply gerotranscendence to your own life?

To give effective EOL care, you need to be at peace with death and its complexities. You should see it as the personal, meaningful, unique experience it is and then be able to share that with the patients, residents, and families with whom you work.

As all people know, death is an inevitable and natural human experience. Death has been shrouded in mystery, however, and envisioned as an experience of great suffering and generally is contemplated with fear. The early settlers in the United States had a different perception. They had a welcoming relationship with death, one that desired a release from pain and recognized the cycles of nature. For them, there was a time to live and a time to die. They were able to accept death as a transition into an afterlife and a reward for a life well lived. Somehow, modern society has lost that important concept. What has been the cause of this transition in thinking?

As I watched my grandmother on the acute unit in the hospital, I saw how different members of my family reacted to the possibility of her death. There were many emotions ranging from acceptance to denial as well as fear, anger, joy, and confusion. Those emotions were real and will be emotions that you, the nurse, will experience as you encounter family members of a dying person. People need to be allowed to cope with death in their own way, even if it is to deny death's reality until the end.

STAGES OF GRIEF

Grief is the normal reaction to a catastrophic loss. What defines the catastrophe? The person experiencing the loss has that responsibility. A catastrophe to one person may not be one to another. Understanding and compassion are essential when relating to people experiencing losses.

Dr. Elisabeth Kübler-Ross, a Swiss psychiatrist, spent much of her life defining the stages of grief. Death, the greatest personal loss a person can have, was the focus of her grief work. If you understand the five stages of grief, you can recognize them within yourself, the older adults to whom you give care, and their families. It is important knowledge to acquire.

Death is hard. It is a one-time experience, which makes death a unique and powerful experience. When a person dies, that individual loses everything they ever had. The dying person loses friends and family members, home, pets, beauty—everything. The stages of grief demonstrate the normal human reactions that people can have when facing a loss. Perhaps the person grieving is a family member of the person dying. His or her loss is also great. In addition to death, the stages of grief are valid with the loss of an extremity through amputation or loss associated with a stroke or divorce; for a

young girl, the loss of a date to the prom can result in a brief grieving process.

Kübler-Ross (1969) identified the five stages as follows:

> Acceptance
> Depression
> Bargaining
> Anger
> Denial

Think of these terms as steps in the process of resolving grief. The person experiencing the loss can go from one stage (or step) to another and then move back up or down the stages. There is no exact formula or prescription to follow because people are individuals and manage their grief in very personalized ways. Nurses need to allow this type of independent grieving.

Denial

When a catastrophic loss occurs, a person's psyche has difficulty accepting it. Consider a young mother who leaves her aging and confused mom outside for "only a moment" while she goes in the house to get her baby. When the young mother comes out of the house, her mother has wandered out into the street, is hit by a car, and eventually dies in the hospital. Some denial behaviors are shock, praying for it to not be true, walking about, or standing and saying, "No, not Mom" over and over again.

Denial is the psyche's way of protecting itself from the harsh, bitter truth. It is as if the young mother were wrapped up in a soft, protective cocoon. This psychological protection is there until the person's psyche can deal with the loss. You have heard of people who "were in a daze" during the funeral of a loved one. That is denial. There is no reason to try to force people out of denial. They will move to the next stage when they are able. During this time, people need to be protected from neglect, injury, and financial abuse. Family members need to understand this stage of the grief process and be willing to take care of other children, prepare meals, and protect the grieving person.

CRITICALLY EXAMINE THE FOLLOWING

List three reasons why anger is a healthy behavior in a person who is experiencing grief:

1.
2.
3.

I will share my answers with you. Perhaps you thought of some reasons that did not occur to me. Compare your list with mine, and come to class prepared to share your thinking.

1. It means the psyche is healthier because the person is no longer in denial.
2. It keeps the people away who say things like "You'll always have your memories of your Mom" or "She is at peace now." Comments like these disrespect the loss and the grief being experienced. People who make such comments often are not comfortable with anger. Their purpose is to "make everything all right," which is not congruent with angry feelings.
3. It is an outlet for the normal frustration one feels when confronted with a catastrophic loss.

Anger

When the psyche has developed the strength to face the situation, it comes out in a way that tends to keep people away, which saves the person grieving a great deal of energy. What else does it do? This is the one time that anger should be encouraged in a person and supported as a healthy behavior when it occurs. Can you think of some of the advantages of the grieving person showing anger?

Anger demonstrates an awareness of the loss and its consequences. This is one step toward adjusting to the loss. It is also an outlet for the outrage the person feels. Assist the grieving person not to hurt himself or herself or others with the anger. The family needs to understand the advantages of the anger so that they can accept what is happening and support the behaviors that occur.

Bargaining

The anger is as if the psyche wants to "scare away" the bad thing that has occurred. As we know, that does not work. When the grieving person realizes that the "bad thing" will not go away, he or she often turns to God or other supernal powers. This behavior often is demonstrated by bargaining.

Bargaining is seen as something like prayers to God stating that the person will donate a great deal of money to a charitable organization, will never sin again, or will actively do good for others. The thinking is that if one trades something of value, like goodness, with God, then God will perform a miracle. This is very heartbreaking for family and friends. Many say they prefer anger over the wrenching episodes of bargaining. The negotiation with God is the final chance to change the situation. If God cannot "fix things," then no one can. This time in the grieving process requires patience and gentleness. People are often exhausted in their efforts to support the grieving person. They do not have much more to give. Yet, more is asked of them. When you teach families about the bargaining stage, reassure them that this is often near the end. Praise them for staying with the grieving person throughout the entire experience. Try to give them strength and courage to see the experience to its conclusion.

Not everyone believes in God or a higher power. Work with grieving people in whatever way they are bargaining. The principles are the same for all forms of grief bargaining.

Depression

Depression never is an easy condition. In the grieving process, it definitely shows progress. When a grieving person is depressed, it means that the individual does not accept the loss but accepts the fact that nothing can change it. The denial, anger, and bargaining did not work. It makes sense that the grieving person would be depressed.

As with all forms of depression, actively assess for suicidal thinking. If you identify it, keep someone with the grieving person and contact the registered nurse (RN). Suicide is a preventable outcome, so be sensitive to its possibility. Depressed people cry, they sleep a great deal, and they have low energy. Teach this to the family members. Ask them to support the grieving person through this last hurtle to acceptance.

Depressed people do not need to be told, "Everything is all right." For them, nothing will ever be all right again. They need quiet love and support while they find a way to continue on with their lives.

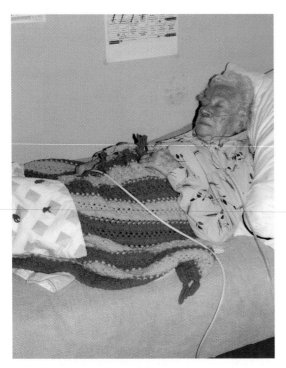

This woman has accepted that she is going to die. As is common with so many people, she does not want to interact with the world anymore. She is done; she has accepted the fact that she is close to death. Notice that she has her call light in hand "just in case." She also must have slowing circulation, as indicated by the afghan, blanket, and oxygen.

Acceptance

When the grieving person reaches acceptance, there is a sense of relief. The individual still is searching for life structure without the loved one who died. The point is that the grief process is over, and living has started again. The grieving person still may call out the name of the deceased person, be found crying after finding a piece of clothing of the loved one, or just sit quietly contemplating the life of the person who died. This is normal.

The grieving process is difficult for the person experiencing the loss and the family members. The management of the experience can be improved when you, the LPN, know the stages of grief and readily share them with appropriate people.

⬤ QUALITIES FOR A NURSE TO BE A PROVIDER OF END-OF-LIFE CARE

Many nurses have difficulty talking about EOL matters with patients. You need to learn new skills and acquire new knowledge to improve the care of older adults who require palliative care (Box 10.2). Some of the new knowledge you need may be communication skills and knowledge of resources and available services.

You, as a nurse, have a tremendous potential to change the care of dying older adults and the support given to their families. It is crucial that you understand human nature as you give care to people who are dying. You need to be able to identify the stages of grief and translate those stages to family members. Because the stages are expressed individually by different people, you need to be able to comprehend the impact on specific individuals and understand the nature of the people involved. Another critical aspect of what you need to know to be an effective palliative care nurse is the ability to identify and meet the holistic needs of individuals, families, and communities.

Tolerance and Empathy

Each individual you encounter in your work is unique. As the care provider, you will need to gain an understanding of people and their differences. This requires that you learn to become tolerant and empathetic to those with whom you associate. Synonyms of tolerance are *compassion, endurance, patience, impartiality,*

BOX 10.2 **Qualities to Develop Before Working With Dying People**

- Motivation
- *Emotional maturity.* Death is serious and individualized and happens only once for each person.
- *Tolerance and empathy.* Nothing goes according to a formula or procedure. This is true of the dying process and people.
- *Communication skills.* You need the ability to empathize with all people involved in the death experience.
- *Confidentiality.* A sense of discretion and respect for patient and family privacy is essential.
- *Flexibility.* You must be willing to do what patients and their families need, not what you think is best.
- *Dependability.* Dependability turns into trust.
- *Good listening skills.* Listening is a wonderful gift you can give to someone who may be feeling frightened and alone.
- *Sense of humor.* Humor in difficult situations can be a plus. It is okay to giggle with patients and families.

and *open-mindedness.* Synonyms of empathy are *understanding, sympathetic, identifying with the patient,* and *providing insight and feeling in your care.* To provide appropriate tolerance and empathy, you must strive to create an environment that meets the physical, emotional, social, and spiritual needs of each dying person.

Sense of Humor

Having a sense of humor with the dying person is a simple way to assist in relieving, reducing, and soothing the symptoms of a disease. You must know the personality and mood of the older adult in your care before making jokes about the situation. You must make sure that it is done at the right time and in the right situation. Think about a time and place when you were suffering and laughter helped with the cure.

Communication

Communication is the key to most situations. When it comes to death and dying, this situation has the possibility of being discussed in a context of hope, meaning, and opportunity. With strong communication skills, uncertainty

FOCUSED LEARNING CHART

Understanding tolerance and empathy

A care provider's goal is to understand the needs of people experiencing an end-of-life situation.

Tolerance	Empathy
Compassion	Understanding
Impartiality	Identify with person
Endurance	Sympathetic
Patience	Be insightful
Open-mindedness	Allow self to feel situation

is replaced with certainty, hopelessness is replaced with faith, and despair is replaced with empowerment.

Good Listening Skills

Being a good listener is the greatest skill any nurse can have. Take time to listen to older adults' stories about their children and grandchildren, stories about falling in love, and possibly stories about losing their loved ones. Older people enjoy sharing their life experiences. It is important to remember when talking to an older person that you need to speak in a voice that he or she can hear. Move in close to the person, touch his or her shoulder, smile, and listen to what he or she has to share.

To listen, you must be fully present and attentive to the other person. You are not listening if you:

- Are in a hurry
- Are thinking about yourself
- Interrupt
- Ask the same question twice
- Do not ask any questions
- Assume that you know what the other person is going to say

A good listener is one who does not think about what to say until after the other person has finished speaking.

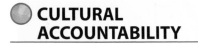

CULTURAL ACCOUNTABILITY

In addition to the previously mentioned qualities that are needed to care for individuals nearing the end of their lives, it is important to be familiar with the cultural diversities of the older adults in your care. A person's culture influences the decision-making process in regard to various treatments.

In many cultures, a family's interdependence, harmony, duty, and obligation to an older family member are obvious. Some cultures believe that it is inappropriate to tell someone that he or she is dying because it would create a sense of hopelessness and sadness. Some cultures believe that a sick individual should not be allowed to make any decisions about EOL care but rather have the family or the eldest son make those decisions. Cultural needs should be addressed immediately on admission to any facility for you, as the LPN, to be aware of the family's and the individual's diverse needs.

END-OF-LIFE DECISIONS

As a care provider for individuals who are nearing the end of their lives, it is crucial that you recognize the importance of being aware of the decisions a person has made about his or her current and future medical care and to honor his or her preferences. According to a study report, 25% of nurses have seen other health-care providers deliberately disregard a patient's advance directive, such as a durable power of attorney, a living will, or a health-care proxy document. To help protect the patient's right to make his or her own health-care choices and to avoid getting yourself or your facility into legal trouble, you need to understand the various laws, your individual duties to the person dying, and the individual wishes of that person.

Gaining an understanding of all of the issues surrounding EOL care is a daunting task. You will run into challenges about knowledge and skills in assessing and managing pain in cognitively impaired older adults. You will experience frustration about physicians being unwilling to consider a nurse's assessment and recommendations. You will find it difficult to deal with the strong emotional attachments that are formed with older adults at the EOL stage. These are all reasons to learn and study EOL issues.

ADVANCE DIRECTIVES

One of the most difficult situations that health-care professionals face when caring for older people is how to assist patients and families who are trying to make decisions about whether to start, continue, or stop life-sustaining treatments. Elderly people as a group account for 73% of deaths each year, making EOL treatment decisions far more prevalent among them. Documents that assist the health-care team in making such complex decisions are advance directives. There are two types of advance directive documents available: the durable power of attorney for health care (also called health-care proxy) and living wills.

The health-care proxy has the authority to make health-care decisions if the individual loses the ability to make decisions or communicate personal wishes (Box 10.3). The proxy can make decisions as the need arises and is not restricted to a decision that was made previously without knowledge of the current situation.

BOX 10.3 Health-Care Proxy

I, _____, of _____, this day of _____, being of sound mind, willingly and voluntarily appoint _____ as my agent and attorney-in-fact, without substitution. This gives my proxy lawful authority to execute a directive on my behalf under Section 75-2-1105, governing the care and treatment to be administered to or to be withheld from me at any time after I incur an injury, disease, or illness that renders me unable to give current directions to attending physicians and other providers of medical services.

I have carefully selected my above-named agent with confidence in the belief that this person's familiarity with my desires, beliefs, and attitudes will result in directions to attending physicians and providers of medical services that would probably be the same as I would give if able to do so.

This power of attorney will remain in effect from the time my attending physician certifies that I have incurred a physical or mental condition rendering me unable to give current directions to attending physicians and other providers of medical services as to my care and treatment.

Signature of Principal _____
State of _____
County of _____
On the _____ day of _____, _____, personally appeared before me, _____, who duly acknowledged to me that he/she has read and fully understands the foregoing power of attorney, executed the same of his/her own volition and for the purposes set forth, and that he/she was acting under no constraint or undue influence whatsoever.

Notary Public _____
My commission expires: _____
Residing at: _____

The other type of advance directive is known as a living will (see Appendix A). This is a legal document that allows individuals to share their opinions and wishes regarding their death. The legal statutes that govern the use of advance directives vary from state to state. You, as an LPN, must clearly understand the advance directive laws where you work.

Advance directives came into use when legal cases such as those involving Karen Ann Quinlan and Nancy Cruzan surfaced in the judicial system. In both of these legal cases, a young woman was kept alive on life-support equipment but had no quality of life at the time and no possibility of improvement in the future. In both cases, the family members decided to remove the life-support equipment and allow their daughters to die. In both cases, the health-care facility refused to remove the equipment, and the parents sued.

In 1989, the U.S. Supreme Court ruled that not even the family should make decisions for an incompetent patient without "clear and convincing evidence" that indicated the person's desire was to die if incompetent. In a five-to-four decision by the U.S. Supreme Court, the following rights were listed for states (*Cruzan v. Director,* 1990):

- The state has a right to assert an unqualified interest in the preservation of human life.
- A choice between life and death is a very personal matter.
- Abuse can occur when incompetent patients do not have loved ones available to serve as surrogate decision makers.

After this court ruling, most state legal systems began requiring an advance directive on admission to health-care facilities to predetermine the actions that should be taken if a patient became incompetent. As an LPN, you need to determine what the law is in your state regarding advance directives. If they are required on admission, you need to know where they are and what they say regarding your clients. It is the role of the nurse to be an advocate for the people to whom care is given. Knowledge about the advance directive and the state laws that govern its use is very important to you.

When one is working with advance directives, there is more involved than just knowing the law. The law represents legal responsibilities. These are serious responsibilities and should not be ignored; however, as with every issue, there is also an ethical component. It is the ethical responsibility of every nurse to ensure that the person signing the advance directive is not coerced and has full understanding of what is being signed. In most states, the nurse is not allowed to witness this document. It is important that outsiders who would not wield undue influence act as witnesses.

Whenever you are giving care to a patient who is in a terminal condition, it is important that you listen as the person talks and provide honest answers to questions. If someone feels

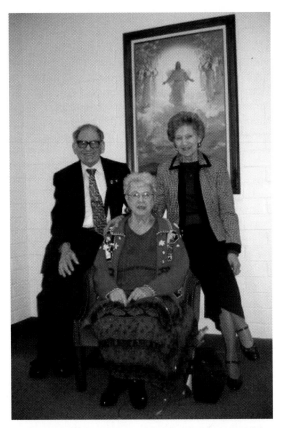

These three friends spent several evenings together to gather information, discuss it, and complete their living wills and durable power of attorney forms. None of them are sick, but all three of them believe it is important to have the forms completed and to discuss their wishes with their family members.

concern over what was written in the advance directive, you should bring that to the attention of the nurse manager. The instructions for completing a living will are provided in Appendix A of this book. In all situations, it is necessary to keep in mind the primary objective of the advance directive: to follow the wishes of the person who wrote it.

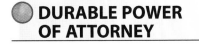

DURABLE POWER OF ATTORNEY

Durable power of attorney is another important legal document. Durable power of attorney is used in cases in which an individual is incompetent. The law allows a competent individual to make all (e.g., health-care, financial, disposition of personal items)

legal decisions for the incompetent person. The classic example is someone with AD. Before persons with AD become incompetent, they can identify someone they trust and who knows their wishes and assign them durable power of attorney. When the dementia increases, the individual's wishes are met.

Not everyone knows that they will eventually become incompetent. When an older person becomes incompetent because of undiagnosed AD or a car accident that causes brain damage, the family may seek a durable power of attorney, and the older person would be unaware of what is happening. The forms for durable power of attorney need to come from a qualified attorney to ensure their legality in the state where the older adult resides.

To ensure protection of the older person's rights, you, as the nurse, need to recommend to families and patients that they seek legal council. After a durable power of attorney has been established, you have a responsibility to identify the type of decision-making authority each person possesses.

IMMINENT SIGNS OF DEATH

As an LPN, it is important for you to know the imminent signs of death. It is easy to assist someone in his or her preparation to die if the person has received a diagnosis of a terminal illness. A terminal diagnosis allows individuals to realign their priorities, mend various relationships, and say goodbye to loved ones. In addition, a terminal diagnosis allows staff the opportunity to prioritize their care and assist persons in meeting their goals and achieving a peaceful life closure.

CRITICALLY EXAMINE THE FOLLOWING

Have you considered what you would like written in your living will? Do you want to be pain-free? What about use of antibiotics? What about use of a ventilator? What about food? Photocopy the living will in this chapter and complete it for yourself. Add the details that are important to you and be prepared to submit your living will to the faculty person or discuss it in class.

Even after a person has gone through the difficult process of writing a living will, that person's family members can change it at any time. This is a point of frustration for many health-care providers, especially nurses. Consider the frustration it causes for the patient and other family members as well.

When death is near, bodily functions slow, and certain signs and symptoms occur, including the following:

- Rapid, weak pulse
- Decline in blood pressure
- Dyspnea and periods of apnea
- Slower or no pupil response to light
- Profuse perspiration
- Cold extremities
- Bladder and bowel incontinence
- Pallor and mottling of skin
- Loss of hearing

One of the last senses lost is that of hearing.

One clear sign of imminent death is TR. Reports indicate that more than three-fourths of dying patients experience this condition. TR occurs in the last hours of life. It is the spiraling down of physiological functions and can be very distressing to the older adult who is dying and to family and staff members. At this time so close to EOL, there is a crucial need for careful and thoughtful intervention to provide the dying person with comfort and to be able to control his or her symptoms.

Dying is an individualized experience. It is something that has never happened to the dying person before, and the individual may need your assistance in making the death a good one. One thing you can do is talk to the person to identify individual attitudes and knowledge regarding death, disease, and support systems already in place. Formal assessments are done by the assigned RN; however, you, as the LPN, are giving the bedside care and need to be prepared to respond to questions that are asked after the RN's assessment. The goal of your assessment is to be able to gain a clear understanding of the older person's experiences with his or her illness. In addition, you need to be able to identify distressing symptoms that need management, convey your concern and empathy to the persons involved, and evaluate any risk that may be expressed owing to current distress or feelings. It is important for you to take immediate action when a problem is detected.

To begin an appropriate assessment or interview with the dying person, you should ask various questions about discouragement or distress. For example, "What hurts or distresses you most, and how can I help?" Another good opening question to ask is what the person worries about most when the illness is at its worst and what has been most difficult throughout the process. Your assessment should review the older adult's various abilities to cope with stress and anxiety. For example, "During periods of discouragement, some people wish all this suffering were over. Have you felt this way? Tell me about it." "You seem to feel as if life is not worth living. Are you thinking of doing something to hasten your death? Tell me about it." "No one thinks about ending their life without a reason; tell me how you are feeling."

ASSISTED SUICIDE

Approximately 2% to 5% of terminally ill people choose to hasten their own deaths (Engber, 2005). Reasons include poor quality of life and failed requests for treatment withdrawal. People have the right to refuse treatments, food, or fluids if they wish to do so. The Patient Care Partnership assures people of that right (see Chapter 5). To make a rational decision about ending life, an older adult needs a clear mind, communication with others, knowledge of alternative treatments, and an understanding of the long-term consequences of actions. The difficulty for most health-care providers is to differentiate between a person's refusal of life-sustaining treatments and providing support to a dying person.

In Oregon, terminally ill people have the right to hasten their deaths by physician-assisted suicide. By the second year physician-assisted suicide was legal in Oregon, 27 people chose this option. Their median age was 71, 16 were men, 26 were white, and 12 were married (Engber, 2005).

CRITICALLY EXAMINE THE FOLLOWING

Answer the questions listed. They are questions that require you to ponder their significance. Perhaps you do not believe that you have enough experience to make such decisions. Remember that you will soon be part of the nursing workforce, and you will need to make some of these decisions. This exercise is an effort to prepare you for them. Be prepared to discuss your answers in class.

How do you feel about assisted suicide?

Would you be a part of such a decision?

Would you work for a facility that supported "slow codes"—passively participating in assisted suicide by not getting to a patient on time—or a facility that openly participated in assisted suicide?

These are questions you will face as you continue to provide care to patients nearing the end of their lives.

CONCLUSION

Now that you have read this chapter, I hope you understand the importance of giving meaningful EOL care to all people but especially to older adults. Dying is a unique experience for everyone. The hallmark of a professional nurse is one who can support the dying person and the family in their personal uniqueness of that special event.

I admire your desire and passion for working with older adults. They are at a fragile time in their lives when they are in need of people who care about them. As the LPN who will provide older adults who are dying with positive EOL experiences, you are one of those individuals.

In this case study scenario, imagine that you have recently moved to Oregon, where assisted suicide has been legalized. You were surprised on your first day when a patient on the unit was going to receive some assistance in her own suicide.

1. Before you moved to Oregon, what resources did you use to learn about the legality, rules, and regulations related to assisted suicide?

2. Every nurse has a right to his or her personal ethical framework of practice. What does your personal framework of practice dictate about what you will do regarding the woman who is assigned to you for assisted suicide?

Solution

1. If I were moving to Oregon and had the potential of working with assisted suicide patients, I would initially contact the state board of nursing for specific Oregon laws. I would also contact the hospital where I would be working and have them send me a packet on their specific protocols regarding assisted suicide. I also may spend some time on the Internet just to see what information is available about the specific topic. You may have additional ideas about gathering information. List them and feel free to discuss your ideas with your class.

2. I do not know how you would respond to this situation. The answer to this question is based on individual standards and beliefs. Take some time to ponder thoughtfully giving this kind of nursing care in terms of your personal ethical framework. Consider your knowledge and acceptance of the death and dying process and your personal reaction to assisted suicide as a health-care principle, and explain your responses in writing. Follow through by sharing those ideas in class in a way you feel most comfortable.

Select the best answer to each question.

1. When an elderly client experiences TR, he or she will display symptoms such as:

   a. Involuntary muscle twitching or jerks

   b. Extreme fatigue

   c. A sudden energy for life

   d. A calm affect causing the body to have no reactions

2. Palliative care is described as:

   a. The type of care aimed at a cure or active treatment of a certain medical condition

   b. The type of care that provides comfort and management of symptoms

   c. The type of care that allows the family to make all of the decisions

   d. The type of care that provides bereavement support to the family for 1 year after death

3. The stages of grief in order are:

   a. Denial, anger, bargaining, depression, acceptance

   b. Denial, communicate, pain, sadness, joy

   c. Denial, affection, bartering, acceptance

   d. Denial, anger, acceptance, joy, peace

4. When speaking to an elderly dying patient, it is important to:

   a. Never talk to the patient, but rather communicate all decisions through family members

   b. Communicate clearly, possibly with a sense of humor, in a manner that the patient will be able to hear what is being said

   c. Explain your frustrations with the patient and his or her care in front of the patient and the family

   d. Be sympathetic rather than empathetic with the patient and the family

5. Four of the eight signs of imminent death are:

   a. Increased blood pressure, warm extremities, bowel and bladder incontinence, and pallor and mottling of the skin

   b. Loss of hearing, dyspnea and periods of apnea, and increased bowel and bladder control

   c. Increased sexual drive, slow pupil response to light, increased awareness of surroundings, and more communicative

   d. Rapid weak pulse, profuse perspiration, loss of hearing, and decline in blood pressure

11

Environments of Care

Kathleen R. Culliton

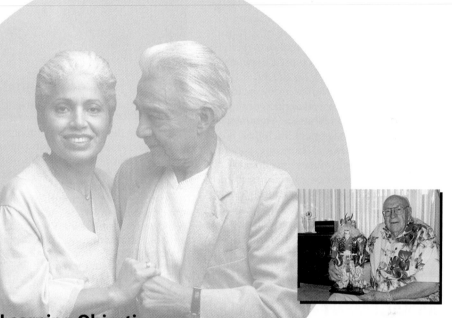

Learning Objectives

After completing this chapter, the student will be able to:

1. Discuss the role of the licensed practical nurse (LPN) as an environmental manager.
2. Describe at least two components of the physical environment that nurses need to consider.
3. Discuss the aspects included in a climate of caring.
4. Identify at least four settings in which nursing care for older adults is provided.
5. Describe how nurses in various care settings meet the needs of older adults.
6. Discuss relocation stress and ways in which a nurse can help an older person adjust to a new environment.

INTRODUCTION

One of the most important tasks for a nurse is to manage the patient-care environment. Florence Nightingale saved the lives of hundreds of soldiers during the Crimean War simply by cleaning the wards, opening the windows, and providing the soldiers with daily hygiene. Nightingale and her nurses also provided direct, caring, "hands-on" nursing to the soldiers under their care. Before Nightingale's interventions, there were more soldiers dying in the hospitals because of the lack of hygienic conditions than there were dying in the battles. Improved health for the men fighting the Crimean War required environmental management and quality nursing care.

The role of a nurse is not that of a housekeeper but that of an environmental manager. To be effective caregivers, nurses must be aware of the influence of environment on the health and functioning of the patient. Nurses are responsible for the manipulation of environmental conditions to improve patient care. In Florence Nightingale's era, environmental management included such tasks as opening windows to clear the patient's room of stale, potentially illness-producing air; managing raw sewage because plumbing was not available; and controlling the population of mice and rats in the hospital. Modern nurses also must understand the effect that the environment can have on enhancing or impeding the progress and functioning of older adults.

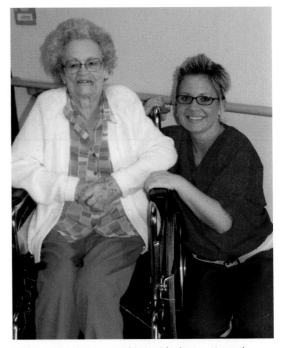

This nursing home resident with dementia and generalized weakness has found herself in a climate of caring. Notice how her clothes match and appear well cared for? Her hair is nicely done, and she is smiling. The LPN kneeling next to her demonstrates the basic symbols of caring. First, she got down to the older woman's wheelchair level so that she could be seen and heard. She is reaching out to her, although she comes short of touching her. She looks well groomed, and she also is smiling. They seem to care about each other.

ENVIRONMENTAL MANAGEMENT

Providing care to older adults must include environmental management. Assessment of the environment is the first step. As a licensed practical nurse (LPN), you need to examine the total environment starting with where the older person is living. There are multiple environments of care in which an older adult might live. If the person lives at home, you might ask the following questions: What is the neighborhood like? Is it a safe neighborhood for an older person? Is there a security system in the home or building?

If an older adult lives in a nursing home or in a hospital, you might ask the following questions: What is the staffing ratio? Is the environment clean and free of odor? Is there a place where the older adult can socialize with family and friends?

If an older adult lives in an assisted living environment, you might ask: How far is it to the dining room? Are there activities that interest the person? Is there a nurse available 24 hours a day?

Assessment of the physical environment includes all aspects of the older adult's living situation that can be seen, heard, touched, or smelled. Each of the physical items in the environment can either contribute to or detract from the optimal functioning of the older person. A room that is too hot may make the older person tired, lethargic, and unwilling to participate in personal-care activities. A room that is too cold may likewise result in lack of activity because the older person is unwilling to get out of bed or to come out from under the cover of an afghan.

A crucial question to ask throughout the assessment of the physical environment is how well the older person functions in the living areas. Is the environment as barrier-free as possible? Can the older person walk unencumbered or wheel a wheelchair through the entire setting? Are there features in the environment to promote physical function? These may include grab bars in the bathroom by the commode, shower, or bathtub seat and handrails by stairs. When assessing how the older person carries out activities of daily living, be aware of possible alterations that may improve function. Lowering a mirror or moving a storage area below shoulder level may improve safety and convenience. The risk of falling can be decreased with adequate room lighting and the use of night-lights. The room where the older person reads should have high-intensity illumination.

Climate of Caring

Another important part of the environmental assessment is evaluating the climate of caring. The climate of caring involves the people in the environment and the environmental tone and atmosphere. The people in an older person's living environment may include family members, neighbors, friends, and paid caregivers.

The people in an environment are extremely important to the older adult's potential for improvement and optimal function. Families, staff members, and visitors can be encouraging and uplifting or depressing and discouraging. A climate of caring includes persons who present a positive but realistic outlook. An older adult's personal space is respected in a caring climate. Such an atmosphere also affords opportunities for privacy, encourages activity and involvement, and facilitates independence.

Safety

In any setting, safety for the older person is a primary concern. Are there any environmental hazards, such as frayed extension cords, malfunctioning equipment, or broken furniture? Falls among elderly people are common. Although not all falls can be avoided, one thing that can be done is to keep the environment free of fall risks. Such risks include clutter, throw rugs, wheelchair leg rests, and poorly fitting shoes or slippers. A pet sometimes can be a fall risk as well.

Stimulation and Personalization

Opinions vary on whether environments for older adults with cognitive impairment should be very stark and nonstimulating or should contain eye-catching and stimulating components. What is more important is a personalized environment for the older person. Personalized items help older adults relate to the environment and maintain a sense of identity. A special picture can be displayed in a hospital room or nursing home. In some settings, such as nursing homes and retirement communities, the entire bedroom or apartment can be personalized with cherished furniture and decorations.

A climate of caring facilitates optimal independence and autonomy for each older person living in the setting. Sometimes the routines and regulations necessary to operate a large health-care facility such as a hospital or nursing home cannot accommodate the individual needs or desires of older adults. The nurse must assess, however, which rules and routines are absolutely necessary and which are the result of a controlling institution or individual staff member. Although a nursing home may need to serve meals at particular times because of regulations and staffing, the rule that all residents must be dressed for breakfast may be unnecessary. This rule does not allow for each resident to take the time personally to do as much of the dressing as possible. Such a rule can force a resident to be dependent on staff for dressing. A climate of caring provides multiple opportunities for individual choice in the environment and encourages the older person to function as independently as possible.

Personal Space and Territoriality

Personal space and territory are important to every human being. Personal space is the area around a person. Some individuals define their personal space very close to their bodies, whereas others define it as a broader area. It is viewed as an intrusion for someone to invade another individual's personal space. In providing nursing care, nurses must frequently invade the personal space of the patient. Nurses must be conscious, however, that they do not do so unnecessarily.

Territory is the space used by a person and seen as owned by the person. Think about a current class. Do the students tend to sit in the same seats during each class session? Technically, you and your classmates do not own the seats, but the tendency exists to define a territory and return to it habitually. The seating arrangement in a dining room in a nursing home or retirement community is frequently consistent for each meal. This consistency tends to occur whether or not seats are assigned. Individuals defend their territory if an unwanted person intrudes. An older person who has a favorite chair at home or in the nursing home may fiercely defend it from others.

Privacy

All human beings need time to be alone. People need to have opportunities for privacy and for human contact. It is difficult sometimes for an older person living in a health-care setting to find opportunities for privacy. Many hospitals and nursing homes have multiple-occupancy rooms so that the patient may never have a chance to be truly alone. As a nurse working with older persons in a congregate setting, you must be aware of the older person's needs for privacy. You should respect that right to privacy by knocking on the door before entering, pulling cubicle curtains during care, and arranging private time for the older adult.

Activity and Involvement

As a person ages, the number of social roles fulfilled tends to diminish. An older woman who was once a daughter, a wife, a mother, a neighbor, an accountant, a Scout leader, and a bridge player may hold none of these social roles at 90 years of age. Because of aging and disability, these roles may no longer be possible. Involvement with others is still a need, however. A climate of caring affords each individual multiple and diverse opportunities for activity and involvement with others.

As a nurse working with older people in multiple health-care settings, you can help to provide

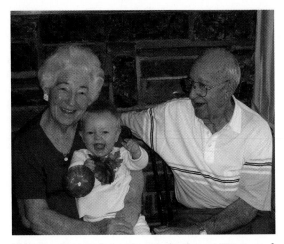

This grandma and grandpa are both past 80 years of age and have lived in their current home since they were a young married couple. They have made it clear to their children that they do not want to leave their home if they become ill. They have a large extended family, and they want to be around them until they die. Many older people have a strong aversion to leaving their homes, which is why home care is such a valuable resource to older adults.

important opportunities for active involvement. It is important to find out the older person's prior social roles, particularly the ones he or she most enjoyed. Activities that include tasks associated with these roles should be encouraged. It also is important to create opportunities for social interaction. By introducing the older person to others in the setting who may share similar interests and by arranging seating for natural conversation rather than against walls, the nurse can be instrumental in encouraging social exchanges.

RELOCATION TRAUMA

Moving from one environment to another is stressful. Anyone who has ever moved from one house to another or from one city to another can appreciate the stress of relocation. It takes time to adjust to and become familiar with a new setting. During times of crisis or illness, one has less energy available to deal constructively with stress. Older adults are particularly susceptible to being overcome with the stress of relocation. Such stress also is referred to as transitional stress. This term refers specifically to the emotional stress that occurs during the time a person is changing from one phase of life to another.

Older people use a considerable amount of energy coping with chronic illness and disabilities.

The onset of an acute illness or some other major crisis requires additional coping. If the crisis or illness results in the need to move to another living situation, the older person's coping abilities may be exhausted. A crisis, superimposed on the day-to-day stresses of living with disability and dysfunction, frequently leaves the older person with little coping reserve to deal with the stress of relocation and transition. When the stress is overwhelming, and the older person is unable to cope with the situation, signs of decompensation appear. These may include disorientation, agitation, acting out, and hallucinations. It is common for an older adult newly admitted to any of the health-care settings described in this chapter to exhibit some of these signs. The movement from one environment to another can be extremely disruptive to the older adult; this disruption has been termed *relocation trauma*.

In addition to identifying and understanding relocation trauma, the nurse can help to relieve relocation stress. Relocation trauma is temporary, and the behavioral signs of decompensation should diminish as the older person becomes familiar with the new environment. You can accelerate the process of adjustment, however.

Limit stimulation and the introduction of new activities and people on the older person's first day in the setting. Orient the older person to the environment slowly so that he or she can incorporate new areas and routines gradually. On the first day, introduce only people and places that are absolutely necessary. For example, placing an older person in the dining room of a nursing home with 20 other residents shortly after admission may be overwhelming.

Look for ways to provide links between the old environment and the new one. The more familiar the new environment is to the older person, the easier the transition is for the person. Bringing favorite furniture and objects, such as pictures, to the new setting increases its familiarity to the older person. Including the older person in planning for the move is ideal. This is not always possible, however, if the move occurs because of an acute illness. If it can be arranged, involve the older person in selecting the items to take to the new location.

SETTINGS OF CARE

Older persons may receive health-care services in a variety of settings. This chapter does not discuss all such settings or services but reviews some of the most commonly used settings of care.

Day Care

Adult day-care centers are available in many communities to provide supervised activities for older adults. Day treatment centers for older people with psychiatric problems and day hospitals for older persons with considerable physical disability are available in many localities. Day treatment centers and day hospitals focus on a

---

FOCUSED LEARNING CHART

Relocation trauma

Symptom of Decompensation	Nursing Care
Disorientation	Temporary condition
Hallucinations	Familiar items such as furniture and photos
Agitation	Involve family and friends
Acting out	Be caring
	Limit stimulation (people, places, and activities) for the first few days

Review the following situation and devise a plan that would have minimized Mrs. B.'s relocation trauma. Be prepared to share your ideas in class.

Mrs. B. was moving from her home of 40 years to a retirement community. She had some short-term memory problems and walked with a slow gait. To expedite the move, Mrs. B.'s son packed for her and sorted through all of her belongings to identify what items to take and what to give away. Because many of her things were very old and worn, her son decided to purchase all new furniture and decorations for her new apartment. The new apartment looked beautiful. After moving, Mrs. B. became extremely disoriented and paranoid, and she accused everyone of stealing her belongings. As the nurse in the retirement community, what would you have taught Mrs. B.'s son about preparing his mother for relocation?

particular type of older person and provide specific services to meet their physical and psychiatric needs. Many day-care centers provide transportation for the older person to and from the center. Fees for day care may be charged on a sliding scale, according to the ability of the older adult to pay. A few insurance policies, including Medicare and Medicaid, cover the cost of day care. Generally, the older person or the family must pay for these services personally.

A typical day in this care setting includes planned activities such as group discussion, current events, exercise, snacks, and lunch. Volunteers may visit a center to speak on community affairs or health-promotion topics or to present entertainment programs that encourage group participation. Many centers have activity directors who plan and schedule events that are appealing, offer a variety of choices for the older adult, and promote group interaction.

Nurses working in a day-care setting provide numerous services, according to the needs of the individual. Assessment of the older person's physical, psychological, and emotional functioning is a critical component of the nurse's role in the day-care center. Health teaching to older persons and their families also may be included in the nurse's role; for example, the nurse may teach ways of administering medication.

Some older people may need assistance with mobility, toileting, or eating. Other older adults may need help in taking medications. Still others simply need encouragement to participate in center activities. Nurses in day-care centers need a solid foundation in gerontological nursing to help them in their daily interactions with older people. This foundation ensures that subtle physical or emotional changes are not disregarded or blamed simply on "old age."

Acute illnesses in older adults can manifest in atypical fashion. A nurse who knows and appreciates normal aging is better prepared to assess subtle changes in older persons and to be alert to the possible implications of these changes. Because so many older adults have chronic illnesses, medication administration often becomes a major responsibility for the nurse in a day-care center. The nurse needs to be skillful at administering medications and needs to know their expected effects and possible side effects. The nurse also can use knowledge of medications to teach the older person and family members the importance of safe and accurate medication use. Do the older adult and family members know which medications are being taken and why they are prescribed? Are the older adult and family members aware of possible side effects, potential drug interactions, and the necessary steps to take if problems are suspected? The nurse, as teacher, has an important role in this setting.

Ongoing assessments of day-care participants are especially important. Frequent contact with the older person allows nurses to see subtle changes in function that may signal serious underlying physiological problems. The nurse's powers of observation and knowledge of the aging process are crucial in detecting actual or impending illness. Is an older person experiencing mobility changes? Are you seeing decreased participation in formerly active participants? Has an older person had changes in weight or affect? If you are making these types of observations, the next question to ask is why are you seeing these changes? Good communication skills may uncover a change in family living conditions, changes in medication, or exacerbation of the effects of a chronic illness.

Day-care centers provide opportunities for socializing and staying involved in the world. Many families use day care to give respite to the main caregiver for the older adult. The stresses of caregiving can have a strong effect on the older person, caregiver, and family. Respite allows caregivers some time to attend to their own needs. Grocery shopping, housekeeping, socializing with friends, and participating in

With the increasing awareness and concern about care for people with dementia, some programs are now available to provide day care specifically for older persons with cognitive impairments. These day-care programs are designed to give care that takes into account the abilities and safety needs of patients with Alzheimer's disease or other dementias.

Home Care

Home health-care agencies provide numerous services for older adults in the home. These agencies provide nursing services, given by licensed nurses and nursing assistants, and therapy services, such as physical, occupational, and speech therapy. Many agencies also provide medical supplies and equipment. Most agencies are licensed and eligible for state or federal reimbursement for services. Medicare, Medicaid, and community funding may pay for limited home health-care services if the older person qualifies for such reimbursement.

Home care may be provided on a daily basis or intermittently, according to the needs of the patient. Nursing care provided in the home has become more complex in the past two decades. It is not unusual for people who need help during their recovery to be discharged from the hospital "quicker and sicker." Older adults with a chronic illness may be receiving home care to avoid frequent hospitalizations.

The LPN in home care works under the instructions of the registered nurse (RN) case manager. In the home-health role, the LPN is assigned basic nursing care, medication administration and teaching, and dressings and wound care. The LPN may be asked to spend 4 to 24 hours in the home to provide respite care to the primary caregivers. The LPN often is asked to work with a certified nurse assistant (CNA) in coordinating care for the patient.

A certain amount of creativity is needed in home-care nursing owing to limitations in the type of equipment and supplies that are available. As in other settings, it is helpful for the nurse to be aware of resources available to the older adult and of ways to gain use of those resources. Nurses who choose home-care nursing can expect a variety of older persons and conditions. Caring for older adults in the home can be very rewarding and challenging. Because a home-care nurse generally visits the older person on a less-than-daily basis, patient and family teaching is very important. Teaching may be needed to help the family ensure a safe environment for the older adult.

enjoyable activities for the caregivers can often mean the difference between continued home care versus institutionalization for an older adult. Nurses in day-care centers are able to use their assessment skills to identify the older person's strengths and weaknesses, help elders to continue to participate in daily living activities, and provide information for older persons and their families about community resources.

Although day-care nurses may perform few technical nursing procedures, they use a variety of different nursing skills. Day-care nurses must have particularly strong physical and psychological assessment skills. They also must be adept in communication and teaching. A day-care nurse also must have a thorough knowledge of community resources and be able to refer older persons and their families to appropriate services in the area.

Education about fall prevention, medication safety, positioning, and transferring techniques for older persons and families may be needed. A family also may need to learn more complex procedures, such as how to change dressings or give injected medications.

The amount of time spent with older persons is often limited by the nurse's workload and the reimbursement for care given. The nurse is responsible for assessing and documenting care needs and providing prescribed treatments. Good communication skills are important to ensure that all members of the health-care team are aware of the older person's needs and progress.

Community-Based Care

Nursing opportunities are available in various settings not linked to formal institutions such as hospitals or nursing homes. LPNs may provide care for older adults in a community clinic, dialysis center, or physician's office. In these noninstitutional settings, the nurse may practice under the direct supervision of a physician rather than RN. Practice in these settings often includes assisting with physical examinations and treatments, and nurses in these settings are frequently an important source of information and clarification for patients. The nurse uses assessment skills and provides information on resources available in the community to meet the older person's needs. Contact with older adults in these settings may be more infrequent than in other care settings.

Hospice

Hospice care is designed to provide care for a dying person and the family. A team approach is central to the hospice concept. Team members include physicians, nurses, social workers, and nursing assistants as well as other ancillary workers. The goal of hospice care is to help dying persons remain at home, if possible, with all the support needed to ensure a "good death." In this case, "good" means that the older person is kept comfortable and able to receive the support of family and loved ones in a familiar setting.

Hospice work allows nurses to give direct patient care and develop a close relationship with the patient and family. As in the care settings previously discussed, the nurse's role as a teacher is especially helpful. Most families are not prepared to meet the needs of a dying family member. The hospice nurse can teach family members how to provide for the comfort of their loved one. The nurse also can identify hospice resources available to help families and older persons cope during this extremely demanding time. Nurses who have not worked in a hospice setting may be reluctant to try this type of nursing because all of the clients are terminally ill. Talking with nurses who work in a hospice often shows, however, that the team support and the closeness to patients and families provide a high degree of job satisfaction.

CRITICALLY EXAMINE THE FOLLOWING

Read the following patient care situation before reading the author's comments. Ponder what you would do and make some notes. Compare your thinking with that of the author. Be prepared to discuss your thinking in class.

You are the staff nurse on a medical unit at Hoover Medical Center. One of your patients is Mrs. O., a 69-year-old, married woman with chronic lung disease. Mrs. O. has been on your unit many times. This time, she and her husband realize that her lungs cannot last much longer, and she expresses that she does not want to be put on a ventilator. Mrs. O. wishes to die at home and tells you that she does not believe she will return to the hospital. She seems to have accepted the idea of death but tells you that she is worried about how her husband will deal with her passing. What suggestions can you offer Mrs. O.?

Author's comments:

Hospice services are available to individuals with terminal illnesses. They are not exclusively for cancer patients. You could talk with Mrs. O. about the services available through hospice, including grief counseling for her husband before and after she dies. She is very receptive to the idea, and you initiate the appropriate referrals.

Assisted Living Environments

As people age, there is a tendency to simplify lifestyles and living space. The size of the home needed to provide adequate living space for a family can become more of a burden than an asset to older adults. Assisted living communities are an increasingly popular way for the elderly person to have a home without homeowner responsibilities. Not having yard work and other maintenance tasks associated with a large home relieves numerous burdens. Assisted living communities generally offer apartments with community dining and activity areas. They have a nurse, an activity director, CNAs, and housekeepers. The goal for these retirement communities is to appeal to a broad range of older adults by offering security and various conveniences and services. Although communities for retirees have been popular for quite a while, assisted living facilities that also provide services for older adults with physical care needs are now increasingly common. Many assisted living complexes have a satellite branch of a home health agency on site.

The goal of assisted living units is to provide older persons with help in performing activities of daily living. Frail older persons who do not require continuous care are able to have help in such activities as meal preparation, grooming and bathing, laundry, and housekeeping. Most assisted living programs require that the older person be ambulatory and fairly independent. Much of the care provided is done by nursing assistants rather than LPNs. The LPN in an assisted living program often provides supervision for nursing assistants, medication administration, basic documentation of care given, and assessment of the older person's ability to function.

The nurse in an assisted living community also must use creative talents to ensure that the environment is as homelike as possible. The nurse must be flexible in tailoring care to the individual needs of each older adult. The nursing assistant in assisted living care may be called a resident assistant and perform many functions that do not relate directly to activities of daily living. Nurses and nursing assistants working in assisted living care often are very involved in activities and social planning for residents.

Some assisted living facilities provide a continuum of care for older adults. Elderly adults can be admitted to their own apartments, but if their health changes, they can also be admitted to the nursing home for care.

For many older adults, the appeal of a continuing-care retirement community lies in the fact that adults are able to stay in a familiar environment regardless of their health status. Nursing in a continuing-care retirement community offers many opportunities. Home visits, health promotion or screening activities (e.g., blood pressure–monitoring clinics), health teaching, and direct bedside care to nursing home residents are a few of the opportunities available to nurses in continuing-care communities. As in assisted living situations, supervisory ability is a valuable asset for the LPN. Retirement community nursing allows nurses to work with older adults who have various needs and abilities. The ability to apply your knowledge of the aging process in this setting helps you enhance the quality of life for the older persons there.

Nursing Homes

The nursing home is an area of practice that has been available to practical nurses for many years. With the growing number of frail elderly adults and old-old (85 and older) adults, the need for nursing home care is great. Some nursing home residents need a full range of nursing care; others may be independent physically but have cognitive changes that require a high degree of supervision to maintain their personal safety. Two categories of nursing home care are defined by federal regulation. The first category is the skilled nursing facility (SNF), and the second is the nursing facility. The nursing facility level was previously referred to as intermediate care.

All nursing homes must be licensed by the state in which they operate. If they wish to receive reimbursement from Medicare or Medicaid for the services provided to residents, they also must meet additional federal requirements and be certified by the federal government. A nursing home may choose not to accept Medicare and Medicaid funding and admit only private-pay residents. Medicare, the federal health insurance program for older and disabled individuals, has two parts that can pay for some services in a nursing home. Most persons older than 65 years have Medicare Part A. This insurance pays for up to 100 days of care in an SNF if the older person is being discharged from the hospital after a stay of at least 3 days and requires skilled nursing or therapy services. The requirements for skilled services are very specific; do not assume Medicare would pay for nursing home care after a hospital stay. Medicare Part B is a voluntary insurance program that many older persons purchase. It pays for some physician and therapy services and some

> ## CRITICALLY EXAMINE THE FOLLOWING
>
> Read the following patient care situation before reading the author's comments. Ponder what you would do and make some notes. Compare your thinking with that of the author. Be prepared to discuss your thinking in class.
>
> As a center staff nurse, you have been invited to the Evergreen Retirement Center's Monday Morning Coffee Club. The center's activity director has asked you to talk with club members about home safety. Make a list of at least four safety concerns for older adults. What suggestions would you give regarding these concerns in speaking to the Coffee Club group?
>
> **Author's comments:**
> Your talk might focus on the following areas:
> 1. *Problem*: Unable to read dials and gauges on thermostats
>   *Solution*: Bright, nonglare lighting to enhance visual ability
> 2. *Problem*: Potential for falls when walking into the home, while using the toilet, and while getting in and out of the shower
>   *Solution*: Handrails and hand guards
> 3. *Problem*: Potential for falls through tripping over items or slipping on unsecured scatter rugs
>   *Solution*: Uncluttered environment
> 4. *Problem*: Hazard of living alone and falling or losing consciousness
>   *Solution*: Daily networking with family or friends

medical equipment, but it does not pay the daily fee for the nursing home.

Medicaid is a welfare program that pays for more than 50% of the nursing home care in the United States. Older people must have a very low income to qualify for Medicaid. Many older persons pay for nursing home care privately at the beginning of their stay until they have spent all of their savings. They then can apply for Medicaid. The Medicaid program pays for all medical services in the nursing home.

In a SNF, licensed nurses provide care around the clock, and an RN is present at least 8 hours a day, 7 days a week. A SNF also offers the services of allied health professionals, such as speech, physical, or occupational therapists, at least 5 days a week. A nursing facility generally does not have the same level of staffing by RNs or therapists as an SNF.

Regardless of category, long-term care facilities offer a team approach to meeting the older person's needs over time. Facilities that receive federal funds are required to offer the services of a social worker and an activity director and dietetic consultant. Licensed nurses can gain input from various sources in planning and delivering care by being actively involved with the interdisciplinary health-care team.

In long-term care, the LPN has traditionally been responsible for supervising the nursing assistants who give hands-on to residents. In many facilities, LPNs mainly give medications or do treatments.

A nurse interested in long-term care has the opportunity to get to know residents well over a long time. Because of the changing needs and physical condition of residents, the long-term care nurse needs very good assessment skills. Long-term care nurses use skills such as monitoring resident responses to treatments,

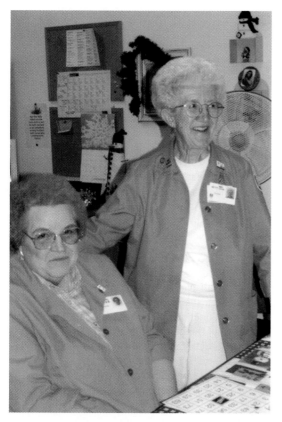

These older women are healthy and able to volunteer at their community's local nursing home. They assist others with making the transition to a new environment and provide many services that otherwise would be unavailable.

CRITICALLY EXAMINE THE FOLLOWING

Read the following patient care situation before reading the author's comments. Ponder what you would do and make some notes. Compare your thinking with that of the author. Be prepared to discuss your thinking in class.

Mrs. H., an 85-year-old widow, was recently admitted to Sunny Acres Nursing Home after falling in her apartment and breaking a hip. She had surgery for a hip replacement and can walk short distances, but she is unsteady and tires easily. She is underweight, eats poorly, and does not want to be in the nursing home. Her family lives out of town and is not sure she can live on her own any longer. You are the nurse in charge at Sunny Acres. What are some of the most important areas you would want to assess for Mrs. H.?

Author's comments:

Because Mrs. H. was functioning independently before her fall and she does not want to be in the nursing home, the first area you assess is her potential for discharge. What is the prognosis for improvement in function? With what does she need help? Could she return to her own apartment with additional services in the home? Would she fit appropriately into an assisted living program? In addition to discharge planning, your assessment includes mobility function, eating patterns and ability, and evaluation for signs and symptoms of depression.

observing for signs of decreasing function, and assessing subtle changes in condition on a daily basis. Accurate documentation; skillful use of the nursing process; and good interpersonal skills in working with residents, staff members, and family members are valuable tools in long-term care.

Care in a nursing home differs from hospital care in many ways. The skills required of the nursing home nurse are no less challenging and the tasks no less difficult than those of the hospital nurse. The goal for a hospital patient is to cure illness in a brief time. For a nursing home resident with multiple chronic conditions, cure is impossible. In the nursing home, care rather than cure is the primary focus. When you make the care given to residents transpersonal caring, the quality of that care improves remarkably.

Acute Care

The final clinical site for working with older adults is the acute care setting. Most hospital admissions are patients 65 years and older. Depending on the source used, it is estimated that 40% to 65% of hospital admissions include older adults. Nursing practice in a hospital setting presents many opportunities and challenges. Usually, LPNs are given responsibility for a set number of patients, and, depending on policy, they may perform various procedures. Most patients are hospitalized only briefly. The emphasis on cost containment and federal mandates means that reimbursement for care is often limited to a set period. The concept of diagnosis-related groups (DRGs) has allowed reimbursement for hospital treatment to be based on a specific number of hospital days for specific conditions. Hospital-based practice requires all of the basic skills an LPN possesses. Acute care also involves brief contact with a large number of patients.

There are several challenges in giving nursing care to older adults in the hospital setting. These challenges include establishing a trusting relationship over a short period, dealing with problems secondary to relocation stress or medications, and resisting the tendency to stereotype patients because of their age. In addition, a major challenge for a nurse working with older people in the hospital setting is to create a safe and caring environment that facilitates independence; this must be done while the tasks required for the cure and treatment of the person are accomplished. Environmental management, as discussed earlier in this chapter, is the most difficult task to accomplish in the hospital setting. The short time frame and the urgency for treatment in many situations do not readily accommodate the slowed responses and abilities of older persons. It is your challenge to slow things down so that the older adult can manage them.

As a gerontological nurse, it is important to understand the special needs of older adults. They have difficulty seeing and hearing. They move much slower, and they need clear explanations as to what is happening. When you recognize these needs of older adults, you have a responsibility to meet the needs and assist others involved in the care of the older adults to slow down and focus on those needs as well.

CRITICALLY EXAMINE THE FOLLOWING

Read the following patient care situation before reading the author's comments. Ponder what you would do and make some notes. Compare your thinking with that of the author. Be prepared to discuss your thinking in class.

Mr. W. is a 90-year-old resident of a nursing home who was admitted to your floor at Hoover Medical Center for treatment of congestive heart failure. He has significant dementia, is incontinent of bowel and bladder, and is very unsteady on his feet. As his primary nurse, what can you do to make his hospital environment more like home?

Author's comments:

You call the nursing home nurse and talk with her about Mr. W.'s habits at the nursing home. You also ask her to send to the hospital any familiar items Mr. W. may appreciate having in the hospital. The nurse tells you that Mr. W. likes to stay up late and is accustomed to remaining in bed until after breakfast. You write this routine into the care plan and pass the information on to the night shift.

▲ PRIORITY SETTING 11.1

As with the other chapters, everything mentioned in this chapter is important. The question is: What is the priority?

As a novice nurse, your priority should be to gain knowledge and experience in as many care environments as possible. I do not mean that you should work 3 months, then change jobs, work 3 months, and then change jobs. You need to know about the different environments of care, however, so that you can:

1. Recognize the best place for you to be employed. It is important to have a satisfying job that allows you to be the most effective caregiver possible.
2. Function most effectively as a member of the health-care team. By knowing about different environments of care, you have more information to share with the team where you are working. This is an important aspect of being a valuable member of the health-care team.

One of the positive things about being a nurse is the fact that there are so many opportunities for different types of work.

CONCLUSION

This chapter has provided a brief overview of the nurse's role in environmental management and the various settings where older adults receive health care. Of special significance for the older adult is the opportunity to receive care from a nurse who is familiar with the aging process and uses that knowledge when giving nursing care in any setting.

Your neighbor, Sally, asks your advice about finding good care for her 80-year-old grandmother. The grandmother, Mrs. G., lives at home alone in an isolated section outside the city limits. She recently was discharged from the hospital after injuring her right arm in a fall at home. The arm is in a cast, which makes it difficult for Mrs. G. to cook and perform other self-care activities. Your neighbor is unable to visit her grandmother daily because of work and child-care commitments and is worried about her grandmother's ability to remain at home. She wants her grandmother to move in with her for at least a month. Mrs. G. insists on staying in her own home, however. Sally asks for your advice. She ends the conversation with the statement, "I just don't know what else we can do to make sure Grandma is safe and taken care of in her home."

Discussion

Based on the previously described situation and your reading of this chapter, what advice would you offer Sally?

Solution

Considering Mrs. G.'s location and her desire for independence, Sally could look into home-care services. The assistance with bathing, grooming, and food preparation could be provided by the home-health agency team, and a plan for home care could be developed. There are no indications that Mrs. G. needs the type of care offered by the other agencies or facilities mentioned in the chapter.

Select the best answer to each question.

1. Mr. D., 75 years old, is discharged from the hospital after a right-sided cerebrovascular accident. He requires at least 6 weeks of further nursing care and physical therapy. The facility most likely to meet these needs is:

   a. A continuing-care retirement center

   b. Hospice care

   c. An intermediate-care facility

   d. A skilled nursing facility

2. Hospice care provides a multidisciplinary approach to caring for people with:

   a. A chronic illness

   b. An acute exacerbation of a chronic illness

   c. A terminal illness

   d. A contagious illness

3. The major benefit of living in a continuing-care retirement community is:

   a. Low household maintenance requirements

   b. Services available for a continuum of health-care needs

   c. A safe environment for older adults

   d. The presence of a hospital in the complex

4. Mr. J., 83 years old, has Alzheimer's disease and has wandered from home on several occasions. Mrs. J. is concerned for her husband's safety and desires some respite services. You recommend that she investigate:

   a. A local nursing home

   b. The local senior center

   c. A home health-care agency

   d. An adult day-care center

5. In the home health-care setting, the LPN can expect:

   a. A limited amount of equipment and supplies to be available

   b. Intermittent contact with clients

   c. To care for clients discharged from the hospital with many physical care needs

   d. All of the above

12 Management Role of the Licensed Practical/Vocational Nurse

Mary Ann Anderson
Tamara Chase

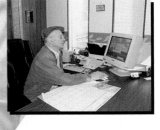

Learning Objectives

After completing this chapter, the student will be able to:

1. Identify three management styles commonly used, and determine the style that is most effective in gerontological settings.
2. Express an overall understanding of communication techniques and their use.
3. Describe two methods for managing stressful communications.
4. Describe the planning hoop and its use in setting priorities.
5. Identify three common errors made in doing employee evaluations.
6. Define "total quality management" and explain its importance.

INTRODUCTION

Administering excellent care to frail and ill individuals through the mechanism of an interdisciplinary team and frequently a mass of bureaucratic paperwork requires management skills of the highest level. This is the challenge of today's licensed practical nurse (LPN): successful administration of managed care to older adults in all settings. Certain skills are crucial for LPNs to master to function successfully in the management arena of health-care delivery. This chapter introduces such skills as they are used in gerontological nursing.

Some people believe that LPNs are not qualified to be managers, yet many are placed on units as charge nurses. I have worked with LPNs over my 40-plus years of nursing and have found your colleagues to be excellent. I remember working night shift as a new graduate when an astute LPN saved the life of a surgical patient. He would have died without her critical observation and intervention. The very fact that you manage patient or resident care makes you a nurse manager. I am proud of you and what you can and will do in this wonderful profession of nursing.

MANAGEMENT ROLES

The management role of the LPN is one that changes constantly to keep pace with changes in health-care delivery. It is challenging to be an LPN prepared to assume the responsibility of management. You need to recognize that the work of a licensed nurse always involves leadership skills, and the scope of responsibility frequently changes.

In some nursing homes, LPNs are directors of nursing, whereas in some hospitals, they are not allowed to administer medications. This diversity in scope of responsibility is important to understand. If a registered nurse (RN) is on the health-care team, the LPN is responsible to the RN. This is always true because of the dictates of licensure. It is possible for an RN and an LPN to have the same job description in an organization, just as it is possible for an LPN to be the director of nursing or shift supervisor. Even if you and an RN have the same job description, you have different licensure; the licensure and its scope of practice are critical for you always to follow.

At the time of employment, the LPN should clarify the scope of responsibility and role expected to be fulfilled. Determining that the duties assigned are not in conflict with the state nurse practice act also is important. As licensed nurses, all LPNs are responsible for knowing the law governing their practice. This responsibility should not be delegated to a supervisor or another nurse.

MANAGEMENT STYLES

Every individual has a personal management style. This comes from the lessons learned while maturing as a person and as a nurse. Nevertheless, to be a successful nurse manager, it is important to understand various management styles and master the styles that are most effective for you.

Three basic styles of leadership need to be understood. Other leadership styles exist, and many leadership theories have been proposed. The LPN nurse manager needs to understand the basic styles and be flexible enough to incorporate other information as it becomes pertinent. The overall objective for understanding the basic styles of leadership is for the LPN to determine an effective but flexible leadership style for professional use.

Authoritarian

In the strictest sense, authoritarianism functions with a high concern for tasks done and low concern for the people who perform those tasks (Anderson, 2009). People with this leadership style work well as assembly line managers in a setting where the employees are not in a job that requires individuality and the machinery is critical to the production of the workload. Does this description cause you to feel concern when considering an authoritarian management style for a gerontological care environment?

The authoritarian or autocratic leader tends to make all decisions in the work environment and order the employees to follow the decisions that have been made. The manager has worked hard to create a power base and does not relinquish it to employees. Generally, this type of manager sees employees as irresponsible and lazy. That opinion of employees is the manager's personal justification for the control placed over them.

An authoritarian manager does not allow for creative thinking or new ideas. No opportunities are presented to try new concepts on a patient or resident care plan unless the idea is the manager's own. This type of manager is more interested in seeing that the work is done rather than that the patients are being lovingly cared for and their individual needs are being met. As an example of this type of management, the workload plan would require baths to be completed by 11:00 a.m. instead of treating the patients as individuals and allowing them autonomy in planning their morning care.

Situations exist in which this type of management style is crucial for success, such as during an emergency. If a visitor or older adult fell to the floor in cardiac arrest, this type of manager would take over, give orders, and, in all likelihood, save the life of the person. The problem with this management style is that life is not a constant series of emergencies. This style does not allow for the creative and caring approaches that are necessary for effective gerontological nursing. Often, older persons miss out on the best possible care, and the employees miss out on opportunities to learn and grow as they implement new care practices. The managers, generally not respected or esteemed by employees, feel frustrated when their work is not valued by others.

Permissive or Laissez Faire

The laissez-faire style of leadership is the exact opposite of the authoritarian style. Essentially, this style consists of an absence of leadership (Anderson, 2009). The manager wants everyone, including himself or herself, to feel good, and he or she works hard toward that end. The basic strategy is to allow the employees to make the decisions, do the planning, set the goals, and essentially manage the organization. This manager sees employees as ambitious, responsible, intelligent, and creative. The laissez-faire manager does not require accountability from employees for their time or for the quality of work done. Initially, this may sound like an ideal management style.

It is important to examine this type of management style in relationship to organizations involved in gerontological health care. Most care given to elderly adults depends on federal approval and on complex payment systems that go through state and federal government organizations. It is difficult to envision the federal guidelines for safety (Occupational Safety and Health Administration [OSHA]) or for nursing home licensure carried out in a permissive or laissez-faire manner. The same is true for quality-assurance programs in health-care environments. Most facilities providing care to older adults require specific attention to the paperwork that keeps an organization in operation. It also is necessary to have layers of responsibility that ensure every person in the facility the best possible care with attention to detail.

In other environments, laissez-faire management is very successful. An example is a group of highly motivated, professional people, such as a group of researchers, for whom independent thinking is rewarded. Conversely, it is difficult to imagine an effective nursing home or hospital unit being managed with this style of leadership.

Democratic or Participative

The democratic management style places strong value on the people on the team. The manager gathers information from the other team members and presents it to the group. All suggestions from the group are considered before decisions are made by the group (Anderson, 2009). This is a very open system of management, yet it identifies the individuals who are responsible for the various projects being managed.

The disadvantage presented by this type of management style is that it takes a great deal of time and energy. Generally, the results are positive, and the employees are very satisfied. This is a style that works well in gerontological environments because it is focused on people and includes the employee, the older adult, and the older adult's family members. It is a system that considers change and improvement continuously and assigns responsibility for such ventures.

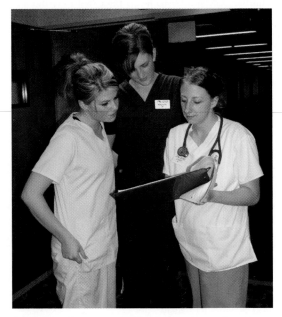

A participative manager always involves others in decisions unless they have to be made in an emergency.

As an LPN nurse manager, you need to evaluate yourself and determine which general management style is yours. Then consider whether it is a style that is best used in the care of older people. If it is not, you need to learn more about other management styles and, with that knowledge, consider making changes in yourself. You may need to find a mentor who has a management style you would like to learn more about and ask that person to assist you. This mentor could teach you, become a role model for you, and assist you in applying the management techniques you want in the real-world setting. Being a manager is a challenging facet of your professional life. Take the time to learn the skills and patterns of thought that you need to function at your most effective level.

⬤ COMMUNICATION

The most important skill for a manager in any situation is communication. Nurses in gerontological care spend 85% of their time communicating with a variety of people who are involved in the care of older adults. Mastering the skills of communication is essential for a successful LPN. Communication involves delivering messages that will be understood; listening to messages that may or may not be confusing; and properly interpreting messages that have been misdirected or are delivered with intense emotion, such as with anger.

For the LPN, the art of communication involves various groups of people. The LPN needs to be able to communicate successfully with the older adult, the family or other members of the person's support group, and the numerous members of the interdisciplinary health-care team. Expertise in communication is demanded every day from individuals who manage, direct, or administer care to older people.

Verbal Communication

Verbal communication is the exchange of ideas and understanding that occurs through the use of spoken words and phrases. For the message to be received, the sender must use words and phrases that are appropriate for the listener. The success of all communication is measured by the question: Was the message properly received?

It should be easy to remember sitting in a class and "listening" to a lecture or presentation when you did not "receive" the message. Perhaps you were too tired to concentrate, or the instructor was boring or had inappropriate

content to share. For communication to occur, being present is not enough. The critical measure is whether the listener actually understood or "received" the message.

Nonverbal Communication

Nonverbal communication is the ability to share messages without using words. It refers, among other things, to a person's body posture (is the person tired and slouched over, or excited and alert), the tone and speed of the voice, the kind of clothes a person wears, and hand and facial movements. Nonverbal communication is considered to be the most honest communication a person can receive. Someone may say, "I'm having a great day. How are things for you?" in a cheerful-sounding way, but an examination of his appearance may indicate something different. The face is not smiling, and the posture is one of fatigue. The person's hands may be clenching and unclenching as a symptom of stress. Another classic example is a resident in a nursing home who is asked each morning, "How are you?" and each day responds verbally, "I'm fine." The person asking the question is busy with the breakfast tray or the linen and does not look at the sad and worried face of the resident who answers with the reply that is expected, rather than with the truth.

The ability to recognize honest communication and respond to it is crucial for a successful nurse manager. The nurse manager must learn to develop the refined skill of understanding nonverbal communication because it conveys valuable information about patients and employees. Nonverbal communication is an honest method of communication and allows the LPN to follow through on problems and concerns that otherwise might not have been recognized.

Communicating With Patients and Residents

The decision to work with elderly adults is a commitment to accept the normal physiological losses that accompany the aging process. That commitment requires knowledge of the normal changes that occur in elderly people (see Chapter 2) and the skill to work with them successfully. A tendency exists in our ageist society to judge older people negatively because of the normal aging processes they exhibit. Normal aging changes that might affect communication are slower speech, presbycusis (difficulty in discriminating sounds), presbyopia (difficulty seeing near objects), and

Understanding nonverbal communication

Critical to learn, to recognize, and to respond to as a nurse manager	The most honest form of communication	Examples
		Posture
		Facial expressions
		Tone and speed of voice
		Personal hygiene
		Type of clothing being worn
		Hand and facial movements
		Symptoms of stress

overall slower movements or responses to what is being communicated. The knowledgeable LPN recognizes these as normal occurrences and responds to them with skill and compassion.

Some people are impatient and negative about the aging process. It is as if they were punishing people who had simply neglected to die young! This is ageist behavior and is unacceptable in any setting. The skills necessary for successful communication with older adults must be firmly based on respect for them as people. If that ingredient is missing, communication is unsuccessful. Consider the following strategies (not every older adult would need every strategy):

• Do not approach the person from the side because you may not be seen, and the person could be startled by your sudden appearance. Approach only from the front.

This factor is important because of the gradual loss of peripheral vision that often accompanies aging.

• Place yourself on eye level with the older person so that a comfortable presence occurs during the communication process.
• Reach out and touch the person if it seems appropriate; this is often the bridge to a trusting relationship.
• Speak at a normal rate and do not shout, even if the older person is having trouble hearing. Shouting does not overcome the problems of presbycusis. Speak in a normal tone and speak slower than usual, but not so slow as to insult the person.
• If the patient is having trouble hearing you, move closer and speak in a normal tone. Moving closer often allows for lip reading or the reading of facial expressions.

POINT OF INTEREST

Presbyopia and *presbycusis* are commonly used words when talking about older adults. It will complement your educational process to take the time to memorize those words and use them as you speak. Work with them and make them a natural part of your vocabulary. Make it fun!

- Pleasantly repeat what is being said, if necessary.
- Do not be impatient or judgmental.
- Place yourself and the older adult in a setting where there is a bright light but no glaring of light.
- Use a setting without disturbing or distracting noises.
- If the older adult gets confused while speaking or responding to a question, give the person time to collect personal thoughts. Do not rush the person.
- Repeat questions or comments in a different sentence structure if the older person is having trouble understanding what is said. Do not keep repeating the same information in the same way.
- Reflect on what the older person has said by repeating it back in a different way; for example, "Do you mean that you are lonely because your wife is in the hospital and not able to visit you here in the nursing home?"
- Listen carefully to the words used and verify what they mean.
- "Listen" carefully to the body movements and other nonverbal communication and verify what they mean.

Your goal is to have the message successfully received. The use of these basic, caring strategies enhances your achievement of that goal and your relationship with the older adults in your care.

Communicating With the Families of Older Adults

Often, the family members of older patients or residents are worried, exhausted (if there has been extensive care given at home), and experiencing feelings of guilt over the condition of their family member or the necessity of admitting their loved one to a health-care facility. Successful communication with this varied group of people is challenging because of their emotional status. The issues involved often go beyond concern over an admission to a hospital or nursing home to such highly charged questions as the right to die, the decision whether to do an amputation, or dealing with a diagnosis such as Alzheimer's disease.

It is crucial for the LPN to recognize the emotional environment of the family members before entering into any communication with them. The goal is still the same: You want the message to be received by the listener. Some communication strategies for families are as follows:

- Listen to them before you attempt to impart information. It is essential that you evaluate the emotional environment to determine if they are able to listen to you. Often, just listening allows for you to learn critical information that you otherwise would not learn.
- Plan to spend time with the family members. They have questions and concerns, and they deserve to have them addressed.
- Family members often feel guilty over some issue with their loved one and need to have that clarified. Families need not feel guilty unless evidence of elder abuse is found.
- Find a quiet place to speak to the family. It should be a place where they can sit comfortably and be together as a group. The nurses' station is never an appropriate place for meaningful communication other than the simple sharing of facts.
- As nurse manager, the LPN needs to facilitate the sharing of information with the family. This could mean arranging an appointment with the social worker or assisting a family member to reach the physician.
- The older adult's family is as important as the older person. Generally, strong personal relationships that are interdependent exist. Always treat the family members with the high level of respect and concern that you use with the older adult.

Interdisciplinary Team Communication

It is unrealistic to give quality care to older adults without the support of an interdisciplinary team (IDT). Generally, the care given to older people in all settings is based on the interdisciplinary approach. It is critical that the nurse manager be an active and contributing part of this team. Generally, nurses are with the patients 24 hours a day, or if the older person is a home patient, the nurse generally sees the individual more frequently than other members of the team. This constant attendance of the nurse to the patient provides a vast amount of personal and pertinent information. It is essential that the nurse manager be active in contributing to the knowledge base and planning of the IDT.

Concern arises over how to share information the nurse has gathered about the older person. It needs to be shared with skill so that the message is received. This process is different in a group

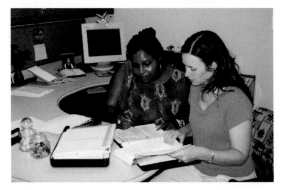

When working with a colleague on patient or resident care or other projects, be sure that your message is received. It pays to check and double check.

setting than it is with an individual patient or family members. The group consists of professionals who have specialized knowledge regarding the older person. There is rarely sufficient time to discuss the patients in a thorough and relaxed manner. A time crunch often exists in IDT planning that establishes a unique atmosphere for communication. The following are strategies for communicating with an IDT:

- Come prepared! There is no time to waste in these meetings, whether in groups or one on one.
- Plan ahead and have priority concerns in your mind or on a piece of paper.
- This is not a team of nurses, and members of an IDT may not understand a nursing concept that is very familiar to you. Because nursing is its own specialty, you may be asked to justify your requests or concerns or to teach the team about a nursing concept.

In most situations, the nurse has the role of patient or resident advocate. This occurs naturally because of the amount of time nurses spend with patients compared with other disciplines. This time allows for personal information and concerns to be communicated. It is crucial that the patient advocacy role be accepted by the nurse so that the patient is protected from the system and its potentially depersonalizing effects.

⬤ ADDITIONAL COMMUNICATION SKILLS

Very specific skills are necessary for successful communication, and each of these skills can be used appropriately in all settings. Such skills are necessary to clarify communication errors, or potential errors, and are commonly necessary in difficult situations. They are important for every LPN to add to the communication skills checklist, and their importance can be compared with that of being expert at cardiopulmonary resuscitation (CPR). You may not use the skills very often, but when they are necessary, you need to know how to use them.

Assertive Communication Skills

The normal physiological reaction to being attacked physically or verbally is "fight or flight." This reaction occurs without thinking about it; it is normal physiology. When a situation occurs in which you are being attacked verbally or feel threatened by what is being said or done, the normal response is to fight back (an argument) or to take flight (avoidance). In the framework of assertive communication, these two normal responses are more formally identified as *aggressive*—fight—or *passive*—flight. The third concept that belongs on a continuum between these two is *assertive*—dealing with the problem.

Ideally, you would use assertive behavior when someone has violated the rights of an individual either verbally or physically. Assertive behavior is the most effective response to that violation. The major rule regarding the concept of assertive communication is simply that the assertive response *must not* violate the rights of the person who just infringed on your rights. What does that look like? An argument is the best example. Someone comes to the nurses' station and criticizes you in an angry, loud manner. There are residents or patients, visitors, and co-workers in the area listening to this *aggressive* communication. It is embarrassing and humiliating to be the victim of a communication delivered in such an inappropriate way. The normal physiological response is either to run away, perhaps crying (*passive*), or to scream back (*aggressive*). Screaming back or starting an argument is a violation of the other person's rights. It does not matter if he or she deserves it; it is still wrong. The *passive* behavior, or running away, does not violate the other person's rights, but it does prevent a resolution of the problem.

Assertive communication requires that the person being violated not respond in a normal physiological fashion to the situation. Instead, it is necessary to resist the normal response and use the skills of communication to promote problem solving. This is done most effectively in a private area. Assertive communication often follows this response format:

"I feel"—Tell the other person how the aggressive attack made you feel. Perhaps you feel frustrated, devalued, angry, or frightened. Many other options are available for you to describe how you feel about what has been said.

"When you"—Describe for the person the behavior that has caused you to feel the way you do. It could be "when you raise your voice at me," "talk about private concerns in public," "demand things from me that I cannot do," "or criticize me in front of others." Many other statements could be used here. The statements used must not be personal statements that attack the other person.

"We should"—Together determine a solution to the problem. This is difficult to do because it is not one of the two normal and usual responses. Use it anyway. Take a deep breath and simply ask what the two of you can do to prevent this from happening again. Be open-minded and expect that there will be more hostility because of the discomfort that comes to the aggressive person with your unusual approach. It is hoped that the two of you can resolve the problem. If not, you still have done a good thing. Another skill that may help you in this type of situation is active listening.

Active Listening

Another communication skill that complements assertive behavior is that of *active listening*. Most people respond to aggressive and negative remarks with defensive communication. While the aggressor is making comments, the person being attacked generally is mentally preparing the defense to the aggressor's attack. These are the defensive comments that often provoke an argument. They follow the script of "It is not my fault; now let me tell you why!"

Active listening requires that the person being verbally attacked listen to what is being said. Because of the natural inclination to prepare a defense, listening is a challenging thing to do. Just listen, and, while listening, try to determine the cause of the problem beyond the apparent anger.

The person who is out of control must be removed to a private setting, such as an office or the clean holding area. This prevents that individual from self-embarrassment in front of

others, and it places you in an environment with fewer distractions.

After the angry person has finished saying all the aggressive things there are to say, he or she will take a deep breath and stop talking. This is where the person uneducated in communication skills presents his or her defense. You, the nurse manager, need skills beyond the ordinary person, however. Active listening is one of those skills. The deep breath is the signal to use the information you learned, while listening, to clarify the problem and negotiate a solution.

Comments such as "You seem so frustrated with…," "It is unlike you to be so upset," or "How can I help?" are effective ones to use. They are not what the aggressive person expects to hear and generally prevent the person from losing control again. They are helpful comments that show caring and problem-solving skills. These are hallmark behaviors for nurse managers. The next move is for the two people involved to sit down and look at the problem rationally and work on a solution. The whole process begins with the nurse being able to stop "self-defending" and focus on listening.

The format for active listening is as follows:

- Remove the conversation to a private setting.
- Listen.
- Do not prepare a defense.
- Listen for the deep breath that means the person has finished speaking.
- Show support for the other person's feelings.
- Negotiate how to resolve the problem.

Some LPNs reading this text may feel concern over being responsible for assertive communication and active listening skills. They are two of many possible communication skills that could have been discussed in this book. They are listed for a very specific purpose. LPNs, in management roles, have very challenging positions that may place them in serious situations that must be managed rather than ignored. Some people will say, "But I am just an LPN!" and feel that their role does not involve managing and solving problems of this nature. If you are a nurse manager, however, you have an obligation to develop the skills necessary for managing these acute and potentially destructive problems.

 PLANNING HOOP

Every day, decisions must be made regarding the workload of the LPN and others that affect the scope of LPN practice. These are decisions that should be made with careful thought and planning, rather than casually and without attention to detail. The decision that may be required of you could be as simple as who will get the first bath as you give morning care, but even this decision may have serious implications for the patients or residents who are receiving your care. Other decisions that may be required of the LPN nurse manager could be counseling an employee whose behavior is unacceptable, making care assignments, confronting a physician or therapist with an alternate plan of care for a resident, or managing daily staffing. None of these tasks—or the many others that are required of a nurse manager—are easy or simple. They require the highest level of skill and attention to manage the process of making such decisions effectively.

To set priorities and make excellent decisions, the LPN nurse manager must understand the importance of planning, which is an intelligent process of thinking based on facts and information, rather than on emotion and wishes. An example is the holiday schedule. Staff members want Christmas Day off to be with their families. You, the manager, want everyone on your staff to be happy, but you have a clear picture as to what would happen if you granted everyone's wishes for Christmas Day! Instead, you need to make a rotation plan for the holidays, or perhaps draw names out of a hat, assign requests according to seniority, or determine some other way for the Christmas Day shift to be adequately staffed.

Planning is a process that never ends. It can be thought of as a hoop with notches where you stop and enter another phase of the planning process; then you continue going around the hoop over and over again. It is unrealistic to develop a plan and think that it will never change. It may be perfect for the moment, a week, or even an entire year; but the complexity of health care and the individuality of patients or residents and staff members require that your excellent plan be continuously re-evaluated. The planning hoop (Fig. 12.1) begins with an assessment.

Assessment

What is the problem or potential problem that concerns you? You know how to do a physical assessment. This is a similar process. Look at the

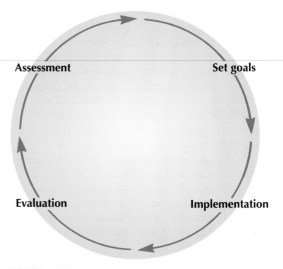

FIGURE 12.1 The planning hoop. An effective nurse manager must learn that planning is critical to getting the total workload done effectively.

problem from "head to toe" and assess what really is wrong. If it is a staffing problem in a nursing home, look at the mix of licensed and unlicensed personnel. Is it right for the needs of the residents?

Is the problem a lack of knowledge? If it is, you need to assess where the lack is, who needs to know the information, and how to teach it most effectively. Do not be distracted by other issues as you do your assessment. Keep focused on the problem you are trying to resolve and learn all you can about it. Otherwise, it would be similar to trying to assess two residents at the same time. One does not get a clear picture of the problem unless a very focused effort is made. The next step in the planning hoop is to set goals.

Goal Setting

Now that you have a complete set of data regarding the problem, you have enough information to set goals. This is very similar to the nursing process. Instead of writing a care plan, you are preparing a plan to resolve a management problem. Make the goals reasonable and achievable. Not everyone can have Christmas Day off. If the problem is an unbalanced mix of licensed and unlicensed personnel, your goal could be to correct the mix through attrition and selective hiring within the next 6 months. If the problem is knowledge, your goal would be to have 100% of your staff attend a class on the information needed by a specific date. The goals should be meaningful and reflect your most careful and organized thinking.

Implementation

Implementation is the test of good planning. Was your assessment done accurately, and are your goals realistic? Perhaps the actual implementation requires you not to hire an RN or LPN when one applies because your staff has too great a proportion of licensed personnel. Or, implementation may mean that you need to find the budget money to pay the staff to attend the education program you determined they needed. In addition, you need a plan for getting everyone to attend. This could involve bonus money or other rewards, and in all likelihood, it would mean presenting the education program several times. Implementation is the actual performance of your plan.

Evaluation

Did your plan work? Was Christmas Day successfully staffed, and did the staff feel that the staffing decisions were made with fairness? Within 6 months, was your staff mix at the level where you needed it to be? How effective was your education program? Did it bring about the change you wanted? Such questions initiate the process of evaluation. A nurse manager cannot just do something and consider the problem solved. Instead, a careful evaluation must be performed so that the cycle of the planning hoop can begin again. That's right; once you have evaluated your plan, you need to do another assessment and begin the circle again!

Many people do not spend a great deal of time planning solutions to the unit's problems. The profession of nursing is filled with "doing" types of people. One of the critical skills of being a manager is to learn to quit "just doing" and begin planning "to do." It is a challenge to take the time necessary to plan because planning does not enter into the conventional description of a "good nurse."

When a person is planning, that person is sitting somewhere quietly thinking. The profession of nursing generally does not see that as productive because beds need to be made, and there are baths and treatments to be given. With those unfinished care issues, how can a real nurse take the time to sit and think? A real nurse manager soon learns that doing the thinking or planning is critical to getting the total workload done effectively. So, fight the urge to be busy when planning is needed. Teach the staff that the time you spend planning is critical to the overall picture of care for patients and job satisfaction for them. Be courageous enough to use the planning hoop to resolve problems and prevent new ones. Because if you do not, you will become a victim of crisis management.

Crisis Management

A crisis manager is a person who does not take the time to plan. This manager waits until the week before Christmas to resolve the problem of the staffing crisis. A great deal of hysteria, excess energy, and distress are involved in solving problems when they occur, rather than foreseeing them and taking the time to plan a solution for the problem. The phrase, "All I do is run around and put out fires!" is indicative of the crisis manager. It is not effective management and can be prevented by the implementation of the planning hoop into your management style. Look to the future and anticipate problems. Then devise a plan for solving them before a crisis happens.

Some situations still will become a crisis for even the best manager. Accept this, solve the problem, design a plan so it will not be a crisis the next time, and move on to the next situation.

⬤ PRIORITY SETTING

Every LPN has learned how to prioritize the work of giving patient or resident care. Traditionally, the sickest patient receives the nurse's attention first, and the least seriously ill person waits until last. This concept assumes that each patient is assessed and observed frequently, rather than being ignored until his or her turn comes to receive care.

Priority setting in management situations has a similar format. The priority of each management problem is determined after the assessment of the situation has been completed. The method for determining priority problems generally is based on determining what is essential for the organization or the person at the time. Staffing for Christmas Day is essential, as is giving pain medications in a timely manner.

The nurse manager needs to think of the entire organization when determining priorities. They often are divided into two categories: (1) concerns that relate to patient or resident care and (2) concerns that relate to the process of running the business of the institution.

Each category should be considered separately, although a great deal of overlap of concerns occurs in implementing problem solutions. Each concern needs to be listed as a *need* or a *want*. Needs should be met before wants. It is helpful to use this method for categorizing your management concerns before prioritizing them.

⬤ MANAGING PERSONNEL

As a nurse manager, you will be involved in, if not responsible for, the hiring and evaluating of employees. This is a critical aspect of your job and one that requires the highest level of professional skill and performance. This work cannot be done by intuition or "best guess." All personnel decisions directly affect the lives of the employees of the institution. These people deserve as much care and attention as the patients.

The hiring process is where the employee begins a career with your organization or, if not employed, will leave with an impression that will be taken out to the community. It should be your desire to have that impression be a good one. Many legal issues are involved in the hiring process. Be sure to clarify them with your personnel manager or administrator. Laws exist that involve the advertisement of a job and how the interview is conducted, and federal rules identify questions that cannot be asked in an interview because of concern over discrimination. Be alert to these rules and follow them.

The purpose of interviewing someone for employment is to find someone who fits with the philosophy and image of your institution. The applicant needs the licensure or certification that the job description demands and the experience to perform the job at a satisfactory level. The interview also allows the nurse manager to determine the shift availability and whether the potential employee is available for part-time or full-time work. An effort should be made to learn the specific interests of the applicant so that plans can be made to use any special skills and knowledge the person possesses. The screening process of the personnel department presumably would eliminate anyone unqualified for the job. Unqualified people do not need to be interviewed.

Interview

The purpose of the interview is to exchange information. Be prepared to give positive information about your facility to all applicants whether they are to be employed or not. You

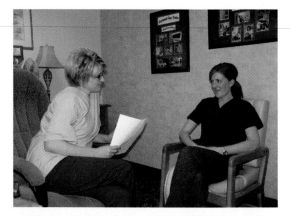

When interviewing someone for a position, establish a friendly and positive atmosphere. Be consistent in the interview process with all applicants, and be honest in your assessment of qualifications.

want applicants to say favorable things about your organization even if they are not selected for the job. During the interview, the nurse manager is expected to determine the applicant's:

- Dependability
- Skill level
- Willingness to assume the responsibilities of the job
- Willingness and ability to work with others
- Interest in the job
- Adaptability
- Consistency of goals with available opportunities
- Conformity of manner and appearance to job requirements

The interview has definite purposes and should be conducted in a professional manner. It is not the place for social chitchat; however, some warm and friendly comments at the beginning of the interview should put the applicant at ease so that the interview can be emotionally comfortable.

The greatest predictor of the applicant's future success is past performance. Is this someone who has worked with older adults previously and enjoyed it? Has the applicant sought additional educational experiences that would enhance work in your type of setting? Was this person a desirable employee at the last place of employment or, if a new graduate, a good student? These crucial pieces of information should be noted on the application and verified in the interview.

It is your responsibility as the nurse manager to set the tone for honesty in the interview. Be specific and direct in your comments. It is helpful to have an interview guide available to use for every interview. This guide is a written document that contains questions, directions, and pertinent information to be shared with the applicant. The presence of an interview guide ensures you, the applicant, and the institution that the same process is being used in every interview. It avoids the gathering of prejudicial information and provides consistency in the interview process.

Questions on the interview guide should cover subjects such as which shifts the applicant is willing to work, whether part-time or full-time work is desired, and feelings about working with older people. It also could contain a brief case study or scenario about a gerontologically focused situation that requires a response from the applicant. The presence of two or three such questions gives you additional information about the potential employee. All applicants must be asked the same questions to avoid discrimination or the appearance of discrimination in choosing future employees. You also need to review the Title VII Civil Rights Act carefully before conducting any interviewing. This federal law prohibits discrimination in any personnel decision on the basis of race, color, sex, age, religion, or national origin. A comfortable format for an interview is as follows:

- Use an opening to establish rapport and put the applicant at ease.
- Share the interview procedure with the applicant.
- Discuss the applicant's interests in being employed at your facility.
- Obtain an educational history.
- Discuss future plans of the applicant, such as upward mobility and future education.
- Share case studies and situations and discuss them.
- Inform the applicant about the organization.
- Allow time for the applicant to ask questions and get answers.
- Close by clarifying how to reach the applicant after the interview, informing the applicant when the decision will be made, and thanking the applicant for considering your organization for employment.

Employee Evaluation

After the nurse manager has made a decision to hire an applicant, a very focused effort must be made to give that person a thorough and extensive orientation to the job, its standards, and its expectations. The quality of personnel hired and retained in the organization determines the success of the organization. The quality of the orientation directly determines the overall success for the organization and the employee.

After the employee has had the opportunity to work with other qualified employees and to establish an effective working routine, the new employee can be allowed to work independently. A resource person should always be available, in some way, to the new employee for the first 3 months of employment. This provision indicates that a sincere effort is being made to ensure success for the organization and the employee.

Each organization has an established process for evaluating employees. The first evaluation may come at 3, 6, or 12 months. Earlier and more frequent evaluations take more of the manager's time but also provide regular feedback for the employee. Overall, it is generally time well spent. Your organization also should have an established written form for evaluating employees. This process should be consistent for all employees to avoid discrimination.

For all employing organizations, a performance appraisal may be based on the following five basic realistic assumptions:

1. The appraisal is intended to help an employee improve the management of the workload.
2. Employee appraisal is a difficult process, but it is a skill that can be mastered with hard work.
3. Few people like the current form (a perfect one simply does not exist).
4. The employee's supervisor makes the appraisal.
5. Information must be gathered on a day-to-day basis.

The challenge to the nurse manager is that the performance appraisal must accurately reflect the person's actual job performance. It cannot contain prejudicial information, hearsay, or undocumented information. It is designed to be helpful to the employee, and by assisting the employee to improve, it is helpful to the organization.

Traditionally, potential evaluation problems can contribute to an inaccurate evaluation. The first one is *leniency error*. This occurs when a supervisor wants everyone to be buddies or to be the manager's best friend. It results when the manager "looks the other way" or gives an employee the "benefit of the doubt" rather than finding out what really happened.

A competent nurse manager cannot afford to be "best friends" with employees. The manager needs to be the manager. It is crucial to success for the manager to be an honest and fair person who does not lose the ability to be objective. The leniency error does not help an employee improve, and it does not contribute to the overall functioning of the organization.

The *recency error* is an indication of a manager who has forgotten the basic assumptions of evaluation and who has not kept records of employee performance over the year. Because of the lack of written record, the manager evaluates only on what is remembered most recently. All employees know when their annual review is scheduled and often find it easy to "look good" during the time just before their evaluation. This type of evaluation process enhances neither the performance of the employee nor that of the organization.

The *halo error* is allowing one trait to influence the entire evaluation. It could be either a strongly positive trait or a strongly negative one. Either way, it clouds the objective evaluation of an employee if only the halo behavior is remembered. Evaluations need to be fair and comprehensive regarding the employee's behavior and skills.

The evaluation process is critical to the growth and stability of the organization. Evaluation standards cannot be successful if they are ambiguous. The process of rewarding a strong employee and counseling a poor employee must be valid. This happens only if the manager maintains a professional and consistent attitude toward the evaluation process.

Negative or probationary evaluations are very difficult for all managers to give. Use the same process you would use for a positive evaluation. Make it fair and comprehensive, and share the information you have in a professional manner. For all terminations, the process of counseling the employee must be carefully documented over time. This is an act of fairness toward the employee and a protection against litigation for the institution.

Making Care Assignments for Older Adults

One of the day-to-day management skills used by LPNs is that of making care assignments for older adults. The skill of making effective assignments is crucial to any clinical area. The goal of making successful care assignments is to match the worker with the older person in a manner that allows for the best nursing care to be administered and received. As the manager, you also need to focus on an assignment that affords the highest level of employee satisfaction. This requires sensitivity, awareness of the skills and attitudes of others, and the ability to form a plan and to follow through on it. Several aspects of making care assignments should be examined.

When making care assignments, you must consider the personal skills of each person you are managing. You have learned how to assess older adults; now your question might be, "How do I accurately assess a nursing assistant's skills?" Dr. Patricia Benner (2001), who developed her nursing theory in her book, *From Novice to Expert*, describes a specific way to identify clinical skills. Benner's theory focuses on intensive care, RNs, and their clinical expertise along the five points of:

- Novice
- Advanced beginner
- Competent
- Proficient
- Expert

Benner's theory was designed for RNs. National research is currently under way to determine if the five points of clinical expertise can identify the clinical skills of certified nursing assistant (CNAs).

As a nurse manager, it is important for you to understand the five points of clinical expertise and how you can use them to identify skill levels for CNAs and other individuals who work under your direction. The five points are:

1. *Novice*—CNAs performing at this level have no prior experience with certain situations. They do not understand the detailed information regarding what is happening. They simply do not have the experience to understand what is going on in the situation. For example, a CNA may have several years of employment as a CNA but may not have any experience working on an Alzheimer's unit. As a nurse manager, you should be aware of such a lack of skill and may want to assign a

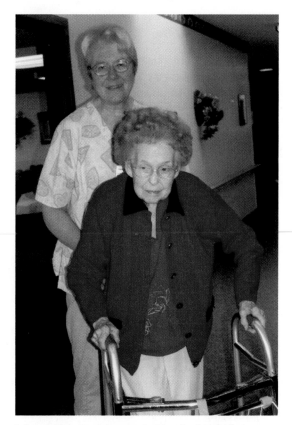

It is worth your time to consider the level of expertise that the CNAs who work with you have achieved. This knowledge influences your scheduling, educational programs, and, most importantly, the quality of care provided to older adults. It is your responsibility to identify and assist CNAs who need more education or experience.

novice CNA to work several shifts with a CNA who is experienced in caring for people with Alzheimer's disease.

2. *Advanced beginner*—CNAs functioning at this level can demonstrate limited acceptable performance. Advanced beginners generally have had multiple clinical experiences, independently or with a mentor, so that they have a general understanding of the clinical situation. Advanced beginners perform tasks using behavior that follows instructions only, rather than appropriate behavior for a specific situation.

As the nurse manager, you may ask a CNA to assist a resident into the shower. When the CNA enters the room, the resident is found confused and combative. Rather than gauging the situation and deciding that this may not be the best time to give this resident a shower, the CNA does everything possible to complete the task of giving the shower. The focus is on the task, not the aspects of the specific situation or the needs of the older person.

3. *Competent*—A competent CNA has an increased level of skill and ability. The knowledge is based on following the positive role-modeling of other CNAs and dealing with various situations in which clinical skills were learned. A competent CNA still focuses on organizing the assigned tasks, however. A competent CNA makes sure the time is managed well in an effort to complete the tasks on the list, instead of basing work decisions on the older person's needs.

As a nurse manager, it is critical that you ensure that the resident's needs are actually being met by the CNA in a timely manner. Otherwise, the individuals you manage may give care based on a schedule and a list rather on than the needs of older adults.

4. *Proficient*—A proficient CNA is much more comfortable with clinical skills and has the ability to deal with different situations as they arise. A proficient CNA engages more with the older adult and family members instead of focusing on required tasks. The focus of nursing care of a proficient CNA is on the needs of the older person rather than on a list. An advantage to working with proficient CNAs is their ability to reprioritize the workload based on patient or resident needs. As a nurse manager, you may delegate several things to a proficient CNA, who then decides in what order they should be completed.

5. *Expert*—An expert CNA has experienced many different situations and has learned from the experiences. These experiences assist the CNA in making decisions based more on intuition (referred to by Benner as "intuitive knowing") than on timetables and rules. An expert CNA knows the older adult's patterns of behavior and is able to anticipate the unexpected. This complexity of skill and thinking assists the CNA in making decisions based on the "big picture" or the holistic needs of the person receiving care.

An expert CNA walks into a room where an older adult is behaving differently and spends time with the person in an effort to identify the problem. The expert CNA takes vital signs and asks questions so there are data to report to the licensed nurse. The expert CNA knows what to do for this patient.

Are you able to identify where your CNAs fit in Benner's five points of clinical expertise?

Do you have a new CNA who is still working at the novice level? If so, that person should be assigned to older adults who require only basic skills that were learned in the CNA class. A novice CNA also should be assigned to an expert CNA who can assist with care when needed and serve as a positive role model. Novice CNAs should not be assigned to give care to challenging patients or residents. They could be assigned to work with another CNA who has the challenging patient or resident and, in that way, have experiences that eventually lead the CNA to the level of expert without hurting an older person in the learning process.

Do you also have a CNA who has worked at the facility for several years, is very familiar with the residents, and has excellent clinical skills? That is the CNA who should be assigned to the most challenging older adults so that these older adults can benefit from the CNA's skills and knowledge. This may not always be the sickest patient on the unit. The assignment could be to the latest admission, in which the older person and the family are having a difficult time adjusting to the transitional stress of the admission.

It is important when developing staffing patterns that a team should not consist of a novice CNA and a novice licensed nurse. A better staffing pattern would be an expert CNA with a novice nurse or expert nurse with a novice CNA. The mix of novice and the levels of expertise that lead to expert are important to acknowledge and use as you manage care.

When you, as the nurse manager, have identified the expertise levels of each nursing assistant, you should praise each one for their special skills and allow them to use those skills. Assist employees to develop skills related to their interests and abilities, and recognize them for the skills they develop. Assign staff members older adults who would benefit from their skill and knowledge. This assignment enhances quality of care and employee self-esteem, which enhances the entire organization.

When working with older adults, it is generally more effective to assign the same employee to an older person for several days in succession. This practice allows the caregiver to learn the personal needs and nuances of the persons receiving care and address them successfully. When a "new" person is assigned to an older person each day, it puts a demand on the older adult to need to explain again that he or she cannot hear out of the right ear, that the older adult wants two cups of coffee on his or her breakfast tray, or that it is the older adult's right knee that does not work very well. Generally, a comfortable camaraderie and sense of teamwork develop between the caregiver and the care receiver that enhance the work of healing when they work together over time.

Sometimes a difficult or demanding older person requires more energy and patience than most employees can provide day after day. When this occurs, the nurse manager should rotate the assignment in a direct effort to avoid burnout of the employees.

Another consideration for making assignments is that of physical demands. Often when caring for older adults or chronically ill patients, a heavy physical demand is made in turning, positioning, and assisting the older person to ambulate. When the nurse manager makes the assignment, the physical, muscular work of the care should be considered so as not to overwork a particular employee. Another consideration is the geographic placement of the rooms. It is unnecessary to make assignments that require an employee to travel to both ends of the hall or in other diverse patterns. Make a strong effort to group the room numbers assigned to avoid unnecessary walking. Most workdays are tiring enough.

Delegation

As the LPN manager, you need to know what is involved in delegating to CNAs. The goal is to delegate tasks while maintaining quality patient and resident care. Your first step is to familiarize yourself with the nurse practice act for the state where you work. This document defines the roles and responsibilities of a licensed nurse. You need to determine if the nurse practice act allows for delegation and, if so, whether there are any limitations as to what you can delegate to a CNA or unlicensed assistive person.

Your next step is to become familiar with the policy and procedures for your facility and the written job descriptions. Any job you assign must be within the employee's job description. After you have identified a task that can be delegated, you need to use sound delegation approaches. Also keep in mind how delegating this task would affect the safety of the older adult. Has the older person been accurately assessed, and are there any safety issues that need to be addressed? The National Council of State Boards of Nursing (NCSBN) has developed guidelines to help nurses ensure safe and proper delegation.

The NCSBN has developed the Five Rights of Delegation, which provides a checklist that nurses can use when making delegation decisions. The Five Rights of Delegation are:

1. The right task
2. The right circumstances
3. The right person
4. The right direction
5. The right supervision

Generally, CNAs can do tasks that assist older adults with basic needs and activities of daily living. They cannot assess, plan, or evaluate any aspects of patient care. If an older person is taking digoxin (Lanoxin) for his heart, the nurse can delegate to the CNA the task of taking an apical pulse and notifying the nurse what the heart rate is when the pulse is taken. The CNA cannot decide if the older adult can have medication based on the pulse the CNA took. In addition, the nurse makes the decision as to when the pulse should be checked again. When working with CNAs, it is very important that the nurse give clear instructions regarding what time the task should be completed and whether the CNA needs to report back to the nurse directly after completing the task. It is wise to encourage CNAs to take notes as you are giving them the information regarding the delegated assignment. When delegating a task to a CNA, you still are responsible for the older adult's care. If you delegate a task to a novice CNA, and the task should have been delegated to an expert CNA, or if you do not give proper supervision, you may be held responsible for the outcome of the care. If you delegate to the appropriate person and provide appropriate supervision, the CNA may be liable for his or her own actions.

As a manager, you should always be willing to delegate certain projects. As organizational needs arise, you may be assigned a project that would not allow you to complete your regular workload. This is a good time to delegate routine work that can be done by someone else.

In your role as an LPN, you will find it necessary to do effective delegation. Does that mean that you delegate the projects that you do not want to do? Does delegating make you a lazy person? The answer to both of these questions is "no." Delegation of routine tasks to someone else frees the manager to work on more complicated unit needs. Because delegation is crucial to effective management, you want to ensure you are doing it as efficiently as possible. When delegating to anyone, your responsibility as the manager is to identify if they have the basic skills or education necessary to complete the assignment. You also should ensure they have the time to complete the assignment by the deadline without requiring them to put aside their regular job responsibilities. Delegating to someone who is interested in the assignment is a good choice.

When the individual for the assignment is identified, you should give him or her clear, direct instructions on what is to be done, including why the individual is doing the assignment. How the person completes the assignment should be an individual choice. This is the really hard part. When you delegate a responsibility in the manner described earlier, just leave it and allow the person to do the work. You can "check in," determine whether the person needs something, or just observe so that you can step in if there is a critical situation. Giving the employee autonomy in deciding how to complete the assignment is a positive factor for the employee and the key to successful delegation. It also is important that you do not oversupervise the employee. If you are going to watch and participate in every step of the project, you may want to ask yourself why you chose to delegate it.

Definite time lines for completion of any delegated project should be discussed, and the manager should check in periodically to ensure that the deadline will be met. Monitoring the assignment periodically allows for questions and discussion regarding the project as the work is being done. Being available for interaction is an important concept. You always should be available to assist the employee if he or she is having difficulty. Taking the delegated project back would be a last-resort behavior because it makes the employee feel like a failure and "demotivates" rather than motivates. When the project is complete, you must evaluate the performance, giving praise and additional information to the employee. This feedback lets the person know what was done well and what may be done differently next time he or she is given a similar assignment. Delegation is an effective way to assist someone to move from novice to expert because of the opportunity to develop new skills and have new experiences.

Providing Education for Employees

This chapter has discussed management concepts needed to supervise employees. Now the question is, "What is the nurse manager's role in providing continuing education to the staff?" What can the nurse manager do to move CNAs from novice care providers to expert care providers? Health care changes on a regular basis, and as licensed professionals, we all are trying to keep up with the changes. It is important for unlicensed health-care providers to keep up with health-care changes as well. As a nurse manager, you need to assist with this endeavor.

Several areas of education need to be addressed. The first is the orientation process for new employees. It is suggested that orientation programs for new CNAs should last at least 3 months. An orientation program should match, one on one, a new or novice CNA with a veteran or expert CNA. The program should provide the new CNA with the information needed to function as an effective member of the nursing team at the end of the orientation period. The orientation information should include the policies and procedures for the facility, information about the daily operation and schedules for the facility, and, most important, detailed information about the older adults and the specific skills needed to give excellent nursing care.

The expert CNA who is willing to be a role model and mentor for the new employee should be a valued employee who consistently demonstrates expert clinical skills and care behaviors. This is a CNA who demonstrates willingness to orient the new employees as well. It is appropriate to demonstrate valuing of employees who participate in the orientation program through some type of a reward.

Novice CNAs must have continuity of instruction throughout the orientation. If the facility has five units, the CNA should spend equal amounts of time on each unit. The time spent should be consecutive days so that the CNA can become acquainted with the staff and procedures on one unit before moving to the next. This approach also provides consistency of care for the older adults who are getting to know the new employee.

At the end of the orientation period, the new employee should be evaluated. The nurse manager must decide at this time if the employee is acceptable for the facility. If you are not satisfied with the employee's performance, a plan of action should be developed to assist the employee in meeting the requirements necessary for successful employment. This also may be the time when the nurse manager may make the difficult decision to terminate the employee.

When a nurse manager hires an employee, an effort should be made to increase and maintain the skills of the employee. There are various ways to accomplish this goal. Mentorship programs match individuals together when one person has the required skills and the other person needs to learn them. These programs generally last for a longer time than orientation and in most cases are less formal. A CNA who is interested in becoming an LPN may be matched with an LPN who is interested in helping the CNA be prepared for nursing school. Or, you may have an employee who works well with people with Alzheimer's disease and their families. This individual could work as a mentor for other employees who would like to possess the same skills.

Some facilities use clinical ladder models to increase employee skills. Different levels of knowledge and ways to obtain and document the skills are identified. When an employee meets the requirements of one level or "rung" of the ladder, there often is a promotion. When employees have met the requirements for an advanced level, they often are recognized with a ceremony and a monetary award, an increase in pay or a set one-time dollar amount. Facilities have found that clinical ladders can assist with employee retention and improve employee morale. The benefit to the facility is better patient care. The improvement in care is a result of the facility seeking to prepare its own expert CNAs, LPNs, and RNs.

● MANAGING THE QUALITY OF CARE

The process of managing and evaluating the quality of health care is not new. Florence Nightingale (1846) urged that all nursing care be carefully evaluated. Because of her innovative nursing-care practices and her ability to measure and evaluate nursing care, she was able to measure changes in the health of patients. At one hospital during the Crimean War, she measured a decrease in patient mortality from 50% to 20% after her nursing-care ideas were instituted. Different outside organizations measure the quality of care given in hospitals and nursing homes. The Joint Commission on Accreditation of Hospitals (JCAH) was founded in 1952 to evaluate health-care services. Two nursing organizations followed this trend in the late 1950s. The American Nurses Association developed and published standards of care for the various nursing specialties, and the National Leagues of Nursing published standards that the public could expect from nursing education. Quality health care is the right of people who enter the health-care system. The aforementioned organizations provide outside evaluation of the health-care system. Other methods for making self-evaluation that involve the LPN also exist.

Total Quality Management

Total quality management (TQM) is a management philosophy that emphasizes a commitment of excellence throughout the entire health-care organization. The principles are widely used throughout many business organizations in addition to health care. The overall purpose of TQM is to improve quality of service and ensure customer satisfaction.

The four major characteristics of TQM are (1) customer/patient focus, (2) total organizational involvement, (3) use of quality tools and statistics for measurement, and (4) identification of key processes for improvement. The LPN is involved in all four aspects of the TQM process.

Most nurses naturally believe that their focus is the customer or patient. This is the overall theme of TQM and calls for all personnel in each department to focus on the needs of the patient. An example would be a smoother admission process, given that that process is often an area that provokes customer complaints. Another example is the housekeeper responding to the patient. This could simply be friendly visiting or putting aside the housekeeper's usual work to go get a nurse for a patient.

The customer focus of TQM is most effective when all employees in a hospital or nursing home respond to the challenge to focus on the needs of the patient. This philosophy eliminates the idea of "That is not my job!" Instead, everyone works toward the overall goal of satisfied customers. A nurse may need to assist the housekeeper in making beds because of the large number of admissions and discharges done in one shift. A physician may need to transport a patient from the emergency department to the unit; respiratory therapists may assist patients to the toilet; the unit secretary may need to transport patients who are being discharged to their cars. The point is that everyone is committed to the idea of customer satisfaction and is willing to fulfill whatever role might be necessary and safe to meet that commitment.

The use of high-quality tools and statistics to measure the level of care that is being given is an important consideration. An organization cannot determine whether the quality of care is being improved unless accurate measurement occurs. This measurement generally is not the responsibility of the LPN but an upper-management or administrative assignment. The LPN may need to complete forms or make reports that contribute to overall measurement of the work being done, but such an assignment would be made by someone else in the system to you, the LPN.

The fourth component of TQM is identification of key processes for improvement. All activities in an organization can be described in terms of people working together. The term *identification of key processes* refers to the efficiency or effectiveness of the work people or teams do together. An example is the *PDCA* cycle. This is the *Plan, Do, Check,* and *Act* cycle. It defines the processes a group or team should be following as they do their work.

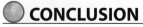

CONCLUSION

Many skills are needed by the nurse manager, but this is just a chapter, not a management textbook. The case study that follows will give you practice in considering management issues. Finally, it is important for you to find a mentor to assist you with the real world of management.

It is 7:35 a.m., and you are the nurse in charge of a 25-bed skilled nursing facility (SNF) unit at the nursing home where you work. The night nurse went home early because she was ill, and you have just discovered that only half of the 6:00 a.m. medications have been distributed. You have a new LPN orienting with you, but she is a recent graduate, and you are not yet sure of her skill level.

You have an 8:00 a.m. meeting with the social worker and a family who is struggling with the decision of whether to allow their mother to die or to place her on stronger life-support mechanisms. The final concern you have is making up the payroll. It is your responsibility to have the paperwork completed on the payroll by 9:00 a.m. If the payroll forms are not in the personnel office, a 3-day delay will occur in paying the employees on your unit. It is the week before Christmas.

As you are struggling to set priorities for the morning, Dr. N. comes onto the unit in a rage and begins talking to you in a raised voice and with an angry nonverbal appearance. This is a physician who is known as a bully with nurses and families, yet you have learned by working with him that he really does care for his residents. You stop everything you are doing to listen to him degrade you with his unprofessional manner. The halls are full of residents and employees who are watching this situation. As the charge nurse, you are responsible for all activities on the unit.

Make a priority list with an explanation for the ranking of each item. Then, in narrative form, describe how you would implement the priority list you have made. Good luck!

Discussion

Priority List

1.
EXPLANATION:
2.
EXPLANATION:

3.
EXPLANATION
4.
EXPLANATION

Solution

1. The medications must be distributed.
   EXPLANATION: The medications are already an hour and a half late. This could have very serious physiological consequences for the frail elderly residents on the unit. This is a critical need.
2. The physician must be managed.
   EXPLANATION: He is preventing you from resolving the other problems on the unit, and some of them are critical. In addition, he is very disruptive to the people (including residents) on the unit.
3. The meeting with the social worker and the resident's family must be held.
   EXPLANATION: This is a very emotional situation for this family, and it is unethical and unkind to ask them to wait or come back at a more convenient time. An issue of this importance cannot be delayed when people are ready to deal with it. It is listed third because the meeting could go ahead without me (the LPN) because the social worker will be there.
4. The payroll forms need to be completed.
   EXPLANATION: It is unfair not to have the employees paid in a timely manner. Yet people are always more important than paperwork. This could wait because paperwork does not bleed, die, or have feelings.

Continued on page 206

Narrative Explanation of This List

I would ignore the physician and his screaming; in the meantime I would call an experienced nurse on another unit. I would quickly explain to her the medication errors and the availability of only my newly hired LPN for assistance. My request would be for her to come to my floor and work with the new LPN to pass the medications that were missed. I am asking her for 30 minutes of her time in an emergency situation. I would not turn this assignment over to the new LPN because I am unsure of her skill level. This is a critical situation that demands immediate correction by someone with a very high skill level.

Because I know the physician really cares about his residents, I would resist the desire to humor him; instead, I would let him know that I had a resident emergency and could see him about his problem after 10:30 a.m. This is not a good example of problem solving with him, but it is an excellent example of setting priorities. He might still be angry with me, but I would be keeping my residents in the best health possible with my decisive action. My hope would be that his natural caring for residents would prevail, and he would cooperate in this situation.

I would notify the social worker that I would be at the meeting but that I might be late. Finally, I would call the personnel office and explain to them that a crisis involving the residents occurred and that the paperwork would be delivered to them by noon. If that did not allow for the employees on the unit to be paid in a timely manner, I would request that an employee from their office come to the floor and do the necessary paperwork.

I would not give lengthy explanations to any of these people. Instead, I would count on my professional reputation to underlie the urgency of the situation. After the day was under control and all of the problems resolved, I would conscientiously go to each person involved and thank him or her for their cooperation and give the explanation each person deserves. I would call the night nurse and let him or her know of the situation and ask the nurse to come in within 24 hours to complete the medication error forms. I already would have made the necessary phone calls to the physicians informing them of the medication errors.

Select the best answer to each question.

1. Every LPN must practice within the definition of the state nurse practice act. The best way for an LPN to determine whether the current job description is within the nurse practice act is to:

   a. Ask the supervisor.

   b. Discuss it with the personnel office during the hiring interview.

   c. Read the nurse practice act.

   d. Ask another LPN.

2. The authoritarian style of leadership is the most effective to use in gerontological settings because:

   a. The work gets done in a timely manner.

   b. Geriatric settings have many emergencies to manage.

   c. Authoritarian leaders are very person focused.

   d. Authoritarian leadership is not strongly compatible with geriatric settings.

3. The most honest form of communication is:

   a. Nonverbal communication

   b. Verbal communications with facial movements

   c. Sitting quietly and listening

   d. The written word

4. Assertive communication is:

   a. Inappropriate for an LPN to use

   b. A meaningful way to share angry feelings

   c. A learned behavior that allows for effective communication

   d. A normal physiological response to stressful communication

5. The purpose of an employee interview is to:

   a. Learn the prejudices of the applicant before employment

   b. Exchange information

   c. Fill the employment quota of minorities

   d. Make new friends

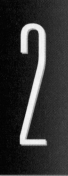

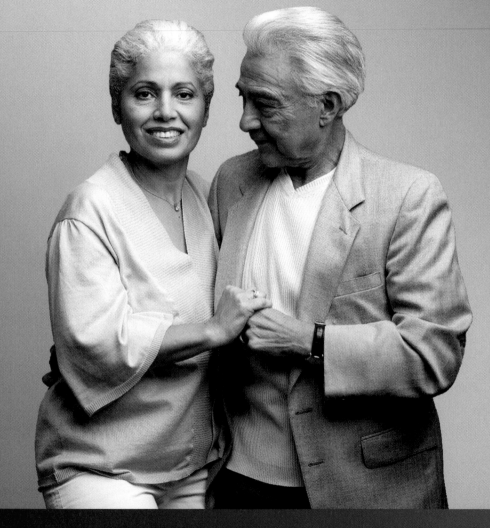

Clinical Practice

13 Common Infectious Diseases

Vickie Anderson
Judith Pratt

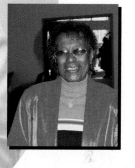

Learning Objectives

After completing this chapter, the student will be able to:

1. Identify causes of common infectious diseases in older adults.
2. Use appropriate environmental and hygienic measures that can reduce infectious diseases.
3. Identify measures that can assist older adults in maintaining a healthy immune system.
4. Identify appropriate immunization protocols.
5. Identify infections that can be precipitated by chronic medical conditions and by the aging process.
6. Discuss the role of the licensed practical nurse (LPN) in the management of infections in older adults.

INTRODUCTION

Everyone wants to be healthy. Even a simple head cold is an irritating and inconvenient event in our lives. As a nurse, you know that there are many more serious infectious diseases than a head cold. When these infections attack older adults, the problems can be grave. This chapter is a challenge to you, the bedside nurse, to protect older adults knowledgeably from the harsh reality of infectious diseases.

Natural immunity toward infectious diseases may not be affected by aging in healthy older adults. Some infections tend to increase with the process of aging, however, and are major health problems in older people. The physiological responses of older adults during an infectious illness differ from those of younger or middle-aged adults. In addition, the course of illnesses leading to recovery or death is different.

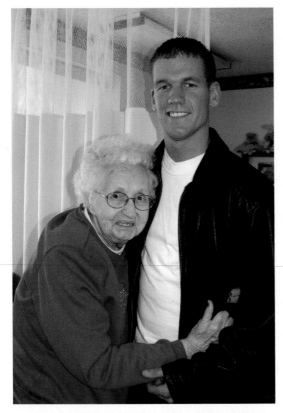

This picture portrays a sharp contrast between the health of the immune system. This grandmother is saying goodbye to her great-grandson, who is leaving for 2 years in the Peace Corps. The great-grandson is 19 and in perfect health. Grandma is 84 and cannot be around anyone with an infectious disease because of her compromised immune system.

This chapter provides information on the prevention of infectious diseases and the treatment of infections when they occur. Items to be discussed are as follows:

- Maintaining a healthy immune system by participating in health-promoting activities
- Preventing infections with scheduled immunizations, keeping a clean environment, and following good hygiene
- Knowledge about common infections caused by food or water, other people, animals, or insects

Infections can affect all the systems of the body and may be precipitated by chronic medical conditions such as diabetes, asthma, or chronic obstructive pulmonary disease (COPD). In this chapter, respiratory, genital and urinary, intra-abdominal, and integumentary infections are addressed.

Many new viruses are being discovered that can cause an outbreak of illnesses, such as the SARS outbreak in 2005 and the H1N1 influenza ("swine flu") of 2009. As a nurse caring for older adults, you need to be aware of your own personal hygiene and become vigilant about washing your hands and taking proper care of soiled materials. Masks, gloves, and gowns should be worn when there is a question about the spread of an infection. Infections can be carried from patient to patient on the hands of a nurse. As a dedicated caregiver, you want to avoid being a carrier of even the most innocent contaminant. The nursing role in the management of infection in older adults includes recognizing, reporting, and documenting signs and symptoms of infection, complying with medical direction for care, and preventing the spread of infection.

MAINTAINING A HEALTHY IMMUNE SYSTEM

One of the purposes of the immune system is to protect the body from the invasion of harmful bacteria, fungi, viruses, parasites, and other

PRIORITY SETTING 13.1

This chapter discusses so many serious diseases that, in my mind, there is only one overriding priority. It is described well in the chapter. I can summarize it by saying, "Wash your hands!"

microorganisms. As the body ages, lymphocyte function and antibody immune responses become delayed or inadequate and put the older adult at risk for infections. The following are ways to support the health of the immune system.

Nutrition

The LPN is responsible for assessing and monitoring an older person's nutritional status. This is an important aspect of maintaining a healthy immune system. (Review nutrition and the reasons for poor nutrition in Chapter 7.) It is important to identify nutritional deficits and potential reasons for these deficits. The LPN must determine, through questioning and observing the person's nutritional patterns, why there may be deficits in eating.

There often are problems with older adults and the food they eat. Food may be too expensive, or it may not taste good because of the decreased sensitivity of the taste buds. Perhaps there is no desire to prepare food, or the older person may be unable to chew or digest food properly. These are just a few reasons for poor nutritional patterns. You, the LPN, are an important team player when reporting nutritional concerns and potential solutions to members of the interdisciplinary health-care team for management.

Fluid Intake

Another challenge related to nutrition is for older adults to maintain adequate fluid balance for wellness. Dehydration following outside activities, an illness, or not drinking enough fluid during the day can lead to potential problems. It is common for older adults to drink insufficient fluids during the day. Fluid intake should be assessed, along with nutritional intake and deficits.

Lifestyle

The need for exercise, rest, and stress management and the need to avoid cigarette smoke and alcohol use are discussed in Chapter 6. Compliance with these activities heightens the abilities of the immune system. As an LPN, you need to assess compliance or noncompliance with these activities frequently and educate the person as necessary. Knowing older adults' lifestyles, living conditions, and economic situations is important when assisting them in maintaining a healthy immune system.

Chronic Medical Conditions

Chronic medical conditions have an effect on an older adult's immune system. Chapter 14 discusses chronic medical conditions and the potential for infections. A classic example is a person with diabetes. You need to educate the diabetic person to take precautions to prevent infections by wearing appropriate shoes, observing for lesions that do not heal, and caring for skin cuts and abrasions.

Urinary Tract Infections

Preventing urinary tract infections is an important aspect of preventive nursing. Older adults should be encouraged to drink adequate fluids and to empty their bladders frequently. If incontinence occurs, older persons should have their skin cleansed and soiled clothes replaced. Older adults' skin is sensitive and can break down, which invites infection. Catheters often are a source of infection; the LPN needs to follow agency protocols in an effort to prevent them.

Respiratory Infections

Respiratory infections may have a significant effect on an older adult. Older people need to be encouraged to receive the yearly influenza vaccination. Pneumococcal vaccines can also prevent severe respiratory infections. Increased fluids keep secretions thin and allow the pathogens to be coughed out of the respiratory tract.

The pneumococcal vaccine builds antibodies to fight against 23 pneumonia organisms. I know an active older adult who enjoyed the many busy things she was doing in the areas of service as a volunteer at the local hospital. She was around patients and welcomed them to the hospital at the front entrance desk. Each winter she would miss several months of volunteer service because she had pneumonia. After receiving strong encouragement from her physician and several older friends, she decided to take the pneumococcal vaccine. She has not had pneumonia since! Often, individuals simply need education to make the decision to improve their health. As an LPN, you are in a perfect position to provide the necessary teaching.

Intra-Abdominal Infections

Intra-abdominal infections are common in older adults. Signs and symptoms of infections may be difficult to differentiate from other chronic diseases in older people. Laboratory results and uncharacteristic complaints may confuse the findings. Older adults may have coexisting conditions or be mentally confused, making the history and physical examination difficult or misleading. Cholecystitis, diverticulitis, and appendicitis are examples of intra-abdominal infections that may be difficult to diagnosis in older people. The LPN is able to help gather verbal information, note signs and symptoms, and evaluate vital signs to assist in diagnosing the condition.

Integumentary System

Changes in the integumentary system accompany the process of aging. Many factors influence changes in the course of aging. Exposure to the sun, diet, heredity, and general health affect the skin. Pressure ulcers and their potential for infection are discussed in Chapter 16. The LPN needs to be aware of other skin infections. Redness, swelling, pain, lesions, and discoloration are some signs and symptoms of skin infections. As an LPN, you must report all signs and symptoms of a skin infection to the registered nurse (RN). If requested, you will obtain a specimen for culture. Culture and sensitivity tests may be necessary to identify the organism causing the infection and to treat it appropriately.

Skin pathogens include the following microorganisms:

- Staphylococcal bacterial infections include impetigo, boils, carbuncles, and cellulitis.
- Streptococcal bacterial infections include impetigo and erysipelas.
- Fungal infections include the cause of "athlete's foot" and thickened nails on the fingers and toes.
- Viral infections include herpes zoster (shingles) and herpes simplex.
- Parasitic infections include scabies and lice.

It is impossible to protect people from the invasion of harmful microorganisms, but an older adult with a healthy immune system will have a better recovery if an infection occurs. Adherence to wellness activities, plus additional measures, can prevent infections and increase positive outcomes.

POINT OF INTEREST

Recently, the CDC changed the term *universal precautions* to *standard precautions* (CDC, 2007, 2007 Guideline for Isolation Precautions: Preventing Transmission of Infectious Agents in Healthcare Settings). This term means you treat everyone's blood and body fluids as if they are infectious.

PREVENTING INFECTIONS

Immunizations

Immunization recommendations change as people age, and health conditions affect immune responses. The need for an older adult to be immunized is not always recognized. Immunization histories may not be part of the person's medical record, or the information simply may not be noted. In addition, the older adult's immune system may need to be "boosted" for the body to continue to have the ability to resist certain infections. The LPN must consider the need for the older adult to have continued protection from preventable disease.

Immunizations should be continued throughout life for vaccine-preventable diseases. A report from the U.S. Centers for Disease Control and Prevention (CDC Guidelines, 2008) claimed that approximately 6000 American adults die from diseases that could have been prevented by vaccines or complications as a result of not being immunized. Immunization histories are an important part of the assessment that you, as the LPN, will perform. New vaccines are being developed, and when completed, they will be added to the list of available treatment options.

Tetanus, Diphtheria, and Pertussis Vaccine (Tdap)

Tetanus, diphtheria, and pertussis are serious diseases caused by bacteria. Diphtheria and pertussis are spread from person to person, whereas tetanus enters the body through cuts or wounds. The signs or symptoms of each disease are as follows:

- *Tetanus* (lockjaw) causes painful tightening of the muscles, usually all over the body. It can lead to "locking" of the jaw so that the victim cannot open his mouth or swallow. Tetanus can lead to death in 2 out of 10 cases.
- *Diphtheria* causes a thick covering in the back of the throat. It can lead to breathing problems, paralysis, heart failure, and death.
- *Pertussis* (whooping cough) causes coughing spells so bad that it is hard for infants and adults to eat, drink, or breathe. These episodes can last for weeks. Pertussis can lead to pneumonia, seizures (jerking and staring spells), brain damage, and death.

Tetanus, diphtheria, and pertussis vaccines (Tdap) can help prevent these diseases. A single dose of Tdap is recommended for people 11 through 64 years of age. Another vaccine, called Td, protects against tetanus and diphtheria but not pertussis. Td is recommended every 10 years for people age 7 and older.

Tetanus-Diphtheria Vaccine (Td)

Tetanus-diphtheria vaccine (Td) is probably the most overlooked immunization. After the initial Td series has been given, a booster is required every 10 years for life. The LPN should evaluate the Td status for all older adults and determine the need for a booster. It is often discovered that some older adults have never had a Td series. All men going into the military during World War II were given Td immunizations, but during this time period, women were not routinely immunized. Not all adults who lived during the 1940s were immunized. The LPN should report the need for the Td series if a person is identified who has never had it.

Influenza Vaccine

The influenza or "flu" vaccine should be given each year to all adults older than 65 years, unless contraindicated. Older adults who have lung disease, diabetes, kidney disease, or other diseases that affect the immune system should be particularly encouraged to get the vaccine. The flu virus changes each year, so the formulation of the vaccine changes each year. Vaccines should be given starting around mid-October. The vaccine is generally available in physician offices, senior centers, home-health agencies, public health departments, and certain places of business.

H1N1 Influenza Vaccination

The H1N1 vaccine was given to help decrease the spread of H1N1 influenza. In fall 2009, many older adults received two flu shots. The first shot was to cover the normal flu season, and the second flu shot was specific to H1N1. In the future, H1N1 vaccine is expected to be added to the regular influenza vaccination.

Pneumococcal Vaccine

Pneumococcal vaccine provides protection against 23 pneumonia organisms. Only one dose is needed if it is given after age 65, but a booster is needed every 5 years after the initial dose.

When chronic health conditions, such as lung disease, heart disease, diabetes, kidney disease, alcoholism, liver disease, cerebrospinal fluid leak, or cancer, are present, the vaccine should be considered at age 50 (CDC Guidelines, 2008). If pneumococcal vaccine was given before age 65, a second dose is required after age 65. The second dose needs to be given at least 5 years after the first dose. The physician or primary care provider determines when the vaccine should be given. The vaccine is available from a physician's office, hospital, or public health department.

Hepatitis A Vaccine

Hepatitis A vaccines are recommended for people traveling to global areas where hepatitis A prevalence is high. In the past, people traveling to some countries would request immune globulin or the "gamma shot." Now, getting the first dose of a two-dose series of hepatitis A 2 weeks before traveling provides significant protection against this disease. For the best protection, an older adult should receive both doses. Immune globulin "gamma" is not necessary with the hepatitis A two-dose series, and the vaccine provides protection for many years.

Hepatitis A is prevalent in some areas of the United States as well, and a hepatitis A vaccination may be warranted. Local health departments should be consulted as needed. The vaccine is available at public health departments.

Hepatitis B Vaccine

Hepatitis B continues to be problematic throughout the world. Older adults traveling to areas of the world where hepatitis B is present should consider being vaccinated. If the person is planning on staying in the country longer than 6 months, hepatitis B immunization should be strongly encouraged. The vaccination is given in a three-part series over 6 months. Patients on kidney dialysis or requiring transfusions for clotting problems are candidates for hepatitis B vaccine. Older adults who provide services to developmentally delayed persons, health-care workers, or safety workers should consider being vaccinated. Hepatitis B has not been specifically categorized as a sexually transmitted disease, but it is a blood-borne pathogen. The LPN may be asked to evaluate the person's sexual history to help the primary health-care provider decide whether or not to vaccinate against hepatitis B. The vaccine is available at hospitals, physician's offices, or public health departments.

Measles-Mumps-Rubella Vaccine

Measles-mumps-rubella vaccine (MMR) is thought of as a childhood immunization. The vaccine may be recommended for persons who travel internationally. Health-care workers and older adults who are actively working with or volunteering to help "high-risk groups" should be

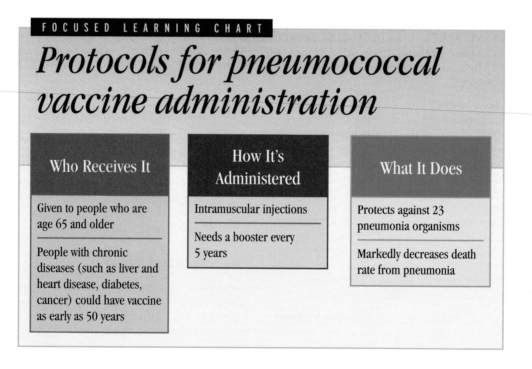

FOCUSED LEARNING CHART

Protocols for pneumococcal vaccine administration

Who Receives It	How It's Administered	What It Does
Given to people who are age 65 and older	Intramuscular injections	Protects against 23 pneumonia organisms
People with chronic diseases (such as liver and heart disease, diabetes, cancer) could have vaccine as early as 50 years	Needs a booster every 5 years	Markedly decreases death rate from pneumonia

considered for MMR immunization. Even if MMR has been given during the person's lifetime, a second dose of MMR is recommended for people in the above-mentioned groups. The LPN assesses the immunization status and reports the findings to the primary care provider, who determines immunization needs. The vaccine is available at hospitals, physicians' offices, or public health departments.

Meningococcal Vaccine and *Haemophilus influenzae* Type B Vaccine

Older people with compromised immune systems, organ transplants, cancer treatments, or splenectomy should be considered for meningococcal and *Haemophilus influenzae* type B (HIB) immunizations. These immunizations also are recommended for older adults who travel to areas of the world where these diseases are prevalent. The LPN assesses the need for the immunizations and reports the findings. The primary health-care provider determines if the immunization is needed. The vaccines are available from the public health department.

● SAFE FOOD AND WATER

Food-borne diseases are very common in the United States. Millions of people become ill each year as a result of contaminated food, and thousands die. Microorganisms find food a great place to live and breed. The signs and symptoms of food-borne diseases may resemble a bad case of "stomach flu," and the older adult may delay seeking medical care. Most food-borne diseases have common signs and symptoms, which are abdominal pain, fever, vomiting, and diarrhea of sudden onset. Laboratory testing (stool culture) is required to identify the infecting organism. The LPN needs to instruct the person on collecting a stool specimen.

Campylobacteriosis

Campylobacter infections are the most common food-borne diseases. Foods most commonly associated with *Campylobacter* infections are undercooked poultry, unpasteurized milk, and contaminated water (campylobacteriosis is also known as travelers' diarrhea). Inadequate cleaning of food preparation areas and poor hand washing before food preparation can lead to infection. Symptoms of *Campylobacter* infection are diarrhea, abdominal pain, fever, nausea, and vomiting. These symptoms occur within 2 to 7 days after exposure. A stool specimen is required for an accurate diagnosis. Older adults are at risk for dehydration complications secondary to the diarrhea. The LPN needs to encourage the elderly person to drink more fluids.

Campylobacter infections may resolve without medical treatment, but elderly adults with dehydration and delayed recovery need to be referred to a health-care provider. The LPN needs to educate all household members about hand washing to prevent the spread of the infection to others.

Cholera

Sporadic outbreaks of cholera occur in the United States related to eating raw or undercooked seafood from contaminated waters. In addition, cholera can be spread by the people preparing foods and by foods that have been washed with contaminated water. The main symptom of cholera is diarrhea, and it may appear in a few hours or up to 5 days after exposure. Stool specimens are required for diagnosis and treatment. Increased fluid intake needs to be stressed because diarrhea puts an older adult at risk for dehydration. Medical intervention may be required. Travel information is available for people who plan to visit global areas where cholera is present. Travelers should be particularly aware of food preparation, water,

---

and certain foods being served. Cholera has been very rare in industrialized nations for the last 100 years; however, the disease is still common today in other parts of the world, including the Indian subcontinent and sub-Saharan Africa.

Although cholera can be life-threatening, it is easily prevented and treated. In the United States, because of advanced water and sanitation systems, cholera is not a major threat; however, everyone, especially travelers, should be aware of how the disease is transmitted and what can be done to prevent it (CDC, 2007, Infectious Disease Information: Cholera).

Salmonellosis

Salmonella bacteria can be found in many foods, such as custards, milk, eggs, salad dressing, and shellfish. Contaminated water and food handlers are the causes of many salmonella infections. Symptoms of infection are diarrhea, fever, and abdominal cramps that usually occur within 12 to 72 hours after exposure (CDC, 2010, Salmonella). A stool specimen is required for the diagnosis of salmonellosis. The concern of salmonella infection in the older adult is dehydration from diarrhea. The LPN needs to educate the person to increase fluid intake. As in all cases of food-borne illnesses, the LPN needs to educate household members to practice good hand washing and to keep food preparation places clean.

Shigellosis

Shigella bacteria are found in many foods, and infections are usually due to contaminated water or poor hygiene practiced by food handlers. Symptoms of infection are vomiting, nausea, cramps, and diarrhea, with blood or mucus or both in the stool. Symptoms may occur 12 to 96 hours after exposure. Shigellosis may require medical intervention in a frail elderly person and other older adults. Increased fluid intake is important, and the LPN needs to give instructions to family members on hand washing and sanitary food preparation.

Other Food-Borne Infections

There are other food-borne infections that are not mentioned in this chapter. Signs and symptoms of food-borne infections are similar, and diagnosis can be made only by a laboratory test. In your role as the nurse, you will want to note the following in a suspected food-borne illness: the time that signs and symptoms occurred, what the person ate in the last few days, where the food was served, and whether other people became ill. This information should be reported to the local health department. The health department investigates all potential food-borne diseases, and they take appropriate actions.

Food-borne infections can be prevented by good hand washing, using safe foods, and keeping food preparation areas sanitary. You need to instruct persons preparing food to:

- Store food correctly
- Protect food from insects, rodents, and animals
- Cook food thoroughly
- Eat cooked food immediately
- Refrigerate uneaten food immediately
- Reheat cooked foods thoroughly
- Wash hands frequently
- Keep food preparation areas clean

POINT OF INTEREST

While I was consulting for an extended-care facility, a call came that three health-care workers had diarrhea, as did two residents. Any more than two cases of diarrhea at one time in a nursing home is an alert for close observation to see if others come down with the same symptoms. Stool cultures were sent to the laboratory, and while we waited for the results, four more residents and two more health-care providers became ill with diarrhea. It was important to stop the spread of this organism. The recommendation was to stop all dining room privileges and have everyone eat in his or her own room. All outside activities with large groups were stopped, and an extra person worked with environmental services to clean all parts of the facility. If anyone had signs and symptoms of diarrhea, they were asked to stay home until 24 hours after their diarrhea stopped. Staff members, residents, and family members were instructed on hand hygiene and the appropriate use of gloves. Shortly afterward, the diarrhea stopped with just two more cases. The organism was Norwalk virus, which is sometimes called the cruise ship virus. Its current and correct name is norovirus. It has killed many older adults in nursing homes because of their weakened conditions.

ENVIRONMENTAL CLEANLINESS

Household Pets

Household pets are a source of friendship and companionship for older adults. Older people need to be aware, however, that pets also can become a source of infection. Pets may become infected and transfer their disease to household members. Animal waste can become a source of infection if it is not properly handled. A pet needs health and medical consideration to protect the older adult from a disease carried by the pet. An assessment of the home always should include mention of household pets and how care of the pet is managed.

Kitchens and Bathrooms

Kitchens and bathrooms are great harbors for infections. Household assessments need to include bathroom inspection of towels, tooth-care items, sinks, tubs, and toilets. Instructions by the LPN include not sharing personal hygiene items such as razors and tooth-care articles. Kitchen assessments involve reviewing food preparation and food storage as discussed

---

CRITICALLY EXAMINE THE FOLLOWING

You are working at the local health department and have been asked to answer the phone while the secretary goes to lunch. You are the only nurse in the department when you receive a call from Mr. Harold Gee. Mr. Gee reports to you that he and his wife began vomiting and having diarrhea a few hours after eating a shrimp salad at a local restaurant. Mr. Gee mentions his wife has a history of heart problems since her heart attack at age 60.

1. What information would you want from Mr. Gee?
2. Why would you report this information to your supervisor as soon as possible?

Note: Health departments have information report forms that are used by the public health nurse when conducting a potential food-borne infection investigation. This form may not be immediately available to you when the call comes. Nevertheless, it is a form you need to know exists.

---

earlier. Personal cleanliness and hygiene may need frequent reinforced instructions. When instructing older adults about hand washing, the LPN should include cleaning under the fingernails. Older adults who love and care for others in the household would not want to be the cause of a loved one's illness.

SEXUALLY TRANSMITTED DISEASES

Many health-care providers are uncomfortable when considering sexually transmitted diseases (STDs) in older adults. A myth of aging is that older people cannot participate in enjoyable sexual activity. The reality is that they can, and many do. With the development of new medications, such as sildenafil (Viagra) and various vaginal creams, there is the potential of increased sexual activity and sexually transmitted diseases in older persons.

Some people who have lived in monogamous relationships and have lost their companion may have sexual relations with one or more persons who have uncertain sexual histories. This factor can have a strong impact on an older adult's overall health. STDs about which you, as the LPN in the community, should have a working knowledge include syphilis; gonorrhea; chlamydiosis; hepatitis A, B, and C; HIV; genital warts; lice; and other viral and bacterial infections. These diseases generally are discussed in basic medical/surgical classes. Their impact and treatment in older adults do not differ from that in younger adults.

As the nurse, you need to teach older adults who are sexually active with more than one partner the signs and symptoms of STDs and to seek medical treatment for them immediately. Older adults tend not to discuss sexual matters with younger people. This is a barrier that you need to overcome through caring and sensitive communication skills. Older adults need to realize the variety of STDs and the symptoms of the most common ones. They should be able to report their symptoms clearly so that the appropriate tests can be performed for accurate diagnosis. Common symptoms are pain, discharge from the penis or vagina, abdominal pain, and genital lesions. Your responsibility is to teach the older adults in your care about STDs, their signs and symptoms, how to get appropriate care, and how to have safe sex.

Obtaining a Sexual History

Prevention of STDs in older adults is the reason for obtaining a sexual history. Some older adults are at little or no risk for STDs, whereas others may be at high risk. Health education, appropriate treatments, and stopping the transmission of STDs begin with the identification of at-risk behavior.

A sexual history is an integral part of a complete patient history profile. The right questions need to be asked to elicit responses that give key information about risk factors and patient behaviors. Open-ended questions are more likely to give responses that have the most pertinent information. "Tell me about your sex life" would give much more information than simply asking, "Do you have sex?"

Patients must be reassured that their responses are confidential. Developing a confidential relationship aids the LPN in building a rapport of trust and confidence with the older adult. It is important to remember that the patient's values regarding acceptable sexual behavior may differ from yours, and you should not make personal judgments.

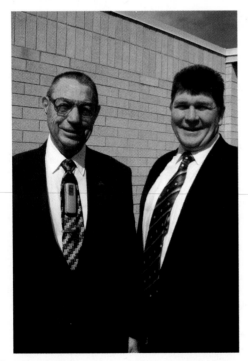

These businessmen are sexual partners and have been together for the last 5 years. The older man is HIV positive, and it is a near-certainty that he will transfer the disease to his partner. They both have excellent, job-related insurance, but the quality of their lives is still questionable.

Some specific questions need be asked and may cause you, as the interviewer, some discomfort. Questions such as "How many sexual partners have you had in the past 3 months?" or "Do you prefer to have sex with men, women, or both?" can seem intrusive. These answers are very important, however, when identifying potential risks for STDs. A complete sexual history should be included on the history form.

HIV and AIDS

Older people are at increasing risk for HIV/AIDS and other STDs. A growing number of older people now have HIV/AIDS. About 19% of all people with HIV/AIDS in the United States are age 50 and older. Because older people do not get tested for HIV/AIDS on a regular basis, there may be even more cases than those that are currently known.

Many factors contribute to the increasing risk of infection in older people. Older people in the United States generally know less about HIV/AIDS and STDs than younger people because elderly adults have been neglected by the individuals responsible for education and prevention messages. In addition, older people are less likely than younger people to talk about their sex lives or drug use with their physicians, and physicians tend not to ask their older patients about sex or drug use. Finally, older people often mistake the symptoms of HIV/AIDS for the aches and pains of normal aging, so they are less likely to get tested (CDC, 2010, HIV/AIDS).

The initial intervention that you, as the LPN, need to undertake is sex education. People age 60 and older generally have not had the benefit of sex education on any level. They did not have the friendly chat with their mom, high school gym teacher, or a sex counselor. An intensive but sensitive interview may indicate that the older adult does not have a full working knowledge of his or her own reproductive system even after having multiple children. This is the place to start if your assessment indicates that there is a knowledge deficit in this area. Be careful to not patronize older adults, or, in other words, do not treat them as though you are the "all-knowing" parent. Be a colleague and a friend. Explore the information together. Share only what is essential for good health unless the learner indicates a desire for more information. Allow the older adult to share the wisdom that comes through the experience of having and raising children.

The second educational concept that you need to teach sexually active older adults is safe sex. Many older people no longer feel a need to protect themselves sexually because they are not concerned about becoming pregnant. Your responsibility is to teach them that safe sex also means protection against STDs, most critically HIV/AIDS. Many older adults have never used a condom. Older adults often associate condoms with birth control, something about which they no longer feel concern. It may be uncomfortable to teach someone old enough to be your grandparent how to use one. The easiest technique may be practicing putting a condom on a banana. It is acceptable to laugh and make the teaching fun. Laughter would assist the older adult who is uncomfortable with the exercise to relax and learn better. Make the point that the only truly safe sex is abstinence or monogamy. Then emphasize that condoms are next in terms of safety and should always be used.

Another point that needs to be explored with sexually active older adults is the type of disease HIV/AIDS really is. In the 21st century, many people view HIV/AIDS as a chronic disease. The common association is with diabetes mellitus. People recognize diabetes as a disease for which there is not a cure and one that requires a careful medication regimen. It also is seen as something with which millions of people live successfully. People such as "Magic" Johnson, a former national basketball star with HIV, help perpetuate the chronic disease myth.

It is crucial that the older adults you teach understand that HIV/AIDS is a killer disease, not a chronic disease. The medications, antivirals, that keep people with this disease alive must be taken every 4 to 6 hours around the clock. It requires setting an alarm during the night because doses cannot be missed. People who think of HIV/AIDS as a chronic disease do not see the gastrointestinal distress and emotional agony that accompany this disease.

The patient care for hospitalized older adults with HIV/AIDS is similar to care for other fragile patients or residents. Be gentle and do not rush the care given. Listen to the needs of the older person, and take the time to demonstrate genuine caring.

When caring for someone with HIV/AIDS, always use standard precautions. It is crucial that you follow the medication regimen closely and report any adverse reactions immediately. Good nutrition and hydration also are important; you can encourage this by sitting with the older adult in a nonrushed manner and providing encouragement to eat and drink. The intake and output in older adults with HIV/AIDS should be carefully noted.

The person with HIV/AIDS is often dying. Review Chapter 10 on end-of-life issues in older adults, and evaluate how you can apply the information to the patient with HIV/AIDS. Do not judge the person to whom you are giving care. Some people are critical of patients with HIV/AIDS and believe that they "deserve" the disease. That simply is not true. Do not be taken in by such thinking.

The responsibility you have as the nurse is to educate the sexually active older adult in an effort to promote avoidance of all STDs, especially HIV/AIDS. If you are caring for a person with HIV/AIDS, you have a responsibility to assist him or her with management of the disease and to deliver quality palliative care.

Human Papillomavirus Infection

There are many types of human papillomavirus (HPV) that can infect the genital tract and anus of women and men. Generally, the resulting genital warts are not painful and, if visible, have a "fleshy" cauliflower appearance. The warts can spread easily and increase in frequency with an increase in the number of sexual partners. A person can be infected with multiple types of HPV at the same time. The LPN must be aware that some cancers of the genital tract are associated with HPV infections. Medical treatment should begin as soon as a diagnosis is made.

Trichomoniasis

Trichomoniasis is a condition caused by a protozoan pathogen. Generally, symptoms are characterized by a foul-smelling, yellow-green discharge. Women may complain of intense vaginal itching, especially at night. Pain and burning on urination are common complaints with this STD. Redness and swelling may be present. Women more often have complaints with this STD than men. All sexual partners should be treated.

Gonorrhea

Gonorrhea is caused by the bacteria *Neisseria gonorrhoeae*. In this disease, symptoms are much more pronounced in men than in women. Symptoms in men are large amounts of green discharge from the penis and burning during urination. Testicular pain is frequently reported. Often, women present with abdominal or pelvic pain. Treatment needs to begin at once after a diagnosis is made. All sexual partners need to be identified and treated.

Chlamydia trachomatis

Many people who are infected with gonorrhea are co-infected with chlamydia. Signs and symptoms of chlamydial infections are similar to the signs and symptoms of gonorrheal infections. As the nurse, you need to assist in identifying sexual partners for treatment.

Syphilis

Syphilis is a complex disease and can manifest throughout the life span if it is not detected and treated. Generally, the description of the disease is based on signs and symptoms at the time the diagnosis is made. The first symptoms appear about 3 weeks after exposure. A chancre, or open painless sore, appears. The chancre can appear anywhere on the body. It is the classic symptom of primary syphilis. The sore resolves without treatment, but that does not mean the disease has disappeared.

A classic rash marks secondary syphilis, most prominent on the palms of the hands and the soles of the feet. You, as the nurse, should report these unique symptoms as soon as they appear so that treatment can be started. These symptoms may last a few weeks or a year without treatment.

If syphilis is not treated in the primary or secondary stage, latent syphilis symptoms manifest as neurological impairment, mental retardation, and memory problems. Syphilis may not be identified until the latent stage, when an older adult exhibits the symptoms of latent syphilis.

Treatment for syphilis depends on the stage. Testing techniques are advanced, and the disease is usually detected early, in the primary stage, when cure is likely to be successful. The exacerbating and remitting nature of the disease, moving from an acute phase to dormancy, makes this a difficult disease to diagnose. That is why a good sexual history is so important.

Genital Herpes

A virus causes genital herpes, and treatment options for virus infections are limited. Herpes usually manifests with blisters on the genital area. These blisters are fluid-filled and very painful. Besides the blisters, other symptoms include itching, tingling, and burning and even achy joints. Transmission of the virus can occur with or without symptoms. As the LPN, you can educate the older adult about the transmission of the virus that causes genital herpes. Antiretroviral therapy is not curative and seems only to shorten the duration of symptoms and infectiousness.

Hepatitis B

Hepatitis B is transmitted sexually and by exposure to infected blood. A unique characteristic of hepatitis B is that a person can be in a "carrier" state. The carrier is always considered infectious. A vaccine against hepatitis B has been available for many years and provides excellent protection against exposure. You, the LPN, need to instruct the older adult about the availability of the vaccine and to use condoms or abstinence to prevent transmission. A small percentage of carriers go on to develop cancer of the liver.

Hepatitis A

Hepatitis A is usually considered an infection caused by food or water, not by a sexually transmitted infection. Men who have sex with men are at risk for hepatitis A, so hepatitis A is mentioned here as an STD in gay men. As mentioned earlier, a hepatitis A vaccine is available, and you should encourage people at risk to receive the vaccine to prevent infection.

⬤ TUBERCULOSIS

In the early part of the 20th century, tuberculosis (TB) was a major cause of death in the United States. In the 1940s, new drugs became available to treat TB. The United States, in contrast to many poorer countries, had the resources to treat all cases of TB, and the disease was almost eliminated in this country before the 1980s. Worldwide, TB is the cause of many illnesses and deaths, however. Resources for TB treatment have been lacking in poorer countries and continue to be problematic for world health organizations.

Few new cases of TB were reported in the 1970s in the United States because of the national "push" to treat the disease. This lack of reported cases resulted in TB services being cut from government funding sources in the 1980s. Suddenly, after this cut, new cases of TB began to occur. HIV was identified at that time, and TB was diagnosed in some HIV patients. Was lack of funding for treatment a reason for an increase in TB? This question continues to be debated by the public health service because treatment protocols for TB have been complicated by a TB strain that is drug resistant. This drug-resistant strain occurred after the period of minimal treatment of TB in the United States.

TB cases reported to the CDC for 2008 represented a decrease in occurrences. In 2005, which was the 13th consecutive year of decline, the TB case rate was 4.8 per 100,000. This reduction is attributed to more effective TB-control programs that emphasize prompt identification of persons with TB, prompt initiation of appropriate therapy, and efforts to ensure that therapy will be completed (CDC, 2010, Tuberculosis).

Older adults have a high probability for exposure to TB compared with when they were younger. In many cases, older adults were exposed but never developed the disease. The TB bacterium may lay dormant in the body for many years and never cause active disease unless the immune system weakens, which can happen as people age. The signs and symptoms of an active TB case are night sweats, weight loss, low-grade fever, and chronic cough.

TB screening should be conducted on all nursing home residents to identify undiagnosed cases for treatment. Staff members and other residents need to be protected from TB if a case is identified. Chapter 15 addresses TB skin testing. Sputum smears also confirm a case of active TB. The LPN may be asked to collect a sputum specimen. The protocols at your facility dictate how the specimen should be gathered. Review the protocols, and ask questions if you are unsure of the procedure.

As a TB nurse, you need to follow the medical orders closely and watch for signs and symptoms of complications with the drug protocols. It is possible that you will be asked to watch the older person take the medications to ensure that the pills are consumed. The medications may cause some side effects in the older person, which is why the patient may avoid taking the medication. Directly observed therapy (DOT) has been found to be successful in ensuring that the medications are being taken as directed. The LPN may do this or choose a responsible family member to observe the medication therapy.

Medication regimens would be ordered specifically for persons with TB in your care. You need to be aware of medication doses, times to be given, and possible side effects.

As an LPN, you need to teach older adults with TB to wear a mask when in public or with people. You need to support the older person because the mask is uncomfortable to wear, difficult to use, may cause an imbalance in blood gases, and may cause the person to be sensitive about needing to wear the mask. The mask needs to be worn until sputum smears confirm that the person is no longer infectious.

Hospitals have special ventilation rooms for patients with TB to prevent the pathogen from being spread to other areas of the hospital. If the person is at home and weather permits, windows and doors should be opened to ventilate the home. Sunlight destroys the TB bacteria, so excursions outside on a sunny day should be encouraged.

⬤ WEST NILE FEVER

West Nile fever is a new infection that has caused older people to become very ill and can lead to death. This infection has been confirmed in all states in the United States and is thought to have been brought to this country by birds traveling on the wind currents from Africa. The mosquito is the vector that transfers the infection from

POINT OF INTEREST

Drug-Resistant Organisms

The misuse of antibiotics has caused drug resistance. This means that the organism has become familiar with the antibiotic, which cannot now kill a specific organism. The organisms that infect our bodies have a great ability to change to survive. They become familiar with the antibiotics that are in the bloodstream. If there is not enough antibiotic in the body or if a wrong antibiotic is used, the organism can change its shape or chemistry so that the antibiotic cannot adhere to the organism and kill it. This is what drug resistance is.

The following is the best advice to decrease drug-resistant organisms:

1. Take antibiotics only when prescribed. It is just as important that if you start the antibiotic, you also finish every pill. Doing so ensures the killing of the organism.
2. Do not take antibiotics if you have a cold or the flu. They will not do any good. Antibiotics do not kill viruses, which are what cause colds and flu.
3. Wash your hands. This decreases the spread of drug-resistant organisms to other people who may have weakened immune systems that could easily be infected by the organism.
4. Do not treat people who have a drug-resistant organism as though they have the plague. Your protection is to wear personal protective equipment when touching an ill person's blood or body fluids.

Let us look at an example: A research study was being done to see if older adults in a nursing home had methicillin-resistant *Staphylococcus aureus* (MRSA) colonized in their nose; if it was present, the symptoms and level of illness were recorded. An 85-year-old mother of six children and grandmother to 17 grandchildren agreed to be in the study.

The test came back positive that she had MRSA in her nose. She was not ill with this organism. After the study identified the MRSA, the nursing home placed her into solitary confinement. She could not go out of her room to participate in the daytime activities and had to eat all meals alone in her room. This was devastating to the woman, who was in the nursing home to enjoy friends and neighbors during the last years of her life. She was very social and enjoyed her time with her friends and with her large family. This woman was also instructed not to hold, touch, or kiss any of her children or grandchildren. She was horrified about having to live as she was being told. More important, this older woman clearly was given the wrong information.

When a person is colonized (not showing any signs of an infection) with a drug-resistant organism, the following principles should be taught:

1. Wash your hands before you leave your room. Basic hand hygiene with an alcohol hand rub kills drug-resistant organisms.
2. If you have a cold or a cough, you need to use tissues and good hand hygiene.

In this case, the proper teaching provided this woman with a return to her usual quality of life so that she could continue to enjoy her life in the nursing home and with her family.

The prevention and control of multidrug-resistant organisms (MDROs) is a national priority—one that requires responsibility from all health-care facilities and agencies. At some facilities, an infected person with an MDRO may be placed into contact isolation. The person caring for this patient needs to wear gloves. If you would like further information on this subject, go to: CDC.gov and look under "MDRO."

Make sure you understand the organism that a patient has and whether it can or cannot be spread. I am sure that having this woman out with her family and friends lengthened her life and added a tremendous amount of enjoyment. Correct education and information can take away the fear of drug-resistant organisms.

birds to humans. The symptoms are fever, chills, headache, aching bones, malaise, symptoms of respiratory infection, and muscle pain. Meningoencephalitis and pneumonia are complications of West Nile fever (CDC, 2010, West Nile Virus). The LPN should advise older adults to protect themselves against mosquito bites by wearing long-sleeved tops and long pants and insect repellent from dawn to dusk. Screens on windows and doors help keep the mosquitoes out of the house. In addition, because mosquitoes breed in standing water, all containers, such as a birdbath, should be refreshed often.

Let us look at the case of an elderly couple who would sit together on their front-porch swing on summer evenings for hours on end. Doing so had been the greatest joy of their older life! Late in August, the husband became ill and was diagnosed with West Nile virus. He lived, but carried the complication of being slower and unable to function at his previous level of good health. When asked why he did not wear mosquito repellent, he said, "Who would ever think that it would be *me* who would get bitten by an infected mosquito?" As LPNs, we need to teach older people that sufficient precautions against mosquitoes could help them to maintain their current quality of life.

Worldwide, mosquitoes are the cause of many serious diseases, such as malaria and dengue fever. All older adults should take precautions when planning to travel to countries where mosquito-borne diseases exist. You need to remind the older person to wear proper clothing and have the individual consult with the physician regarding the most appropriate insect repellent.

ANTHRAX

Anthrax has been suggested as a potential bioterrorism infectious agent. The anthrax bacterium has existed in the United States for centuries, and, except in a few populations that are exposed to infected anthrax animals, there has not been an outbreak of this disease. Anthrax can be found in wild and domestic animals. The general population is not at risk for anthrax infection except in the case of bioterrorism. Anthrax infections can occur on the skin, in the lungs, or in the intestinal system. Skin infections may manifest as a depressed black eschar at the site of infection. Lung symptoms are similar to a respiratory infection. Intestinal infections resemble food-borne illnesses. It may be necessary to treat the infected person with an antibiotic.

AVIAN (BIRD) INFLUENZA

Various nations and the World Health Organization (WHO) are vigorously conducting research on a newer infection known as avian influenza. The infection first was identified in Asian countries but now has been identified in several nations in Europe. Causes and treatments of avian flu are unknown. Most evidence suggests that avian flu is related to unsanitary conditions where chickens are raised. People who care for the chickens or are eating the infected chickens are most at risk for the disease.

A great fear is that the virus causing avian flu will mutate and begin to spread from person to person instead of bird to bird. Avian influenza viruses do not normally infect humans. There have been instances, however, of certain highly pathogenic strains causing severe respiratory disease in humans. In most cases, the people infected had been in close contact with infected

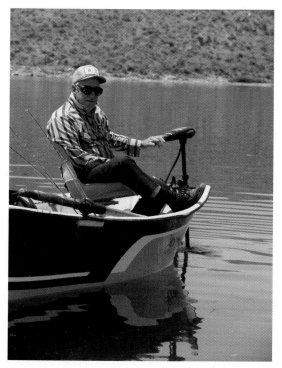

This 65-year-old man fishes year round. When it is "mosquito season," he protects himself with a long-sleeved shirt and an upturned collar. It still is possible to get bitten by a mosquito, but he is minimizing the danger by being cautious.

poultry or with objects contaminated by their feces. Nevertheless, there is concern that the virus could mutate to become more easily transmissible between humans, raising the possibility of an influenza pandemic (WHO, 2010). Health departments in each community would provide instructions on recognizing symptoms and treatments for avian flu if this infection were to come to your community.

PANDEMIC PREVENTION

The severe acute respiratory syndrome (SARS) epidemic in 2003 is an example of how quarantine and quick reaction can prevent a pandemic. Scientists worked around the clock to learn about the transfer and treatment for the disease. Borders to countries were closed. People were checked for fever or other symptoms of SARS before being admitted to a country. Many people cancelled their travel plans and stayed home. All of these things assisted in controlling the disease from spreading. SARS, avian flu, and H1N1 are examples of newer infectious diseases that frequently appear. You need to keep yourself educated regarding infectious diseases and teach what you know to the older people within your care. In addition, be aware of your own use of standard precautions. Focus on your hand washing and your care of soiled materials. Masks, gloves, and gowns should be worn whenever there is a question of the spread of an infection. Err on the side of caution. Always protect yourself as well as others from any potential infection.

CONCLUSION

This chapter has discussed infections that have the potential to cause illnesses, including serious illnesses leading to death. The LPN has an important task to perform by assessing signs and symptoms of infectious diseases. The immune system changes with aging and may make it more difficult to recognize an infectious process. The LPN often is responsible for assessing older adults. Remember to consider the subtle signs and symptoms that could indicate an infectious process, including elevated temperature, lesion, redness, swelling, and pain. The LPN needs to consider other changes the older adult may exhibit, such as confusion, lethargy, and loss of appetite. It is important for the LPN to be a critical thinker while performing an assessment on older adults.

Mrs. B. is 95 years old and was recently widowed. Mrs. B. and her husband immigrated to the United States from Germany 45 years ago. She has been in generally good health and is being treated for osteoporosis and a mild elevation in blood pressure. Mrs. B. has reported a persistent dry cough for 1 month. Her health history does not reveal any other health problems. Mrs. B. uses a walker to help her ambulate. She enjoys a close relationship with her daughter and church friends. She has lived alone for nearly a year because her husband resided in an extended care facility until his death. Mrs. B. insists on being as independent as possible but does allow family and friends to visit her and help her with some personal and household tasks. Mrs. B. prefers speaking in her native language, which is German.

Just before his death, it was discovered that Mr. B. had infectious TB. Mr. B. was plagued with a persistent cough and recurrent pneumonia for the last 5 months of his life. A full-scale contact investigation was initiated at the extended-care facility and among close family members.

A PPD (Mantoux) skin test was done on Mrs. B., and she was found to have a 16-mm induration. A chest x-ray revealed right upper lobe fibronodular calcification. It was suspected that Mrs. B. had a case of infectious TB. Medical orders were written for a sputum test to confirm the suspicion of TB, for a liver function profile laboratory test, and for medical treatment to be started. Results of the liver function test were normal. The sputum test came back 4+ for acid-fast bacilli. Mrs. B. did have active TB. The appropriate medications were started to treat the disease.

Mrs. B. is to wear a high-efficiency particulate air (HEPA) filter mask when in public places or anytime she is with other people. The mask is necessary only until her sputum smears become negative for acid-fast bacilli. You are the LPN assigned to Mrs. B. as her home health nurse.

Discussion

1. What nursing care should the LPN implement?

2. How can the LPN help Mrs. B. maintain social contact with family and friends?

Solutions

What nursing care should the LPN implement?

1. The LPN should incorporate appropriate respiratory isolation measures until Mrs. B. is no longer infectious. The HEPA filter mask is worn for personal protection. If the weather permits, windows and doors should be open for sunlight and ventilation. The sunlight kills the TB bacterium, and the ventilation can disperse any airborne bacteria.

2. The LPN should observe Mrs. B. taking all her medication. This is called DOT, or directly observed therapy. It means that the LPN would need to visit the home daily or designate a reliable family member or neighbor to ensure the medications are taken correctly. The objective of DOT is to ensure compliance with the medical regimen and avoid building any drug-resistant TB bacterium.

3. The LPN needs to educate Mrs. B. continually on the importance of taking all the medications. You need to teach Mrs. B. about the side effects of the medications. With any medication, you need to watch for generalized rashes, hypersensitivity, and shortness of breath that are associated with medication dosing. You are responsible for medication compliance and for observing for complications. Immediately report all changes to the RN case manager.

How can the LPN assist Mrs. B. with maintaining social contact with her family and friends?

1. As the LPN, you need to help Mrs. B. to not feel socially isolated because of the need to limit visitors for infection control measures. You do not want her to become depressed or lonely. Make your own visits unhurried and pleasant. Make the effort to bring stories that would interest her. Reinforce the fact that this is a temporary situation, and she can expect to return to her usual activities as soon as her sputum smears return negative. When appropriate therapy begins, Mrs. B. could become noninfectious within 2 weeks.

Continued on page 228

2. You need to instruct Mrs. B. on how to wear a filter mask when in public or with others. The mask is uncomfortable when worn, even for short periods. It can impair ease of breathing and may promote feelings of claustrophobia. Changes in blood gases may occur when the mask is worn for any length of time. Mrs. B. may feel self-conscious when wearing the mask in public. She may prefer to stay at home until she is no longer infectious. As her nurse, you need to listen to her and support her in her feelings. Teach her the importance of wearing the mask despite the discomfort. Ensure that she has access to the telephone and telephone numbers of her family and friends. (The numbers may need to be written in large print.) Does Mrs. B. have access to the Internet? E-mail is an effective way to communicate with people. If her communication needs are met, she would only have to wear the mask minimally.

3. Mrs. B. may experience feelings of anger, loss, guilt, or uncertainty or a host of other feelings associated with her disease. You need to be sensitive to her feelings. In many cultures, TB is a "taboo" disease because it is seen as a disease of the poor. TB is an emotionally charged disease, and you are the person to give social support to Mrs. B. to assist her in managing her feelings.

Select the best answer to each question.

1. All of the following are signs and symptoms of food-borne illness *except:*

   a. Sudden onset

   b. Abdominal pain

   c. Vomiting and diarrhea

   d. Cough

2. Which of the following items would not need to be taught to an older adult to prevent a food-borne disease?

   a. Storing food safely

   b. Maintaining a clean kitchen

   c. Washing hands before and during food preparation

   d. Wearing a HEPA filter mask when preparing food

3. In assessing the immunization status of an older woman, the LPN needs to ask:

   a. "Do you have trouble seeing red-green colors?"

   b. "Have you had a DPT immunization in the past 5 years?"

   c. "Have you had a pneumococcal vaccination?"

   d. "How many sex partners have you had in the past 3 months?"

4. Many older adult diabetics are at risk for infections because they are not eating correctly.

   T   F

5. TB testing should be done on all long-term nursing home residents.

   T   F

14 Common Medical Diagnoses

Mary Ann Anderson

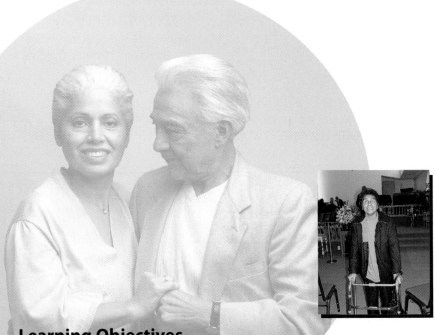

Learning Objectives

After completing this chapter, the student will be able to:

1. Identify differences between acute and chronic stages of common medical problems in older adults.
2. Describe at least two common physiological changes in each body system that are normal aging changes.
3. Describe nursing care appropriate for long-term care of an older adult who has one or more of the common pathologies discussed in this chapter.
4. Apply the concept of gerotranscendence to the common medical diagnoses of older adults.

INTRODUCTION

Congratulations! You now are at the point where you will learn how to enhance and personalize the bedside nursing care you will give to older people. The points of emphasis are specifically on the physiology and psychology of older adults. You will recognize what makes gerontological nursing a specialty after reading this chapter and the chapters that follow. Be open to the uniqueness of giving holistic care (care that involves the entire person) to older adults. Frame the care that you give within a transpersonal caring format. The knowledge you will learn will be valuable to you throughout your entire career.

Older people develop multiple health-care and medical problems that often complicate nursing and medical treatment plans. Older adults statistically have at least three chronic diseases or health-care problems by the time they reach 65 years of age. In contrast, younger people frequently see a physician or enter a hospital with a single health problem.

This chapter provides information in the following four areas:

- The differences between the acute and chronic states of a problem or medical diagnosis. More emphasis is placed on problems related to chronic rather than acute situations because of the frequency of chronic problems in older adults.

▲ PRIORITY SETTING 14.1

This chapter provides an excellent explanation of chronic disease. The priority here is for you to focus on the chronic disease information and learn and understand it. Because you will spend 75% of your career caring for older adults and because older adults statistically (on average) have three chronic diseases, you need to know about them. Learn the information in this chapter and build on it as you spend time in clinical areas. Ask questions of other nurses and the older persons with chronic diseases. Learn to understand how the diseases affect older people and their families, learn how to manage the illnesses, and learn how to assist the older person in managing the diseases because they (the diseases) are there to stay.

- The differences between nursing care for acute and chronic medical conditions. For more detail regarding the acute phase of illness, the student is referred to the many texts that are available to explain signs and symptoms of the acute phase of medically diagnosed illnesses.
- The effect of the normal changes of aging on medical symptoms. These symptoms are discussed in terms of the specific effect that aging has on a health problem.
- Application of the concept of gerotranscendence to common medical illnesses of older people.

Five body systems have been selected for discussion in this chapter. The changes in these systems are commonly found with older adults in any setting. Frequently seen medical conditions are included as examples of the disorders that affect each system. Often these conditions do not occur alone. For example, two or more cardiac problems may be present at the same time, and arthritis often occurs with other chronic conditions.

ACUTE VERSUS CHRONIC CONDITIONS

Acute medical problems develop rapidly. The person experiencing an acute problem notices symptoms for a few minutes to less than a month. The acute symptoms may be caused by some previous chronic condition, such as congestive heart failure (CHF), or by a change in body function that is related to aging. For example, changes in kidney function could induce acute renal failure. An acute problem also may be due to an infection.

Traditionally, chronic conditions exist for at least 6 months and create some disruption in biological, sociological, and psychological function. Examples include physical and emotional conditions that are not limited to older people. Chronic health problems are common, however, in older adults. Approximately 80% of older people who live in the community have at least three chronic conditions. Arthritis, heart conditions (including hypertension), and sensory changes occur most frequently.

There are numerous ways to distinguish between acute and chronic medical conditions. Acute conditions may be thought of as requiring more immediate and often more sophisticated or technical levels of treatment. The goal with an acute condition is to cure the problem.

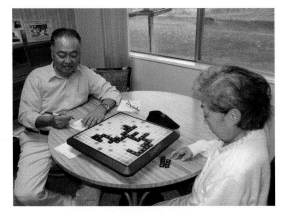

This woman has adapted to severe rheumatoid arthritis. She is unable to walk or straighten out her hands or legs, yet she lives a full and satisfying life. A major reason for her ability to manage is the support and love she receives from her family. In this picture, she is playing Scrabble with her husband. For them, it is legal to do words in both English and Japanese!

Chronic conditions develop over time and often are not noticed by the person with the problem until major deficits become manifest. These conditions tend to require more help from the informal system of caregiving, specifically from the family or a home-health nurse. Often an older adult develops a partnership with members of the informal system to gain more control over the chronic disease. Cure is not the goal with chronic conditions. From a nursing standpoint, the goal is to provide care that is helpful in managing chronic diseases. This care should be focused on assisting the older adult to function at the highest possible level in the physical, social, psychological, and spiritual arenas of life. Achievement of this goal should provide a higher quality of life for the individual and decreased morbidity (disability). An alternative goal is to work with an individual to enable him or her to die with dignity; this is a realistic goal that needs to be acknowledged when working with people who have chronic, debilitating diseases. Chapter 10, which focuses on end-of-life care in the elderly person, can assist you in understanding this goal.

Nursing care requires observation of the patient's physical functioning, which makes this one of your responsibilities. In the acute phase of illness, it is essential that the nurse note responses to medical treatments such as medications or surgery. New signs and symptoms may arise because of such treatments. All changes must be reported because the new symptoms may be critical in determining whether to continue treatment, or they may indicate complications.

Nursing care for people with chronic diseases also requires the nurse to observe the person's physical functioning. In addition, it is important to have the observations of informal caregivers. The most critical information comes from the chronically ill person's observation of personal symptoms and overall condition. For treatment to be most effective, the person must be tuned in to the body's responses to treatment or to changes in total body function.

Various stressors may exacerbate a chronic but stable disease in the short-term and in the long-term. Such stressors include uncertainty about the future, such as relocation or transition stress; starting a new treatment; or the development of an acute condition. For example, a person with emphysema may develop pneumonia, and although penicillin may cure the acute condition, the pneumonia may cause a flare-up of the previously controlled chronic emphysema.

Many nurses and other health-care workers have difficulty working with people with chronic conditions. There is a tendency to look for time lines, to place limits on how long the condition may last, or to predict when it might get worse. It is crucial for you, the licensed practical nurse (LPN), to recognize that each chronic condition has its own pattern. Some conditions, such as cancer, may get progressively worse. For a patient with a cerebrovascular accident (CVA), the recovery and return of ability depend on the part of the body affected. There is no accurate prediction or measure of recovery because of variable factors that differ from person to person. Other conditions may not change over months or years. This situation can be seen with multiple sclerosis, in which a person goes through a period of remission or absence of symptoms that lasts for a prolonged period.

A person with a chronic health problem, such as hypertension, may have to learn to cope with a disease in which there are no visible signs of pathology. Some people may not realize the disease is even present. Medications for hypertension often have side effects that cause people to stop taking their drugs. Other people stop taking their medication for hypertension when they feel good or believe the condition has been cured. This creates a very dangerous situation for the person. It can occur with physical and emotional conditions and is something that the knowledgeable nurse frequently assesses and works to deter. Chronic diseases require chronic, or long-term, treatments.

Understanding the differences between acute and chronic diseases

Older adults have both acute and chronic diseases

Acute	Chronic
Develop rapidly	Exist for at least 6 months
Need immediate care	80% of community living elders have three chronic diseases
Often, more sophisticated care	Develop over time until major deficits are manifest
Goal is to cure the problem	Require assistance from informal caregivers (family, friends)
In older adults, the acute disease treatment may exacerbate one or more chronic diseases	The goal is not cure, but management

Working with people with chronic conditions is a challenge for the nurse. It is common for people with chronic diseases to become discouraged. This type of nursing care calls on your creativity to assist the older person to conserve time and energy to participate in activities that have meaning for the individual. Fatigue should be prevented, and ways must be found to help the chronically ill person learn to cope with loss and change. Use of a self-care model in providing nursing care can help patients maintain their remaining abilities. The nurse, patient, and family form the team that is needed to encourage self-care. A crucial part of the team's function is maintaining good communication. This begins with an understanding of the past history of the older person. One part of that past history comes from a review of systems.

● REVIEW OF SYSTEMS

To determine pathology and functional ability, a review of systems is used as part of the history and physical examination. This review covers all of the body systems in an orderly fashion. One purpose of the review of systems is to uncover symptoms that may be associated with the current health problem.

Another goal is to identify chronic conditions that may have persisted for years and to learn how the person has managed those conditions over time. The review of systems also is a method of gathering data that can help in deciding on the appropriate type of treatment for each individual. For example, some medications may be inappropriate if the person has problems with falling.

The review of systems is especially useful for an older adult because:

- Older people frequently have nonspecific, atypical symptoms. The review helps to identify possible causes for present problems. It is a method of defining the usual and unusual for the individual.
- Changes of aging may affect two or more body systems simultaneously. The review can help to show how an interaction between systems occurs.
- Older people often have a complex history. The review can help to tie the past into the present problem.

For the review of systems, each system and the usual questions asked are listed. Any positive response to a question is followed by other questions to determine the extent or duration of the problem and treatment, if any. It is desirable to have information about treatments used in the past and the effectiveness of those treatments. Treatments include medications bought over-the-counter (OTC) in addition to those prescribed by a physician.

Pulmonary System

- History of frequent colds or upper respiratory infections?
- Cough? Productive or nonproductive of sputum?
- Appearance of sputum (not saliva)?
- Dyspnea, whether on exertion, changing position (orthopnea), or during the night (paroxysmal nocturnal dyspnea)?
- Immunization history (pneumococcal vaccine [Pneumovax] and influenza)?
- Exposure to anyone with tuberculosis and knowledge about the purified protein derivative (PPD) test for tuberculosis?

Cardiovascular System

- History of hypertension?
- History of murmurs, irregular heartbeat, or palpitations?
- Fainting or falls, especially when changing position?
- Chest pain (at rest or after exercising) or presence of edema?
- Easy bruising? Varicose veins? Anemia? Blood clots (if so, where)?

Gastrointestinal System

- Food and fluid intake: Typical 24-hour food intake? Number and size of glasses of water and other fluids? Who prepares the meals? Any food intolerances? Likes and dislikes? Vitamins taken? Use of alcohol or tobacco?
- Stomach or abdominal discomfort before or after meals?
- Problems with bowels and frequency of use of laxatives (what types)? Presence of hemorrhoids (any bleeding, pain, itching)?
- Nausea or vomiting (under what conditions)?

Musculoskeletal System

- Pain, stiffness, or discomfort in joints (when and in what situations)?
- Pain or cramping in muscles (when and in what situations)?
- Weakness of arms or legs? Swelling in joints? History of broken bones or other injuries to muscles or bones?
- Ability to walk? Distance traveled before stopping and reason for stopping?
- Use of assistive devices such as cane or walker (if so, under what circumstances)?
- Type of daily exercise or activity?

Genitourinary System

- Difficulty holding urine and under what conditions?
- Burning, pain, or bleeding on urination?
- Sense of fullness in bladder even after urinating?

Women

- Number of pregnancies? Any problems?
- Symptoms associated with menopause?
- Vaginal drainage? Itching? Burning?
- If sexually active, any pain or discomfort?

Men

- Nocturia? Dribbling after urinating or difficulty starting to urinate?
- If sexually active, any problems?

Neurological System

- Falls or fainting with or without dizziness? Steady or unsteady gait?

- Periods of amnesia or forgetfulness?
- Inability to hold onto objects?
- History of stroke?
- Difficulty with vision or hearing? Ask to describe.
- Loss of feeling or numbness in legs or arms?
- Headaches?

Endocrine System

- History of increased thirst, urination, or hunger?
- Dry skin, loss of hair, or thinning of hair?
- Intolerance to either heat or cold?

This review of systems provides only a base-line of information. As a physical examination is performed, the patient frequently remembers other symptoms or events to be added to the history. Often, the first contact with any patient does not provide all the information that may contribute to an understanding of the patient's health problems. The person may believe that symptoms were not important at the time, or the symptoms may simply have been forgotten, so the review remains incomplete. Consequently, the review of systems is always left open for additional information that may help with the planning and the continuity of care.

⬤ CHRONIC ILLNESSES COMMONLY FOUND IN OLDER ADULTS

This section provides some background infor-mation about chronic conditions frequently found in older adults. The primary focus is on continuation of care rather than on immediate treatment and nursing care.

Cardiovascular Conditions

Coronary Artery Disease

The term *coronary artery disease* (CAD) indi-cates that the heart muscle is not receiving a blood supply adequate to meet its needs. CAD includes angina pectoris, myocardial ischemia and infarction, arrhythmias, CHF, valvular diseases, and hypertension. Examples of three of these conditions are discussed to show how some of the changes of aging may compound a person's ability to manage the condition. The first example includes angina and myocardial infarction (MI).

A heart attack (MI) may be the first indica-tion of CAD for an older person. This condition is found in men and women older than 65 years. The mortality rate for adults older than 70 years is about twice the rate for younger individuals. Cardiovascular disease is the leading cause of death and disability in older adults. For an older person, the symptoms of MI are often atypical. Instead of chest pain, there may be delirium or a change in behavior, fainting, stroke, dyspnea, or gastrointestinal symptoms such as nausea and vomiting. Chest pain occurs even less often in a person older than 85 years.

Because of the atypical symptoms, the diag-nosis of myocardial ischemia or MI may be difficult to make in older people. The electrocar-diogram (ECG) may not be as specific in diagnosing MI in older people as in younger people because of age-related changes such as ventricular hypertrophy. The cardiac enzymes, especially troponin, may not be elevated as much as in a younger person because of decreased muscle mass. Younger people usually have a more extensive MI, however, because of lack of collateral circulation. Nurses who work with older people need to be alert to the possibility of MI even when the usual signs do not appear.

Medical management for an older person is essentially the same as that for a younger person. Coronary artery bypass surgery has been shown to be effective in older adults. Decreasing risk factors such as obesity, smok-ing, and hypertension also helps decrease the probability of a heart attack. One goal of medical care is to avoid complications. CHF, arrhythmias, thrombi and emboli, and extension of the infarction are common complications. These may be prevented by close monitoring during the acute phase after MI. The use of beta blockers, lipid-lowering therapies, and aspirin helps to decrease mortality.

Some people restrict their activity after MI and become less capable of self-care. Decreased activity can lead to *deconditioning*. This decon-ditioning may compound aging changes in the musculoskeletal system, such as decreased muscle mass and decreased muscle strength. The ability to balance activity and rest to avoid inca-pacity requires a strong cooperative effort among the patient, family members, and health-care personnel. Referral to cardiac rehabilitation may help the person to identify individual abilities and limitations and avoid deconditioning. Older people are capable of recovery and may return to their usual lifestyles. Sometimes alterations in lifestyle may be necessary, however.

Congestive Heart Failure

Most patients with CHF are older than 60 years. CHF is defined as the inability of the heart to pump blood to meet the metabolic demands of the body. The common causes of CHF in older adults include hypertension, heart valve calcification, MI, CAD, cardiac hypertrophy, arrhythmias, thyroid disease, and anemia. An acute episode of CHF can be brought on by treatment for other conditions. Overaggressive intravenous fluid replacement (too much, too fast) and medications such as beta blockers are common causes of CHF. The symptoms of dyspnea and frequent nighttime wakening often lead to fatigue and decreased activity.

The goal of medical treatment is to reduce the workload on the heart and improve the ability of the heart to pump. Because patients with CHF have a weakened heart muscle, the pathology of CHF is decreased cardiac output. The use of drugs, such as digoxin, is a primary treatment. Digoxin, which is used to strengthen the force of the contraction of the heart, is most frequently used when atrial fibrillation occurs with CHF. Some older people have taken digoxin for many years. Periodic blood level evaluation of this drug is necessary to prevent toxicity and ensure that the drug is still needed. Other drugs include diuretics and drugs that increase dilation of the blood vessels. A side effect with these drugs is falling, which results from a decrease in blood pressure with change in position (orthopnea).

Nursing responsibility in chronic CHF includes monitoring the older person for:

- Presence of edema in feet, legs, sacral area, lungs, abdomen, and around the eyes. Look for increased fluid in any dependent parts and weight gain, especially when appetite is decreased. Often, people gain weight because of fluid retention but lose actual body weight. This type of weight gain and loss can lead to decreased endurance and increased workload on the heart. A weight record is helpful to monitor fluctuations daily to weekly, depending on severity or level of control of CHF.

- Blood pressure changes with change in position (postural hypotension). Blood pressure and pulse should be checked after 5 to 10 minutes of rest in a flat position, again within 1 minute of sitting, and again 1 minute after standing. Also ask the person whether dizziness occurs with these changes. A decrease of 20 mm Hg in blood pressure on changing position is significant. Patients need to be taught how to control balance before walking and how to use support equipment, such as a cane. The medication may need to be changed, or the patient may not be drinking sufficient fluid. Postural hypotension may result from a physiological change of aging in which the body does not respond to pressure changes. This is due to changes in pressure receptors in blood vessels. The cause of postural hypotension may be any or all three of the preceding possibilities.

- Maintaining a balance between rest and activity. This balance is crucial to prevent fatigue and accompanying inability in self-care. Most patients find that they benefit from a daily routine that allows for short periods of activity followed by rest. During the acute phase of CHF, activity should be minimal. An example is sitting in a chair for 30 minutes three times a day. As cardiac function improves, increased activity is possible. The activity level should be determined by the physician and closely monitored by the nurse.

- Maintaining an adequate diet to prevent loss of lean body mass. The patient's appetite may be decreased, or fatigue may be so great that five instead of three meals a day are needed. A reduced-salt diet (2 to 3 g/day) may be prescribed, although many people do well on a diet with no added salt and no foods that are high in salt. Decreased sodium intake may make food unappetizing and can cause anorexia. Use of spices instead of salt (e.g., cinnamon, thyme, lemon) and commercial salt substitutes may improve the taste of some food.

◗ POINT OF INTEREST

When digoxin doses are too high, a common side effect is confusion. This often is not recognized as a cardiac symptom and consequently is not always treated.

Hypertension

A blood pressure greater than 160/90 mm Hg is regarded as hypertension (HTN) for any age group. HTN is the leading cause of death and morbidity in the United States. The prevalence of HTN increases with age, and about 40% of adults older than age 65 are affected. Men, African Americans, and obese people tend to be at greater risk. Most research now supports the need to treat a systolic blood pressure greater than 160 mm Hg and diastolic blood pressure greater than 90 mm Hg. Several factors associated with aging may predispose an older person to HTN. Stiffening of the aorta, increased cardiac afterload (the force needed to pump blood from the ventricle), and increased peripheral vascular resistance may be present. Changes in the baroreceptor reflexes may be indicated by fluctuation of blood pressure during physical activity or emotional experiences. Other causes of HTN may include changes in the kidney and endocrine system secondary to aging.

Blood pressure measurement is one of the most important parts of the physical examination. Following are some guidelines for obtaining an accurate blood pressure reading in older adults:

- Allow the person to sit quietly for 3 to 5 minutes before taking a blood pressure reading. Older adults, especially when physically deconditioned, require more time to adjust to a baseline function even after a minor stress, such as walking into an examination area.
- Select the cuff size appropriate to the person: the regular adult cuff may be too large or too small. Use of a pediatric cuff for people with small arms and a large adult or leg cuff for obese people is essential for accuracy. The cuff should be about 20% larger than the diameter of the arm.
- An auscultatory gap is often found with older adults. To avoid an inaccurate systolic reading, palpate the brachial artery and inflate the cuff in increments of 10 mm Hg while palpating. When the pulse disappears, inflate the cuff another 20 to 30 mm Hg, and then listen for the sounds as you deflate the cuff. The first sound may be followed by a gap of 20 to 30 mm Hg before the sounds are again heard.
- If this is the first contact with the older adult, take readings on both arms to determine whether there are differences of more than 10 mm Hg. For example, if there is an arteriosclerotic plaque in the right subclavian artery, the blood pressure is lower in the right arm. The correct reading is then obtained from the left arm.
- Determination of orthostatic hypotension is needed, especially when monitoring the effect of antihypertensive drugs. (See previous note under Congestive Heart Failure regarding technique.)
- If you have difficulty hearing the last sound for diastolic pressure, take the reading of a muffled sound as diastolic pressure. Make a note of this in your recording. One technique that can facilitate the diastolic reading is to elevate the arm above heart level.

Another nursing-care technique for someone with HTN is monitoring medications to ensure the maintenance of regular doses. This monitoring also will tell you the person's willingness to continue taking the drugs. The usual reason for a person to discontinue the drug or alter the dosage schedule is the experience of unpleasant side effects. The specific side effect varies with the class of drug. Examples of side effects that may cause the person to stop taking the drug include constipation, drowsiness, depression, cough, dizziness related to orthostatic hypotension, anorexia, and, in men, impotence. In addition, some people stop taking diuretic medications if frequent trips to the bathroom interfere with their sleep or their daily activities.

When a person has had a consistent systolic pressure reading of 150 mm Hg or greater and then has a normal reading (120/80 mm Hg), further checking may be required. The decrease may be caused by side effects of medication. It also could be an indication of a heart attack. The usual symptoms of MI may not be present, but the person would be more fatigued and have less strength or energy to do things.

Teaching good health habits related to diet and exercise is also a nursing function. Some people may be placed on dietary restrictions, such as no added salt, reduced cholesterol, or reduced calories. Severe restrictions usually are not needed, but basic teaching is needed to alert older adults and their families to factors that can help control blood pressure. If these measures are successful, medications may not be needed.

Efforts to reduce blood lipid levels in people older than 75 years of age are still considered questionable by some practitioners. Measurements of fasting cholesterol and high-density lipoprotein (HDL) are minimal laboratory tests to determine lipid levels. An older person may have more difficulty than a younger person in changing a lifetime pattern of eating. Use of a food diary may help with this change. Periodic contacts with nursing staff should check not only adherence to the diet, but also the person's reaction to the changes that have occurred. Emotional support provided in this way increases compliance with difficult dietary changes.

The use of regular exercise in controlling blood pressure is just as important for older people as it is for younger people. The physician may prescribe aerobic exercise, especially walking, as an adjunct to control blood pressure and weight. Regular exercise may be just as beneficial as medication for some people. When people do not exercise regularly, they tend to start too fast. Instructions should be given for a minimum of 5 minutes of warm-up and stretching and a gradual increase in the amount of time spent in aerobic walking. Usually, the older adult can start with 10 minutes of aerobic walking two to three times a week. The time and frequency of aerobic activity can gradually be increased by 5 to 10 minutes each week. The person should be taught how to take a pulse to ensure that the pulse does not go beyond that person's maximum limit during the peak workout time. The maximum is based on resting heart rate and age. A cool-down period of at least 5 minutes after exercise also is needed.

Peripheral Vascular Disease

The maintenance of good vascular supply to the extremities is crucial for older people. When blood vessels are affected by arteriosclerosis and aging changes, the nutrition of tissues is impaired. Arteries and veins may be involved at the same time. A depleted oxygen supply results with retention of waste products in the body.

Evidence of decreased vascular function is indicated by skin ulcers resulting from venous stasis. Venous stasis is marked by changes in the skin, such as thinning and dryness or overgrowth of epidermis. A permanent brown discoloration may appear because of small hemorrhages (petechiae). Any slight trauma to the area can break the skin and begin an ulceration. Prompt treatment is needed to avoid infection. Even when an ulcer is healed, the area is always at risk for further breakdown. Concern about the condition may cause the person to limit activity. Functional problems—for example, limited ability to ambulate—may result.

Prevention of further trauma and interference with blood supply is the guide for nursing intervention. Patients can be taught to:

- Keep the legs elevated when sitting, unless arterial insufficiency is also present.
- Avoid constricting clothing, such as hose with elastic bands.
- Avoid extremes of temperature (hot or cold).
- Keep the legs uncrossed when sitting.
- Use cotton socks or stockings and properly fitted shoes.
- Report any break in the skin as soon as possible.
- Avoid applying tape or any irritants (salves) to the area.

Neurological Conditions

Cerebrovascular Accident

The third leading cause of death for older adults is a CVA or stroke. A stroke occurs when the blood flow to part of the brain is stopped. There are two ways this can happen. First, when a blood clot gets stuck in one of the vessels that goes to the brain, the person has a stroke at that site. Second, if a blood vessel in the brain bursts, that also is a stroke. Both situations cause the blood to cease flowing.

Strokes happen despite increasing emphasis on prevention. One risk factor for stroke is advanced age. Other risk factors include hypertension, diabetes mellitus, transient ischemic attacks, and heart disease such as MI or CHF. Each year, 160,000 people in the United States die as a result of a stroke. The mortality rate has declined over the past decade; however, about 40% of people who have a stroke die within 1 month. About 60% of people who survive must cope with some disability and physical impairment. Such coping may involve sensory or motor abilities, memory, or language and other communication skills.

Strokes can be classified in several ways, as follows:

- *Type:* Thrombosis (large vessel or small vessel), embolism, or hemorrhage
- *Location of ischemia or infarction:* The posterior or anterior circulation, such as the brainstem, pons, cerebellum, medulla, or cortex
- *Rate of development of the stroke:* Slow (sometimes called stroke in progress) or sudden and massive
- *Brain hemisphere:* Right or left hemisphere, or dominant or nondominant hemisphere

The last classification is used herein for the discussion of treatment and continuity of care.

After the patient has been stabilized, usually in the hospital, planning for discharge and follow-up care is needed. Rehabilitation should begin as soon as possible, preferably in the hospital. Such an early beginning helps prevent the development of some of the physical complications of a CVA. Two common complications are contractures and skin breakdown. Continued care aids in regaining prestroke abilities, providing emotional support, and maintaining physiological defense mechanisms, such as resistance to infections.

Classification of stroke on the basis of the involved hemisphere is important because it points to the type of nursing care required. The goals for care and the way the nurse interacts with the patient are particularly affected. Frequently, a patient with a right hemisphere stroke exhibits the following characteristics:

- Has problems accurately determining level of abilities
- Has problems in learning because of a shortened attention span
- Is easily distracted from tasks
- Is unable to transfer learning from one situation to another
- May show poor judgment about the lack of ability that occurred because of the CVA and take risks leading to injury
- Is unable to determine distance or rate of movement of people or objects because of poor spatial perception
- Retains language abilities and can convince others of abilities that do not exist, such as stating, "I can walk," when in reality the person cannot safely do so
- May have visible deficits such as weakness or paralysis on the left, or nondominant, side of the body

In contrast, a patient with a left hemisphere stroke tends to have more visible disabilities, such as:

- Problems with language and physical function
- A need for adaptation of all activities of daily living if the dominant hand is affected
- A tendency to be more cautious in behavior than a patient who sustained a right hemisphere stroke—the tendency is to take few risks and deny the extent of one's abilities (rather than extent of disability)
- A tendency to engage in repetitive behavior, such as washing the same body part over and over again
- Weakness or paralysis on the right, or dominant, side of the body

The goal of care for a patient with a left-hemisphere CVA is to improve his or her physical ability. Physical, occupational, and speech therapies should be included as part of the interdisciplinary team plan of care. Fatigue may require scheduled rest times, but a limit should be placed on the length of time allowed for rest.

Other losses also occur that are independent of the hemisphere involved. Neglect of one side of the body may first be exhibited in failure to eat food placed on one side of the tray

Patients who have had a right-hemisphere stroke are a challenge for you, the LPN, and the family. As the nurse, you have to help the patient and family cope with many frustrations. A major one is conflict between the patient and caregivers that may result from the patient's denial of disability or from impulsive behavior (acting without thinking). The patient may be totally unaware of the effect of this behavior, and the family must be constantly alert to the potential for injury to self or others. This type of behavior may persist throughout the remainder of the person's life.

or by failure to turn toward a visitor. Homonymous hemianopsia (loss of vision in the left or right visual field) (Fig. 14.1) or bitemporal hemianopsia (loss of the peripheral or temporal area of vision) may cause each of these symptoms. Therapy is to teach the person consciously to look at a "total picture" of self and surroundings.

Prevention of complications is a major component of post stroke care. After a stroke, a person is frequently at risk for infections (respiratory and urinary), falls, malnutrition, repeated strokes, and deconditioning secondary to lack of activity. Prevention of complications includes all of the following:

- At a minimum, administering immunizations for pneumonia, influenza, and tetanus
- Keeping a routine for urination
- Monitoring fluid and food intake
- Monitoring medications
- Maintaining mobility and independence at optimal levels

Older people tend to drink inadequate amounts of fluid. Teaching the older adult and family members ways to ensure consumption of 1500 to 2000 mL of water per day is useful. Some people fill a quart bottle with water every morning and drink from that throughout the day, periodically refilling it. When encouraging fluids, however, be sure the person does not have difficulty swallowing. People with swallowing difficulties after a stroke frequently have more difficulty with fluids than they do with swallowing solids.

The person's appetite may be affected by an inability to use a knife and fork. Occupational therapy should help with instruction on new ways for self-feeding. Meal plans may need to be altered to help the person lose weight or control sodium or cholesterol levels. Medications often are used to control HTN, cardiac arrhythmias, and blood clotting. When a person begins to feel better, it is common to believe some medications are no longer needed. Compliance with medications must be frequently assessed. Accurate determination of blood pressure in the home or physician's office is essential. Listening to the apical heartbeat instead of relying on radial pulse is advisable. Laboratory work to follow prothrombin time and international normalized ratio (PT/INR) is critical (see Chapter 21). Following a set schedule to maintain a balance between rest and activity helps to minimize fatigue and to promote activity. Many older people who live at home may need continued follow-up after discharge from the hospital or nursing home. Home health care is important for the older adult to maintain optimal health.

Homonymous hemianopsia

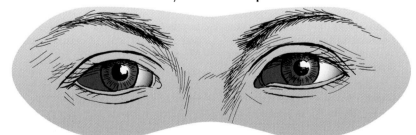

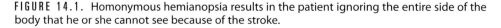

FIGURE 14.1. Homonymous hemianopsia results in the patient ignoring the entire side of the body that he or she cannot see because of the stroke.

CRITICALLY EXAMINE THE FOLLOWING

It is important for you to understand clearly the difference between a right-sided and left-sided CVA. Take the time to outline a teaching plan for the family members (spouse and adult children) of a person with a right-sided CVA. There are some very important concepts that need to be taught to these family members. How can you do the teaching without causing them more distress? Write a teaching plan to submit to the faculty person. Title it at the top and put your name on it. Then make two columns. One could be "Concepts to Be Taught," and the second could be "Method of Teaching." Select three of the problems listed in the text under right-sided CVA and plan a creative and sensitive way to teach them to the patient and family.

Parkinson's Disease

Parkinson's disease (PD) is found more often in men than women. The condition can begin as early as the mid-40s, but it usually appears between 60 and 80 years of age. This is a chronic, progressive disease that is marked by slow movement, rigidity, unstable posture, and tremors at rest. There are some known causes for Parkinson-like symptoms, but the cause of PD is unknown.

The primary treatment for PD is medication. This condition also requires active involvement of the patient affected by the disease and the family. Education of the patient and family should be a primary objective for every nurse. Important information to be taught includes the following:

- Defining the disease and its problems
- Side effects and individual reactions to medications
- Methods to promote independence and activity while providing for safety

Some people with PD become very depressed and withdraw from social contacts. The person with PD can help to prevent depression by identifying times when fatigue occurs. The beneficial effect of medication may "wear off" close to the time for the next dose. Activity planned around these times of fatigue and decreased drug effect would help to maintain physical and social function.

As the disease progresses, the person is at risk for several complications. Infections, gastrointestinal problems, and injury from falls are most common. Respiratory infections occur when swallowing is affected. Aspiration of food and fluids can lead to pneumonia and malnutrition. Urinary tract infections may result from urinary retention and from inadequate fluid intake. Eye infections may result from seborrhea (a dandruff-like skin problem).

Constipation is a common gastrointestinal problem resulting from a lack of bulk-type foods and fluids. Problems swallowing can lead to anorexia. Nausea and anorexia are common side effects of the medications. Consumption of semisolid foods or those with the consistency of pudding and foods with a high water content, such as fruits, may help.

A person with PD tends to be physically unstable. Many falls can be prevented by the use of a cane or walker. Safety devices should be installed in the home, such as handholds in the bathroom and banisters in the stairway. Floor coverings and furniture should enable a barrier-free route for walking. Shoes that fit well, are lightweight, support the foot, and do not cause either slipping or too much friction are needed.

The goal is to maintain the person's function for as long as possible. A secondary goal is to support the family as they help to manage the daily activities of the elderly person. Coping with the changes that usually occur is difficult for most families. Referral to support groups and helping with problem-solving are two important nursing functions.

Sensory Losses

Many adults find that visual and hearing losses begin around 50 years of age. The eyeball changes shape for most people so that they become farsighted and require glasses for near vision, such as when reading. This aging change is referred to as *presbyopia*. Changes in the shape of the lens and a yellow discoloration may alter the person's ability to focus and to distinguish colors.

Three common pathological visual conditions experienced by older people include cataracts, glaucoma, and macular degeneration. Clouding of the lens, resulting in cataracts, is the most common pathological visual condition. Blurred vision and difficulty with nighttime driving may be the first clues of cataract formation. Current techniques for 1-day surgery have relieved the problem for most people who experience cataracts. Other eye conditions require more adjustment, however.

Glaucoma is a major cause of blindness and results from increased pressure in the eye that destroys the optic nerve. Central vision is usually retained, but peripheral vision is lost. People speak of having "tunnel vision." This condition is generally controlled with medications instilled in the eye daily. All people older than 40 years of age should have a yearly examination for increased intraocular pressure (>22 mm Hg).

Macular degeneration destroys the point of maximum sight—the macula. Blindness does not result, but the person loses central vision. Peripheral vision is retained around that central blind spot. Increased magnification helps many people. Some people learn to adjust head positions to use peripheral vision. Use of zinc and vitamin B supplements has been effective for some people in decreasing the extent of this degeneration.

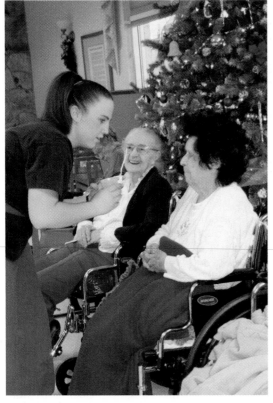

These women reside in a nursing home and have multiple chronic diseases. Both of them have visual losses. The first woman is blind, and the second woman is legally blind but can see shadows and shapes. With the holistic care they receive in the nursing home, they are safe and satisfied with their lives.

Hearing loss increases with aging and is noted more among men than women. This condition may be due to an aging change called *presbycusis* that occurs without previous injury or other known cause. Hearing difficulties have social and emotional consequences because communication with others suffers. Many people tend to talk more loudly to individuals who are hard of hearing. Speaking loudly results in sounds becoming more muddled, so that comprehension is worse. Some people are helped by the use of hearing aids, whereas others cannot be helped in this way because of the type or extent of hearing loss. Adjustment to a hearing aid may be difficult because of lack of finger dexterity. The inability to tune out distracting noises also may discourage individuals from using the aid.

People with visual or hearing loss should be informed about available services. Centers for the visually impaired in large cities can provide materials to assist people with using their remaining vision. Often, people can be taught ways to compensate for the loss. Audio amplifiers are available for hearing-impaired individuals. These devices can provide greater amplification and are especially useful in open-room areas.

Following are general guidelines for nurses working with visually impaired or hearing-impaired older adults:

- Face the person before beginning to speak. Avoid sitting in front of a window or light so there will not be any glare. Glare reduces the ability of a person to read lips.
- Speak clearly and slowly so that words are distinct.
- Try not to exaggerate your speaking voice.
- If possible, use a low pitch when speaking.
- Touch the person to indicate where you are.
- Identify yourself by name and explain why you are there.
- Keep the patient's glasses and hearing aid clean.
- Refer to local, state, or national resources for assistance (e.g., centers for the visually impaired, audiologists, Lions Club for help with glasses).

Pulmonary System

Chronic Obstructive Pulmonary Disease

Chronic obstructive pulmonary disease (COPD) is a pathological condition resulting from exposure to irritants (especially tobacco smoke) and is not limited to older people. Chronic bronchitis, asthma, and emphysema are included in this very broad category. COPD is the fourth leading cause of death for people older than 65 years. The primary signs and symptoms are cough and shortness of breath. The lungs become hyperinflated, and the diaphragm flattens. The person must use abdominal and intercostal muscles (accessory muscles) to breathe. Use of these muscles requires more energy than use of the diaphragm.

Some older adults who develop a barrel chest appear to have developed COPD. This appearance may be due to increased residual volume of air because of destruction of the alveolar walls. In this condition, there is less lung surface for diffusion of gases. Alternatively, the person may have a severe kyphosis of the thorax. This condition should not be confused with COPD.

Different forms of COPD have distinct symptoms; however, the end result for all forms is chronic lung disease that has a strong negative impact on physiological and emotional function. Often, there is one event, usually an infection, that causes the person to recognize the chronic nature of the condition. There is no typical pattern to the disease process except that COPD is progressive, and serious complications do occur, especially repeated infections. Hypoxemia may result with any form of COPD.

The adjustments that a person with COPD has to make in lifestyle, habits, and work can be overwhelming. Prevention of complications is the primary goal of long-term care. Each person (and family member or significant other, when available) needs to have knowledge about the disease process and how to aid in self-care. Teaching self-care includes the following:

- Ways to prevent infections with balanced diet, balanced rest and activity, avoidance of situations in which spread of infection may occur, and use of influenza and pneumococcal immunizations
- How to recognize signs and symptoms of infection, such as increased cough, change in sputum, and decreased tolerance for activity
- Instruction in self-medication, including the use of oxygen, the purpose of each medication, and side effects to be expected
- How to keep track of the medication schedule and medications to avoid, such as cough suppressants
- Explaining the need for adequate hydration (2000 mL/day unless other conditions, such as heart disease, rule this out)

- How to distinguish between anxiety and airway obstruction, and measures to control both
- How to develop a support group or how to locate one

Musculoskeletal System

Osteoarthritis and Degenerative Joint Disease

Osteoarthritis is the major chronic condition reported by older adults. The incidence of arthritis increases with aging. Destruction of the joint cartilage occurs, often followed by overproduction of tissue at the joint margins. The result is a visible enlargement of the joint, especially in the knees and fingers. The cause of the most common form, degenerative joint disease or primary osteoarthritis, is unknown. Inflammation of the joint usually does not occur. Primary arthritis is permanent and progressive. It also can fluctuate or vary in intensity, however. Secondary osteoarthritis develops from a combination of physical stress on joints and a medical problem such as diabetes or inflammation. Gout and rheumatoid arthritis are examples of this form.

A patient with degenerative joint disease usually reports joint stiffness in the morning with limitation of motion and muscle aches, cramps, or spasms. The extent of these symptoms varies from person to person. Some people have very little joint pain or stiffness. Others may experience joint pain most of the day. There is no specific treatment.

The goals for treatment include the following:

- Control of pain with nonsteroidal medications, such as ibuprofen
- Weight loss if the person is overweight
- Maintain activity
- Cope with physical and lifestyle changes

To reach these goals, it is usually helpful for the person to understand the nature of the condition and to avoid the use of ineffective ("quack") treatments. It also is important to learn to identify events or activities that increase and decrease pain to promote self-care.

Another crucial aspect of care is to teach the older adult to use medications to prevent pain rather than to control pain after it has started, that is, take pain medication before activity or on a routine basis. Meal planning is another challenge. Meals should meet but not exceed caloric needs. (This can be a problem for people with low income, minimal sources of emotional support, or lack of energy or motivation to change eating habits.) The nurse should teach the patient and family to plan activities around the time of day when the person feels best and there is less pain.

A physical therapist can teach the proper use of moist heat, physical therapy exercises, and equipment (e.g., a walker) to decrease pain or stress on joints. A walker or other equipment may need to be examined to ensure that it is appropriate for the person's needs. The nurse should focus on teaching the older adult self-expression to maintain self-esteem, decrease depression, and promote social interaction. Referral to an arthritis support group and use of teaching materials from such a group may be helpful to older persons and their families.

Osteoporosis

The term "brittle bones" has been used to describe osteoporosis. Actually the bone is not brittle, but bone mass is decreased because bone is reabsorbed faster than it is formed. This situation results in greater risk for fractures. There are two forms of osteoporosis: type I and type II. Type I osteoporosis is found primarily in women after menopause and is thought to be related to lack of estrogen. White women with fair complexions and women (white and Asian) with small body build are especially at risk. Type II osteoporosis can occur in both sexes with increasing age. (See Box 14.1 for other risk factors.)

Type I affects the spongy (trabecular) portion of bone, such as the ends of long bones. Type II affects compact bone found in the middle portion (diaphysis) of long bones and trabecular bone. Regardless of type, the person may be unaware that he or she has osteoporosis until minimal trauma results in a fracture of a rib or wrist.

BOX 14.1 Risk Factors for Osteoporosis

Positive family history for osteoporosis
Inactivity or immobility
Low calcium intake (<800 mg/day)
Gastric or small bowel resection
Smoking
High intake of alcohol
High intake of caffeine
Long-term use of corticosteroids or anticonvulsant drugs
Hyperparathyroidism
Low body weight

A major goal when working with someone with osteoporosis is to maintain safety. Injury resulting from a fall, especially a hip fracture, is one of the most frequent consequences. The resulting loss of mobility and restriction of activity create emotional problems and place the person at risk for other physical problems, such as skin breakdown and constipation. In addition, treatment is long and costly.

A major nursing responsibility is to teach the person and family to identify hazards in the home and community. Simple techniques that can be used to help maintain safety are the use of grab bars by the toilet in the tub or shower and the use of a sliding board or tub chair for bathing. The house should be carefully examined for safety hazards such as "trippers" (e.g., scatter rugs, electric cords, uneven pavement, and pets). The person should be taught to maintain postural balance by rising slowly and avoiding sudden movement or hyperextension of joints such as neck and hip. Another area in which teaching is beneficial is the identification of risk factors—for example, limiting use of caffeine sources to one a day. Limiting the use of tobacco and alcohol may help decrease the progression of osteoporosis. Increasing the consumption of sources of calcium, such as fortified low-fat milk, yogurt, and cottage cheese, also increases the intake of vitamin D. Do not recommend cottage cheese to someone with CHF because of the high sodium content.

Metabolic and Endocrine Diseases

Type 2 Diabetes

Type 2 diabetes is more common in older adults than type 1 diabetes. Although the pancreas continues to produce insulin, the amount is insufficient for carbohydrate metabolism. The reason for this pathology is unclear. Some researchers believe that the body becomes resistant to insulin as the percentage of body fat increases and lean body mass (muscle) decreases with aging. This belief has been supported by the effect of weight loss on control of hyperglycemia.

There is no cure for type 2 diabetes, but it usually can be controlled with diet alone. When the person is overweight, a reduced caloric intake coupled with regular exercise is recommended. Oral hypoglycemic drugs may be used if control is not achieved with diet and exercise. Some older adults may need insulin when control is not achieved. In most instances, medications should be avoided because they may cause hypoglycemia.

In older people, type 2 diabetes manifests with different symptoms from those of younger people. Older people tend to have anorexia, dehydration, confusion or delirium, incontinence, and decreased vision. In addition, it is not unusual for the older person to have high triglyceride and cholesterol levels along with high glucose level.

The usual precautions for diabetes are needed for people with type 2 diabetes. The types of complications associated with diabetes mellitus, such as skin lesions and renal and neurological problems, also may be typical of aging. Teaching about skin care, protection of the feet, periodic eye examination, dental care, and recognition of infections is just as important for people with type 2 diabetes as it is for people with type 1 diabetes who require insulin. The nurse also needs to teach older adults with type 2 diabetes how to follow a regular schedule involving medication, diet, exercise, and blood glucose monitoring.

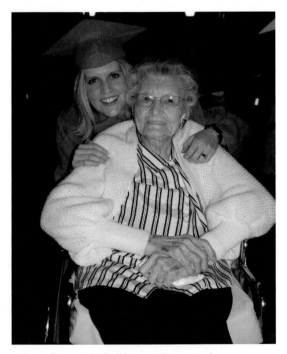

Older adults with diabetes mellitus can live reasonably normal lives if they are willing to attend to the details of managing their disease. If they are unable to do so, they need a caregiver to manage the disease for them. This woman was able to attend her granddaughter's college graduation because of her determination to live well with diabetes.

Hypothyroidism

Hypothyroidism is common especially among older women. The presence of a low thyroid level is often overlooked because of the similarity between the symptoms of hypothyroidism and characteristics of aging. Symptoms of hypothyroidism, which are thought to be typical among older adults, are fatigue, memory loss, slowing of thought processes, slowed speech, intolerance to cold, loss of equilibrium, constipation, and sleep apnea.

The current belief is that older people benefit from treatment with thyroxine, even if they have subclinical hypothyroidism. Caregivers often attribute behavioral changes in an older person only to aging. Even small deficits of thyroxine or small increases in thyroid-stimulating hormone can result in slowed reactions. This should be a clear safety alert for every nurse.

Although hypothyroidism is common among older women, the symptoms often are ignored because they are confused with characteristics of aging. People must be taught how to recognize signs and symptoms of overmedication or undermedication for this disease. It is especially important to monitor respiratory and cardiac function. People usually begin to notice improved function within a few days of starting treatment.

GEROTRANSCENDENCE

Each of the diseases discussed in this chapter requires a great deal of commitment and courage to manage and live with successfully. The people who are most likely to commit to self-management are people who have embraced the concept of gerotranscendence. Most individuals do not know about the concept and don't go about saying, "Look at me, I have achieved gerotranscendence!" Instead, gerotranscendence is something that comes from within after living a life that successfully follows Erikson's developmental stages. A person who has gone through Erikson's stages has managed life well and with successful human interaction. Such individuals have loved and been loved, have avoided despair despite life's tragedies, and have been industrious and successful. Consequently, such people are ready for the losses of old age and the inevitability of death. I have heard many psychologists say that the family and friends who can talk about death openly are the ones who are very close to each other. This comfort with oneself and with the inevitability of death is one aspect of gerotranscendence.

An older adult who has succeeded in Erikson's developmental plan can accept death because of a life well lived. The individual generally can continue living with singular or multiple acute and chronic diseases because there are few regrets in his or her life. Such people accept illness and work to manage it; they also accept the inevitability of death and plan for it.

I have a friend who is 64 years old with multiple serious chronic diseases. Within the last 3 months, she has been diagnosed with an aggressive cancer that has spread. She is undergoing chemotherapy and will also have radiation. She has purchased a burial plot, picked out and had a head stone put into place, and written her obituary. She is affluent and is now working on her will to update it. She made a list of items that she wants to go to friends and each of her nieces and nephews. With those things done, she now plays with and makes plans to do things with her three grandchildren that include her only child and her husband. She has achieved gerotranscendence as she accepts her illnesses and the fact she will eventually die, and she has moved on to enjoy her life.

The way for older adults to achieve gerotranscendence is to have support from caring nurses like you throughout their lives. The way for you to achieve it later in your life is to be aware of Erikson's theory and apply it for yourself and to teach it to people who come into your life. It is worth the effort.

CONCLUSION

Although all of the conditions in this chapter have been discussed separately, you probably have noted that there are similarities in approaches that can be used. Involvement of the patient has been stressed throughout. The need for exercise, high-quality meals with lowered caloric intake, and prevention of complications are three common themes. The following case study serves as an example of thinking out a unified approach to the care of a person with chronic conditions.

Mrs. O. is an 82-year-old widow who has lived alone since the death of her husband last year. She was able to care for herself with all activities of daily living and had help with light house-keeping, shopping, and banking. During the past 6 months, her energy and endurance have less-ened and she has gained 10 lb. Her appetite has not changed, and her food intake is reported to be the same. Her social activities include church and contact with her four children and grandchil-dren at least once a week. Mrs. O. has been told that she has beginning cataracts in both eyes, which need to be checked every 2 months. The only symptoms she has noted are blurring of vision and increased glare, especially at night. She has been treated for several medical prob-lems, including osteoarthritis, HTN, and CHF. Her current weight is 175 lb, and her height is 5'6".

Her mental status has been intact, and she takes pride in her good memory. She has lived a successful life and seems prepared to manage her illnesses and eventual death as she talks about them freely.

An appointment with her physician resulted in hospitalization for 4 days. The following were reported on admission: BP = 187/98 mm Hg; P = 90 (apical) irregular beat; R = 24 with some dyspnea on exertion. The physician heard inspi-ratory crackling in both lower lung bases (poste-rior) up to the mid-scapular area. He made a tentative diagnosis of acute CHF with atrial fibrillation. After 4 days in the hospital, she was sent home. Digoxin (Lanoxin) was ordered at 0.25 mg q.d., and Mrs. O. was given a no-added-sodium diet and was told to decrease the amount of fat in her diet.

Discussion

1. What nursing approaches, especially monitor-ing through home care or physician office visits, can you suggest that may have helped to prevent this acute attack and hospitalization?
2. What chronic health-care problems might interfere with total self-care? What activities needing increased assistance might you anticipate?

3. What positive characteristics of Mrs. O. could be used to help her monitor her own health condition?
4. What referral sources can you think of that could be helpful to Mrs. O.?

Solution

1. You should consider the desired effect of her digoxin and any OTC drugs she may be taking. Consider the possible side effects of each, and whether there are any interactions among the medications. In addition, consider how fre-quently blood pressure needs to be checked (probably every 1 to 2 weeks after a medication is started; consider the use of a home-health nurse to monitor this or use of a senior center if there is one where blood pressure monitoring can be done). Check for edema, especially in the lower extremities, sacral area, and lungs. The area of edema depends on whether heart failure is right-sided or left-sided: Right-sided failure results in edema in the lower extremi-ties, sacral area, and abdomen; left-sided failure results in fluid in the lungs. In each case, the location of edema is related to where the

backup of pressure occurs. Monitoring also should include a review of food actually eaten: 24-hour diet recall, keeping a diary of food eaten, and looking at salt content and quantity of food and fluids. Even after a person has been on medications for some time, reviews of diet, activity, ability to take medications as pre-scribed, and ability to pay for the medications (to avoid skipping doses) are needed. One criti-cal factor to monitor is weight. People with CHF may have increases in weight because of fluid retention and not because of an increase in lean body mass. They may look healthy because of that weight, but fluid accumulation decreases their ability to function by putting more stress on the heart; cardiac output avail-able for daily activities and endurance is decreased.

Continued on page 248

2. You should discuss the effect of gradual loss of vision with possible development of cataracts. How does this affect a person's ability to take medications as ordered, to shop, to use transportation, to use the telephone, and to feel safe, especially at night? When the person also is hampered by osteoarthritis, a vicious circle may develop. Chronic pain may limit activity, which creates more stiffness and decreased range of motion. As a result, the person needs to exert more energy to do even simple housekeeping and leads a more sedentary lifestyle—so the cycle continues. When these limitations are superimposed on the chronic conditions of HTN and CHF, the person may gradually lose not only the ability but also the desire for self-care. These psychosocial losses are added to the physiological losses, and the need for assistance with activities of daily living is increased. You also might want to discuss the differences between acute and chronic pain and the effect of chronic pain on daily activities, perception of self-care abilities, involvement in social activities, and the effect that complaints about this type of pain have on social interaction.

3. One could make some assumptions that would need to be checked out about involvement with family. The case history indicates that Mrs. O. has been able to be self-sufficient, and that she has some support from family members. Family tends to be the first line of defense for older people, and only if family help is unavailable do they rely on community support or formal and governmental agencies. The history of the individual is usually a good indication of what that person will do as an older adult, provided that there is some support when problems occur. Apparently, Mrs. O. has good cognitive ability and is capable of learning. Teaching and helping her to establish a program of monitoring herself (such as weight, food intake, type of food, shopping for inexpensive food) and teaching her ways to simplify housekeeping, conserve energy, and develop a daily schedule to do energy-requiring activities when she has the most energy could be very effective. Involvement of the patient in developing this program of care is essential. Allow the patient to be part of the decision-making process.

4. Look at community resources in her area. Investigate the county agencies on aging, home-health agencies, nutrition programs, transportation resources, and availability of neighbors or friends as well as family. What help is available to assist with visual problems? Is a program available to help with control of arthritic pain, such as water aerobics? Is physical therapy available? Talk to or visit some of these resources to determine if they would help Mrs. O.

Select the best answer to each question.

1. Chronic health conditions differ from acute conditions in which of the following ways?

   a. Chronic conditions begin at an earlier age.

   b. Acute conditions tend to take time developing.

   c. Chronic conditions require active work by patient or family.

   d. Acute conditions occur only once and then disappear.

2. A review of systems helps the nurse identify which of the following?

   a. Possible interaction among health-care problems

   b. Whether the person has been taking care of his or her health properly

   c. How much the patient can remember about past health history

   d. To whom the patient should be referred based on a system need

3. When a person has right-sided neglect caused by a stroke, one way to ensure the patient's continued attention to both sides of the body is to do which of the following?

   a. Observe for equal length of both arms

   b. Observe the condition of the skin and mucous membranes on the affected side

   c. Continue to teach the patient to strengthen the unaffected side and to avoid overuse of the affected extremities

   d. Continue to approach the patient from the unaffected side to encourage communication

4. A major concern with older adults who have chronic conditions such as osteoarthritis is lack of activity. Which of the following is an unwanted result of decreased activity?

   a. Diarrhea

   b. Poor hygiene

   c. Loss of sense of touch

   d. Deconditioning

5. An older person with a chronic condition such as HTN may not take prescribed medications routinely. The main reason for this is which of the following?

   a. Inability to remember a medication schedule

   b. Lack of symptoms that indicate blood pressure is high

   c. Fear of becoming dependent on the medication

   d. Conflicting information about the purpose of the medication

15 Physiological Assessment

Kathleen R. Culliton

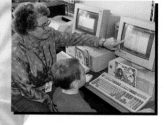

Learning Objectives

After completing this chapter, the student will be able to:

1. Describe two unique aspects of physiological assessment for older adults.
2. Describe at least three normal aging changes for each body system.
3. List two tools that are commonly used to evaluate functional status.
4. Discuss the importance of nutrition to the physiological well-being of the older adult.
5. Describe at least two important components to include in a home assessment.

INTRODUCTION

This chapter provides you with the opportunity to learn how to do a holistic assessment. Holistic assessments go beyond the physical assessment and include all aspects of the older person's life. The ability to perform a holistic assessment requires a high level of thinking and a sophisticated ability to process information. This is your chance to learn and then to do something significant for the older adults in your care. This chapter outlines the parts of a physical, functional, discharge, and wellness assessment. The interrelationship between physical health, psychological well-being, and safety (Fig. 15.1) is highlighted. You, as the licensed practical nurse (LPN), need to be prepared to make a complete and thorough holistic assessment of the older patient in an effort to improve the person's overall health and happiness.

PHYSICAL ASSESSMENT

The techniques for physical examination included in this chapter are not all-inclusive of the techniques used to conduct a total examination. This assessment outline assists you, however, in completing a head-to-toe physical examination of an older adult. It is important to remember to report any abnormal findings to the registered nurse (RN) or the physician.

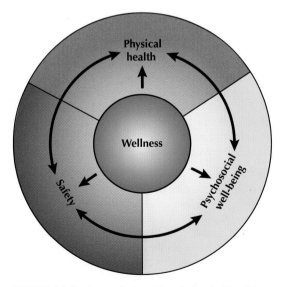

FIGURE 15.1. Interrelationship of physical health, psychosocial well-being, and safety.

HISTORY

When taking a history on any system, there is information you need to have an accurate record of the person's overall health. You need to know the person's:

- Exercise plan
- Eating patterns, including recent weight loss or gain

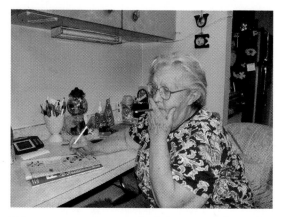

This woman smokes a pack of cigarettes a day and seldom leaves her house. Based on this information, what other questions should you ask her about her health as you take her history?

- Consumption of alcoholic beverages, caffeine, and water
- Sleep patterns
- Smoking habits, or lack of them
- Stress management techniques
- Sexual activity
- Medication record, including prescription and over-the-counter medications

After you have obtained the previously listed holistic information, you need to take a history and do an examination of the person's physiological systems. The following information serves as a guide. If you identify aspects of the assessment or history that you do not understand or know how to do, discuss your concerns in class or privately with the faculty person. I am sure you have been taught how to do a history and physical examination on middle-aged adults. What you are learning in this chapter is not extremely different, yet it includes the aspects of a history and physical examination that relate to people who are growing older. It is important that you learn to adapt from one age group to another as you work in nursing.

The following information is presented in a very didactic manner. That is for ease and efficiency in your study of the material. It is specific and straightforward; I have tried not to deter you along the way with stories or casual information. Read this material and master it! A nurse who can do an excellent history and assessment of a specialized group of people, such as older adults, is very desirable as an employee. Even more important is that you will have the skills and knowledge to "pick up" on a subtle symptom, such as "painless" heart attacks, infections without a fever, or increased white blood count (WBC), all of which many older adults have. Subtle symptoms are important to know because they may save a life.

The material in this chapter is divided into three basic skills for doing an assessment: history, inspection, and palpation.

REVIEW OF SYSTEMS

Head, Neck, and Face

History

Evaluate the older adult's medical history for head injury, increased level of stress, thyroid dysfunction, neck injury, or infection.

Physical Examination

The assessment of the head and neck is the same for older adults as for younger people.

Inspection

Observe the older individual's head position. Note the size, shape, symmetry, and proportion of the head. If it appears abnormally large or small, measure the circumference or distance around the head. Evaluate hair distribution, pattern of baldness, and dryness of the scalp. Note if lice are found in the hair. The presence of lice demands immediate intervention. Assess the face for color, symmetry, and distribution of facial hair. Evaluate facial muscles by having the older adult demonstrate different facial expressions: raise eyebrows, close eyes, puff out cheeks, smile, show teeth, and frown. Note any wrinkles or dryness of the skin. Note the size of the neck. The trachea should be aligned with the midline of the suprasternal notch. Observe for symmetry of the neck muscles. Note venous distention, involuntary muscle tension, or swelling in the neck. Assess the active range of motion (ROM) of the neck by having the older adult tilt the head backward, forward, from side to side, and in a circular motion. ROM of the neck should be completed without limitation or pain.

Palpation

Palpate the alignment of the trachea. Palpate the cervical muscles, and note any tenderness. Palpate the carotid pulses one at a time. What does the pulse feel like? Is it bounding? Weak? Or does it have a vibration-type movement? As the older adult moves the neck, palpate over the spinal area for crepitus. Crepitus is a slight grating sensation that occurs when you palpate, and it is not normal.

Abnormal findings include edema of the face (especially around eyes), involuntary facial movements (tic, tremor, droop), lack of symmetry, unusual size and contour, and tenderness.

Nose and Sinuses

History

Ask the older adult to describe any problems with the nose or sinuses. Note that epistaxis (nosebleed) is more common in older adults than in younger adults.

Physical Examination

Inspection
Observe the size, shape, and color of the nose. Note any flaring of the nostrils during breathing and any nasal drainage. Ask the older person to tilt the head so you can examine the nasal cavity for swelling, drainage, polyps, and bleeding. The nasal mucosa should be moist and dark pink. Frequently, men have an increased amount of nasal hair. Assess the movement of air through each nostril by occluding the nostril not being examined and asking the older adult to inhale and exhale through the nose. Assess the older adult's ability to smell by asking the person to identify different common smells (almond, vanilla, cinnamon, coffee). It is abnormal for the smell to be perceived differently in each nostril.

Palpation
Palpate the nose for tenderness or masses. Abnormal findings include swelling of mucosa, bleeding, discharge, perforation, polyps, and deviation of nasal septum. It is uncommon to find nasal blockage, infection, crusting, and dryness.

Eyes

History

The nurse needs to discuss the following: vision changes, pain, excessive tearing or discharge, diplopia, infection, and cataracts. Ask whether the person wears glasses. When are the glasses worn? When was the last ophthalmic examination?

Physical Examination

Inspection
Assess the external eye and visual acuity. Examine the eyes for position and alignment. Note the symmetry of the eyebrows, eyelashes, pupils, and irises. Changes in the appearance of the eyelids can be due to systemic diseases such as hyperthyroidism, myasthenia gravis, or palsy. The eyes should be evaluated for redness, swelling, and discharge. Pupils should be equal in size unless they have been unequal throughout life or have become unequal as a result of surgery or trauma. They may react more slowly to light than they did in the person's youth. Normally, the pupils are black, equal in size, round, and smooth. If the older adult has cataracts, the pupils may appear cloudy.

Before testing visual acuity, you, as the nurse, need to make sure that adequate light is available. If the older adult wears glasses, the lenses should be checked for cleanliness and alignment because those two factors can affect visual acuity. The line of the bifocals may cause double vision if the glasses are misaligned. Evaluate distant vision with a Snellen's eye chart. Test each eye separately, with and without glasses. After testing separately, test the eyes together with and without glasses. Any person with 20/40 vision or less should be referred to a physician or nurse practitioner. To test near vision, use a newspaper or other conventional reading material; measure the distance from the face to the reading material. Have an alternate plan if the person cannot read. A possibility is to have the person look at an artistic picture and describe the details to you.

Ears

History

The nurse needs to help determine the effect of hearing loss on the older person's life. Does the older adult use any corrective devices, such as amplifiers or hearing aids? The following are some questions that can be used to elicit a history: Have you experienced pain from your ears? Have you had dizziness? In what situations? How long did it last? What relieved the dizziness? Have you had any discharge from your ears? What color? What consistency? Did it have an odor? Have you experienced a sudden or rapid change in your hearing? What were you doing when it occurred? Does it come and go?

Physical Examination

Inspection
Observe the older individual in conversation. Does the person lean forward or cup a hand to the ear to hear? Is a loud speaking voice used? Does the person request repetition of what has been said? If hearing loss is identified, speak to the person in a normal tone of voice and speak

toward the better ear, if there is one. Assess the ear for size, shape, symmetry, redness, inflammation, swelling, discharge, and lesions.

Palpation

The surface of the skin of the ear should have a smooth texture. Palpate around the ear and ask the older adult whether any pain or tenderness is present.

Mouth and Throat

History

The first aspect of history taking related to the mouth is to establish whether the older adult has any dental complaints. The following questions can be used to elicit a history.

Do you have any pain or discomfort? Are any of your teeth especially sensitive to hot or cold temperatures? Have you noticed any swelling in your mouth or throat? Do you have any difficulty chewing or swallowing? How does food taste? Is your mouth dry?

Do your dentures fit properly? Do you have any sores or lesions in your mouth or throat? How often do you brush your teeth, dentures, or tongue? Do you use dental floss? If so, how often? When was your last dental examination? What was the result? Do you clean your dentures at night in a cleaning solution?

Physical Examination

Inspection and Palpation

Inspection and palpation are used concurrently during the oral cavity examination. Use a gloved hand and a gauze pad to perform this part of the examination. If the older adult wears dentures, remove them before starting the examination. Evaluate the fit of the dentures to the gums or alveolar surfaces and the dentures themselves. Dentures are considered to fit improperly if there is inflammation and ulceration of the palate, mucosa, and alveolar ridges. Examine the dentures for cracks, missing pieces, and rough edges. Dentures should be stable and remain securely fixed during chewing. Underlying tissues should be pink and adhere tightly to the bone. There should not be food, debris, or excessive denture adhesive on the inside of the denture. If the older adult does not have dentures, examine the teeth. Note the number and position of teeth. Are they in good repair, or can you see cavities and broken teeth?

The gums should be pink, moist, and smooth. Inspect for signs of inflammation and lesions. The hard palate should be pale. The soft palate should be pink. Inspect for inflammation, lesions, pallor, and any purulent drainage or a white coating on the tongue. The uvula should be midline and red. It should move up as the older adult says "Ah." Tonsils, if present, should be small, pink, and symmetrical. Check the gag reflex with a tongue blade. The top and bottom of the tongue should be examined. A smooth, painful tongue may indicate vitamin B_{12} deficiency. The tongue and mucous membranes should be pink, moist, and free of swelling and lesions. The tongue should relax on the floor of the mouth. Varicose veins on bottom surfaces of the tongue are common. Ask the older adult to stick out the tongue to examine it. While you hold it out with a piece of gauze, inspect all sides of the tongue and the floor of the mouth. Report any white, scaly patches. The lips should be moist, smooth, and pink. Check the corners of the mouth for cracks. These cracks are a prime spot for *Candida* (yeast) infections.

Neurological System

History

Does the older adult have any problems with headaches? Shaking or trembling? Confusion or memory loss? In assessing the neurological system, the nurse also should ask if the older adult has experienced seizures. Is there an existing seizure disorder? What type of treatment has been received? What were the circumstances occurring before, during, and after the seizure?

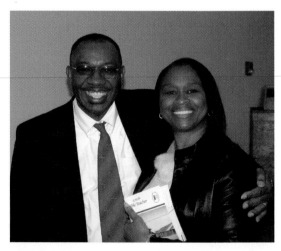

When taking a history on an older adult, it generally is helpful to obtain information from the family as well as the individual being assessed. In many older people, long-term memory may be based on facts that have been altered to "make the story better."

Physical Examination

Inspection

Examine the older adult's level of orientation. Is the person alert, lethargic, or nonresponsive? Oriented to place, time, and person? As the older adult answers questions, observe the face for symmetry of movement when smiling, talking, grimacing, or frowning. Evaluate the older adult's appearance throughout the examination. Is the person dressed appropriately? Is the person wearing multiple layers of clothing? If so, are they appropriate for the weather outdoors? Is there body odor? Does the person appear well groomed? Is the older adult's behavior appropriate? Evaluate the strength and symmetry of the older adult's upper and lower extremities. This is commonly done by asking the person to squeeze your hands. Ask the person to walk across the room and observe the gait for symmetry, balance, and coordination during ambulation. Note any weakness.

Peripheral Vascular System

History

Following are key history questions related to peripheral vascular functioning: Do you have diabetes? Do you wear garters or girdles? Do you wear ankle-, knee-, or thigh-high hosiery? When you take off your hosiery, is there an indentation in your leg that does not go away for several minutes? Do your shoes fit tightly? Do you have pain in your calves after walking? Do you ever experience pains, aches, numbness, or tingling in your calves, feet, buttocks, or legs? Are there any activities that you cannot do because of pains and aches in your extremities? What aggravates your pain? What relieves the pain? Does walking or climbing stairs cause pain? Do you ever notice change in the color of your extremities—red, blue, or pale? Have you noticed any hair loss over any part of your legs? Does your family have a history of problems with the legs? Do you sit for long periods with your legs crossed? Do you experience swelling of your legs at the end of the day? Does swelling return to normal in the morning?

Physical Examination

The physical examination of the peripheral vascular system includes inspection, palpation, and auscultation. The nurse should always compare one side of the body with the other when using these assessment methods.

Inspection

Skin color should be evaluated with the older adult lying down. Inspect the upper and lower extremities. Venous insufficiency is indicated if the legs are cyanotic when they are dependent (hanging down) or when petechiae or broken pigmentation is present on the skin over the legs. Chronic venous insufficiency is common in elderly people. If the legs become pale when they are elevated and turn dark red when they dangle, arterial insufficiency is indicated. The signs of chronic venous insufficiency are distended tortuous veins, hair loss, hyperpigmentation, cool or normal skin temperature, and pretibial edema or pedal edema that is worse during the day but improves at night when the older adult lies down to sleep. The signs of chronic arterial insufficiency include thin, shiny, atrophic skin; hair loss over feet and toes; thick and rigid toenails; and cool skin.

Edema of the legs and feet should be noted. The nurse may choose to record the width of the edematous area by using a measuring tape. When measuring the legs to assess edema, be sure to measure at the same place on each leg. If you wish to monitor changes in edema, lightly mark the location on the leg you are measuring with a felt-tipped marker and measure in the same place each day. Stasis ulcers are rare with varicose veins, but they commonly occur with deep vein insufficiency. Venous stasis ulcers are located on the sides of the ankles. Arterial ulcers may involve toes or places where the skin has been bumped or bruised.

Palpation

Check the skin temperature of the older adult's arms and legs by using the back of your hand. Increased temperature can be caused by a localized response to inflammation. Cool temperature indicates decreased blood flow. Peripheral pulses should be evaluated by using the pads of the index and middle fingers. The pulse is evaluated for rate, rhythm, amplitude, and symmetry. Normal vessels feel smooth and resilient. In most older adults, increased resistance to compression may be palpated because of rigid and tortuous artery walls. The nurse should practice palpating the pulses of a young person and an older person to be able to differentiate the changes associated with aging. Pulses should be evaluated one at a time (carotid, brachial, radial, femoral, popliteal, and dorsalis pedis). They should be regular, strong, and equal bilaterally. Lack of symmetry between extremities indicates possible impaired circulation. If you have difficulty finding a pulse, feel throughout the area where it is expected to be and vary the pressure of your finger. Be sure you are not feeling your own pulse. The rate you feel should be different from your own heart rate. If you had difficulty finding a pulse, you can mark its location with a felt-tipped pen after it is found.

Cardiac System

History

Older adults should be asked questions for assessment of cardiac disease risk factors, including smoking and exercise: Do you have any problems with dyspnea (shortness of breath)? Does your shortness of breath increase with activity (i.e., dyspnea on exertion)? Do you have chest pain? When does it occur? What are you doing when it occurs? Is the chest pain relieved by rest?

Physical Examination

Inspection

A cardiac physical examination procedure is the same for older and younger persons. The older adult should be evaluated while lying down, sitting up, and standing. Observe the neck and chest to detect any visible pulsations, lifts, or heaves. The heartbeat is usually not visible, but it may be if the individual is emaciated. It is abnormal to observe the heart beating on the chest wall of an older adult who is obese or of normal weight. Note any cough, shortness of breath, venous or abdominal distention, or cyanosis of mucous membranes and nailbeds. The legs, ankles, and feet should be observed for edema.

Palpation

Feel the front of the chest over the heart for any thrills, heaves, or lifts. A thrill is a palpable vibration. A lift or heave is a pulsation that is more

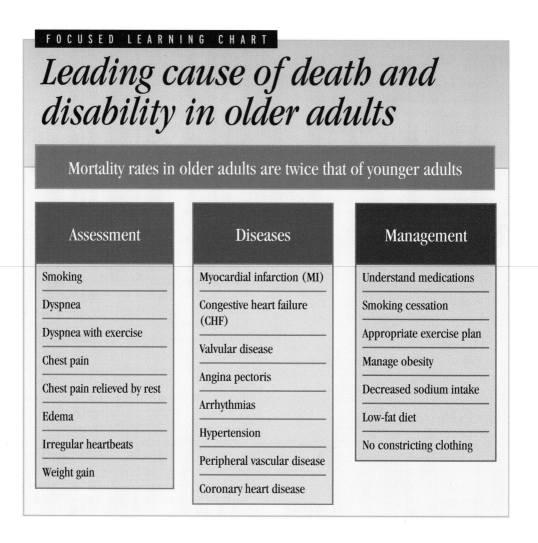

FOCUSED LEARNING CHART

Leading cause of death and disability in older adults

Mortality rates in older adults are twice that of younger adults

Assessment	Diseases	Management
Smoking	Myocardial infarction (MI)	Understand medications
Dyspnea	Congestive heart failure (CHF)	Smoking cessation
Dyspnea with exercise	Valvular disease	Appropriate exercise plan
Chest pain	Angina pectoris	Manage obesity
Chest pain relieved by rest	Arrhythmias	Decreased sodium intake
Edema	Hypertension	Low-fat diet
Irregular heartbeats	Peripheral vascular disease	No constricting clothing
Weight gain	Coronary heart disease	

forceful than anticipated. There should be minimal changes in the pulse when the older adult changes positions between lying, sitting, and standing. Press on the nailbeds and observe for the return of a pink color; this is called capillary refill and should occur quickly. It is abnormal for a refill to take longer than 2 seconds. Skin temperature should be palpated for unusual coolness or heat. The blood pressure should be checked using the orthostatic technique that you learned in Chapter 14. Orthostatic hypotension is a common problem with older adults.

Auscultation

Older adults have more rapid and less distinct heartbeats. Many older persons live normal, everyday lives with chronic atrial fibrillation. Any irregularity of the heartbeat noted while listening to the heart should be reported to the RN or physician. Infrequent extra beats (ectopic) are fairly common. Another common abnormal finding is a heart murmur. A heart murmur is caused by thickened and rigid heart valves and decreased strength of myocardial contractions. It sounds like a hum or click and results from turbulent or backward flow of blood through the heart. If detected, it should be reported.

Respiratory System

History

Questions that are used to assess an older adult's respiratory status include the following: Do you have any difficulty breathing? Do you get short of breath with exercise or exertion? Do you have a cough? Is your cough dry or productive? What color and consistency is the mucus that you cough up? Is there any blood in the mucus?

Dyspnea or difficulty breathing is not a part of normal aging. It is often related to congestive heart failure (CHF), pneumonia, anemia, and other lung diseases. It is present in only one-half of older persons with pneumonia. The first signs of pneumonia often include a nonspecific deterioration in health, such as slight cough, altered mental status, and tachycardia.

Ask the older adult if there is any history of lung disease. If so, what effect does it have on activities of daily living (ADLs)? Is oxygen used? Ask questions to determine if the older adult is using oxygen safely in the home. Other questions that can be used to elicit history of lung disease are as follows: Do you live in an area that has air pollution? Have you or any member of your family ever had tuberculosis? What is the date of your last chest x-ray study? Have you had the pneumonia vaccine (Pneumovax)? If so, when did you receive it? Have you had an influenza shot this year? Have you received one within the last year? Have you had a tuberculosis skin test? When?

Physical Examination

Inspection

In the older adult population, barrel chest, slight use of intercostal muscles, and slightly prolonged respirations may occur normally. If these signs and symptoms occur suddenly, they should be considered abnormal. The respiratory rate for normal older adults is 12 to 24 respirations per minute. A rate of 24 or greater is considered tachypnea. Observe for the use of accessory muscles and nasal flaring. A rate of less than 12 respirations per minute is considered bradypnea. Overt signs of the lower oxygen levels resulting from bradypnea include decreased consciousness, confusion, and lethargy. The character of respirations also should be evaluated. A normal respiratory rate is even and unlabored. The older adult's skin, lips, and nail color should be inspected for cyanosis and pallor. Posture while sitting and standing should be noted. Posture affects the ability to breathe.

Palpation

The anterior and posterior chest should be palpated for masses and tenderness of the ribs. The tracheal area should be palpated for any deviation.

Auscultation

An older adult can become dizzy from hyperventilation if asked to take deep breaths for a long time. Allow the person periods of normal breathing between deep breaths. Listen fully to inspiration and expiration. Softer vesicular sounds and diminished breath sounds in the bases of the lungs are normal. Listen for abnormal (adventitious) sounds. These sounds are superimposed on the normal breath sounds. Crackles are often heard when the older adult has CHF or pulmonary edema. Crackles result from air passing through moisture and sound like hair being rubbed between the fingers. Scattered crackles in dependent lung segments of some older adults should not be mistaken for bronchitis or CHF. If the crackles disappear after coughing, they are not pathological. If they are present after coughing, pathology may be present. Wheezes are a whistling noise caused by air passing through a narrowed airway. This happens with bronchospasm and swelling of the bronchioles. It is commonly heard in chronic obstructive pulmonary disease and in older adults with asthma. Pleural friction rub is due to inflammation between the membranes lining the chest cavity. It sounds like leather rubbing together.

Gastrointestinal System

History

In taking a gastrointestinal (GI) history, the nurse needs to focus on nutritional status, bowel habits, and medications. Ask the older adult or family member to give a 24-hour recall of the older person's diet. Evaluate the reported intake for nutritional balance. Is it full of fatty foods? Is it low in fiber? Does it have a high starch content? Calculate the amount of fluids the older adult drinks in a 24-hour period. The older adult needs 2000 to 3000 mL of fluids per day. Continue with more health history questions: How do you tolerate eating and drinking? Do you have problems with swallowing? Do you have the sensation that food is stuck in your throat? What is your bowel routine? Do you have abdominal pain? Do you use laxatives? Have you used laxatives in the past? How long did you use them? What kind of laxatives? How often were they used? Have you experienced any recent injury or infection?

Physical Examination

Inspection
Inspect the skin of the abdomen and note any lesions caused by rubbing of belts or corsets over the years. Check for fungal rashes in skin folds of adults who are obese or incapacitated. Does the abdomen look rigid? If so, refer the individual to the RN or physician. Abdominal rigidity can indicate bowel obstruction.

Auscultation
Listen to the abdomen with your stethoscope. Mentally divide the abdomen into quadrants that intersect through the umbilicus. Auscultate each quadrant until you hear bowel sounds, or if there are no bowel sounds, listen continuously for 5 minutes. Bowel sounds are decreased in the older adult because of decreased gastric motility that accompanies normal aging. While the history was being taken, did the older adult complain of pain in the abdomen? Ask the older adult to point to the area of pain. Right lower quadrant

FOCUSED LEARNING CHART

Adventitious (abnormal) breath sounds

	Crackles	Wheezes	Plural friction rub
Pathology:	CHF or pulmonary edema	COPD Asthma	Inflammation between membranes lining chest cavity
Caused by:	Air passing through moisture	Air passing through narrowed airway	Inflammation
Sounds like:	Hair being rubbed through fingers	Whistling noise	Leather rubbing together
Report to RN if:	Coughing does not relieve crackles	Present	Present (is very painful)

pain may indicate appendicitis. Left lower quadrant pain may indicate diverticulitis. Tenderness at the base of the xiphoid process may indicate stomach pain, hiatal hernia, or referred pain from the aorta. Palpation provides further information.

Palpation

Relaxation of the abdominal muscles enhances palpation. If the older adult is obese, palpation may be difficult. If you palpate a mass in the abdomen, it could indicate diverticulitis, fecal impaction, mesenteric thrombosis, or cancer.

Integumentary System

History

History taking is the most important aspect of the skin assessment. The most common skin complaints are pain, pruritus (itching), paresthesia (numbness), and dermatitis. The nurse needs to find out as much as possible about any skin problem mentioned. Questions to ask include the following: Do you have any skin problems? What kind? How were they treated? Are you allergic to any drugs or environmental allergens? What are they? How long have you had the allergy? Have you been exposed to an infectious disease? What is your history of sun exposure? What is your skin care regimen? Evaluate all medications that the older adult is taking. Anything that can cause an allergic reaction, no matter how long the product has been used, should be discussed. Common allergens are soaps and topical medications.

Physical Examination

Inspection

Look at the older person's skin in a well-lit room. Skin folds should be evaluated for dampness, irritation, and fissures. Common skin folds are under the breasts and inguinal areas. Observe the scalp, behind the ears, the fingernails and toenails, genitalia, buttocks, and face. How clean is the older adult's skin? Is there an odor present? Assess skin color for variations that are not uniform and have changed since the previous examination. Note any pallor, jaundice, cyanosis, erythema, petechiae, and ecchymosis. Older adults with deeply pigmented skin tones should be evaluated for changes in color such as duskiness, graying, and blackish areas. Jaundice in a person of color should be evaluated on the hard palate and the soles of the hands and feet. Check pressure points over bony prominences, especially on individuals who are debilitated or immobilized. Pay particular attention to the areas over the scapulae, back of the head, earlobes, hips, heels, coccyx, and elbows.

The Braden scale is a common assessment tool used to evaluate the risk of pressure ulcer formation. This is a helpful assessment to complete on every older individual who enters a health-care setting. It provides baseline information on the older person's risk for pressure ulcer formation. Individuals at high risk should have preventive measures implemented from the start. The Braden scale (Fig. 15.2) also can be used for periodic assessment of the older person. If the older adult's risk for pressure ulcer development increases over time, new and more aggressive interventions for prevention should be implemented.

Evaluate the skin for lesions. Some lesions are normal. Table 15.1 describes normal and abnormal skin lesions. Note the consistency of the lesions. If there has been a change in color, consistency, edges, or growth, the lesion may have changed from normal to abnormal.

Palpation

Check the skin for turgor. Gently pinch the skin on the forehead or anterior chest to see how quickly it returns to place. Poor turgor may be a normal aging change. It also could indicate dehydration or malnutrition or both. Palpate skin texture and note the temperature. Notice if the skin has become rough, dry, or coarse. Normally, the skin is smooth with some dryness. Check the skin temperature with the back of your hand. During this evaluation, note the symmetry of temperature and texture.

Musculoskeletal System

History

The most common musculoskeletal complaints are related to the joints. Complaints include pain, stiffness, redness, limitation in movement, and joint deformity. If the older person complains of pain, determine where the pain originates and where it radiates. The most common soft tissue problem is pain in and around the shoulder joint. If the older adult has a sudden onset of low back pain, report it to the RN or physician. This pain could indicate a compression fracture of the spine.

Braden Scale
FOR PREDICTING PRESSURE SORE RISK

Patient's Name _____ Evaluator's Name _____ Date of Assessment

SENSORY PERCEPTION Ability to respond meaningfully to pressure-related discomfort	**1. Completely Limited:** Unresponsive to painful stimuli (does not moan, flinch, or grasp), due to diminished level of consciousness or sedation. OR Limited ability to feel pain over most of body surface.	**2. Very Limited:** Responds only to painful stimuli. Cannot communicate discomfort except by moaning or restlessness. OR Has a sensory impairment which limits the ability to feel pain or discomfort over ½ of body.	**3. Slightly Limited:** Responds to verbal commands, but cannot always communicate discomfort or need to be turned. OR Has some sensory impairment that limits ability to feel pain or discomfort in 1 or 2 extremities.	**4. No Impairment:** Responds to verbal commands. Has no sensory deficit that would limit ability to feel or voice pain or discomfort.
MOISTURE Degree to which skin is exposed to moisture	**1. Constantly Moist:** Skin is kept moist almost constantly by perspiration, urine, and so on. Dampness is detected every time patient is moved or turned.	**2. Very Moist:** Skin is often but not always moist. Linen must be changed at least once a shift.	**3. Occasionally Moist:** Skin is occasionally moist, requiring an extra linen change approximately once a day.	**4. Rarely Moist:** Skin is usually dry, linen requires changing only at routine intervals.
ACTIVITY Degree of physical activity	**1. Bedfast:** Confined to bed.	**2. Chairfast:** Ability to walk severely limited or nonexistent. Cannot bear own weight and/or must be assisted into chair or wheelchair.	**3. Walks Occasionally:** Walks occasionally during day, but for very short distances, with or without assistance. Spends majority of each shift in bed or chair.	**4. Walks Frequently:** Walks outside the room at least twice a day and inside room at least once every 2 hours during waking hours.

FIGURE 15.2. Braden scale for predicting pressure sore risk. (From Braden, B. J. & Bergstrom, N. [1992]. Pressure reduction. In G. Bulechek & J. McCloskey [Eds.], *Nursing Interventions* [2nd ed., p. 63]. Philadelphia: W. B. Saunders, with permission.)

	1.	2.	3.	4.
MOBILITY Ability to change and control body position	**1. Completely Immobile:** Does not make even slight changes in body or extremity position without assistance.	**2. Very Limited:** Makes occasional slight changes in body or extremity position but unable to make frequent or significant changes independently.	**3. Slightly Limited:** Makes frequent though slight changes in body or extremity position independently.	**4. No Limitations:** Makes major and frequent changes in position without assistance.
NUTRITION *Usual* food intake pattern	**1. Very Poor:** Never eats a complete meal. Rarely eats more than ⅓ of any food offered. Eats 2 servings or less of protein (meat or dairy products) per day. Takes fluids poorly. Does not take a liquid dietary supplement. OR Is NPO and/or maintained on clear liquids or IVs for more than 5 days.	**2. Probably Inadequate:** Rarely eats a complete meal and generally eats only about ½ of any food offered. Protein intake includes only 3 servings of meat or dairy products per day. Occasionally will take a dietary supplement. OR Receives less than optimum amount of liquid diet or tube feeding.	**3. Adequate:** Eats over ½ of most meals. Eats a total of 4 servings of protein (meat, dairy products) each day. Occasionally will refuse a meal, but will usually take a supplement if offered. OR Is on tube feeding or TPN regimen, which probably meets most of nutritional needs.	**4. Excellent:** Eats most of every meal. Never refuses a meal. Usually eats a total of 4 or more servings of meat and dairy products. Occasionally eats between meals. Does not require supplementation.
FRICTION AND SHEAR	**1. Problem:** Requires moderate to maximum assistance in moving. Complete lifting without sliding against sheets is impossible. Frequently slides down in bed or chair, requiring frequent repositioning with maximum assistance. Spasticity, contractures, or agitation leads to almost constant friction.	**2. Potential Problem:** Moves feebly or requires minimum assistance. During a move, skin probably slides to some extent against sheets, chair, restraints, or other devices. Maintains relatively good position in chair or bed most of the time but occasionally slides down.	**3. No Apparent Problem:** Moves in bed and in chair independently and has sufficient muscle strength to lift up completely during move. Maintains good position in bed or chair at all times.	

FIGURE 15.2. (Continued)

TABLE 15.1 Normal and Abnormal Skin Lesions

	Normal Skin Lesions
Lesion	**Description**
Seborrheic keratosis	Raised; vary in size; tan to black in color; appear warty or greasy; frequently appear on trunk
Senile purpura	Vivid purple patch; well demarcated; eventually fades
Senile lentigines	Brown; irregularly shaped patches; age or liver spots; occur most frequently on back of hands, forearms, and face
Cherry angioma	Bright; ruby red elevated area; frequently found on trunk; common; insignificant; increase in size and number with age
Sebaceous hyperplasia	Yellowish, flat, solid elevations with central depression; looks like a small doughnut; common on face, forehead, and nose; more common in men
	Abnormal Lesions
Senile or actinic keratosis	Precancerous; superficial patch covered by a persistent scale; common on sun-exposed areas
Squamous cell carcinoma	Firm, red-brown nodule; may arise from senile keratosis; common on sun-exposed areas and in fair-skinned individuals
Basal cell epithelioma	Starts as pearly colored solid elevation on face or ear; ulcerates leaving a crater with an elevated border and depressed center
Malignant melanoma	Brown-black lesion; may have flecks of red, white, or blue irregular border, irregular surface; arise from moles or appear as new pigmented, irregular lesion
Lentigo maligna melanoma	Less aggressive form of malignant melanoma specific to elderly adults; arise from lentigines that enlarge laterally

Source: McGovern, M., & Kuhn, J. K. (1992). Skin assessment of the elderly client. *Journal of Gerontological Nursing* 18(8), 40–41, with permission.

Physical Examination

Inspection

If possible, observe the older adult while the person is participating in ADLs and instrumental activities of daily living (IADLs). (See Functional Assessment section in this chapter.) Doing so allows the nurse to assess ROM, muscle mass, and level of independence in self-care. Some decline in ROM is expected. There is a general rigidity of the lower extremities.

Observe the older adult's ability to walk. Have the person ambulate a specified distance to determine endurance. It is normal for older men to have a slight anterior-flexion of the upper body while the arms and knees are slightly flexed. Note the kind of shoes worn by the older adult. Intervention is necessary if the person has an unstable gait yet wears high-heeled shoes. Have the older adult transfer in and out of the bed and chair, on and off the commode, and from the commode to the bathtub. Observe for symmetry of movement. Determine if the person

needs assistance. Some older people may be independently mobile with the use of a wheelchair. Assess their ability to maneuver the wheelchair in the environment. Check the older adult's feet for lesions and deformity because these can interfere with gait and mobility. As with physical examination of all of the systems, report all abnormal findings of the musculoskeletal system to the RN or physician.

Reproductive System

History: Female Patient

Although questions about sexual functioning and the reproductive organs may be uncomfortable for the nurse and the older adult, it is important to ask them. Ask the older woman if she knows about breast self-examination (Fig. 15.3). If not, education on the subject is needed. Do not be surprised if the older woman is familiar with breast self-examination and does it regularly. Many older women are more compliant than younger women in performing this examination. Inquire about symptoms of breast cancer. Does the person have any pain, nipple discharge, lumps, skin discoloration, or change in breast shape? Is there any family history of breast cancer or other cancerous conditions? Determine if the older woman has used estrogen or other medications that affect the breasts, such as digitalis, thyroid drugs, and antihypertensives. Has the older woman ever had an abnormal Papanicolaou (Pap) smear? If so, was she treated? Did she receive any medications for menopausal symptoms? Has there been any unusual bleeding since menopause?

Some common physical complaints that older women experience with intercourse include vaginal dryness, pain, and limited mobility from arthritis. These complaints should be addressed, and ways to deal with them should be suggested. Lubricants and using different positions during intercourse, such as the side-lying position, can help the older woman manage these concerns. Note the discussion in Chapter 12 on sexually transmitted diseases.

History: Male Patient

The older man should be evaluated for symptoms of benign prostatic hyperplasia. Is there any change in the urinary stream? Any dribbling of urine? A sense that the bladder is not completely empty after urinating? Is there urinary frequency? Urgency? Burning during urination? Does the older man experience nocturia? How often? Review his medications and note whether he takes diuretics or an anticholinergic that might worsen benign prostatic hyperplasia. Does he realize the importance of checking his breasts periodically? Although male breast cancer is rare, it is possible for older men to develop breast cancer.

Physical Examination

Inspection
During the examination process, you should inspect the external genitalia on older male and female patients. Assess for skin or mucous membrane lesions, rashes, discoloration, hair loss, inflammation, discharge, asymmetry, and circumcision.

Urinary System

History

In gathering information about the urinary tract, the nurse needs to discover the chief complaint and the nature and extent of the older adult's underlying problem. The most common complaints are urgency to void, leakage when changing position, pain on urination, frequency of urination, voiding small amounts, and incontinence caused by coughing, sneezing, and laughing. The subject of urinary incontinence frequently causes the older adult to feel embarrassed. Incontinence may cause the older person to withdraw from usual social contact for fear of having an accident. It is also a major risk factor for pressure ulcer formation and urinary tract infections. Despite the difficulties and embarrassment that may be associated with discussing incontinence, it is a serious problem that can have multiple untoward effects.

If the older adult reports any complaints related to the urinary tract, determine the person's normal urinary and bowel habits before the symptoms began. Assess the past medical history for childbirths, previous surgeries involving the lower abdomen and pelvic floor, renal disease, and bladder cancer. Evaluate the older adult's medications. Diuretics and antiparkinsonian drugs can affect the urinary system. Periods of prolonged rest or immobility can cause urinary stasis. Urine that is allowed to pool in the bladder creates a favorable environment for the development of infection. To empty the bladder fully, it is important for the older adult to be able to use the sitting-with-legs-dependent position. Full bladder emptying may not be possible on a bedpan. Decreased fluid intake results in low urine volume and infrequent urination. This situation can create pooling of the urine and increase the risk for infection. It also can lead to dehydration, elevated blood glucose levels, and electrolyte imbalance. These conditions may manifest in the older adult through alterations in mental status.

Physical Examination

Inspection
Assess urine amount and color for the presence of any sediment.

Palpation
Palpate the abdomen for distention of the bladder and signs of pelvic discomfort or masses.

⬤ FUNCTIONAL ASSESSMENT

For an older adult, a functional assessment is as important as a physical assessment. Very often, the older person demonstrates changes in function as the first or only sign indicating the onset

BREAST SELF-EXAMINATION

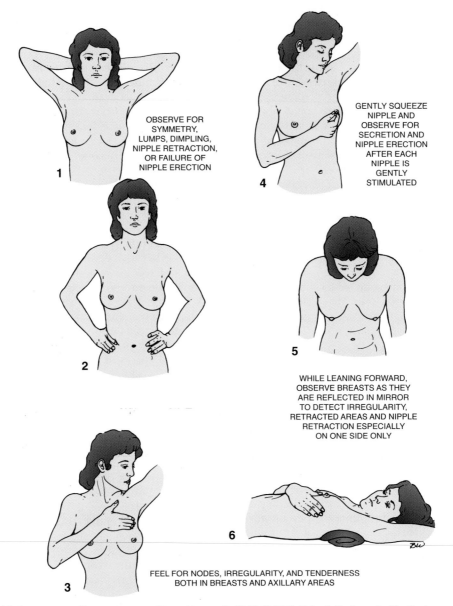

1 OBSERVE FOR SYMMETRY, LUMPS, DIMPLING, NIPPLE RETRACTION, OR FAILURE OF NIPPLE ERECTION

2

3 FEEL FOR NODES, IRREGULARITY, AND TENDERNESS BOTH IN BREASTS AND AXILLARY AREAS

4 GENTLY SQUEEZE NIPPLE AND OBSERVE FOR SECRETION AND NIPPLE ERECTION AFTER EACH NIPPLE IS GENTLY STIMULATED

5 WHILE LEANING FORWARD, OBSERVE BREASTS AS THEY ARE REFLECTED IN MIRROR TO DETECT IRREGULARITY, RETRACTED AREAS AND NIPPLE RETRACTION ESPECIALLY ON ONE SIDE ONLY

6

FIGURE 15.3. Breast self-examination. (From Venes, D. [Ed.]. [2009]. *Taber's Cyclopedic Medical Dictionary* [21st ed., p. 310]. Philadelphia: F. A. Davis, with permission.)

of illness. Although the older person has many chronic illnesses, these typically are not problematic until function is affected.

Functional assessment encompasses a holistic approach to evaluating the older adult that includes physical, cognitive, and social function. Physical function comprises the individual's current health status in addition to how well the person performs ADLs and IADLs. Cognitive function includes the individual's memory, judgment, and thinking abilities. Cognitive function is discussed in Chapter 17 and is not included in this section on functional assessment. Social function involves a psychosocial approach to determine how the individual interacts with the environment and with others.

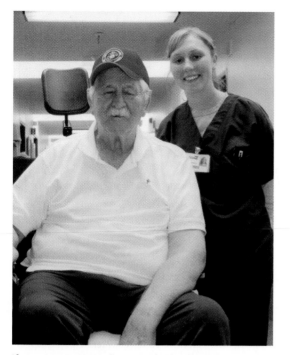

If you were assigned to assess this man on admission to the nursing home where you work, what observations could you make even before talking to him? His right arm is hanging without good positioning or apparent control. Does this man have a muscle or enervation problem in the arm, or has he possibly had a left-sided stroke? He is in a wheelchair. Why? His complexion is slightly ruddy. Is it from the broken vessels that often occur with excessive alcoholic consumption? He is not smiling.

Functional assessment involves evaluating the older adult to determine what the person can do (strengths) and cannot do (deficits). What the health-care team members see as a deficit may not correlate with what the older adult views as a problem. The older adult's true abilities, as assessed by the nurse, and the older adult's perception of these abilities must be considered.

Functional assessment assists in setting realistic goals. Cure as a goal is inappropriate for an older individual with chronic, irreversible conditions. The goal for such a patient would be to maximize functional strengths and compensate for deficits to achieve and maintain optimal independence in function.

In almost any health-care setting, the nurse is the health-care professional who spends the most time with the older adult. The nurse has many opportunities to observe the client's physical functioning. A decline in functional ability may represent a change in an underlying chronic disease or the onset of a new acute illness. Monitoring functional status helps track improvements and setbacks. It also indicates when additional services are needed. Use of a formal tool to evaluate functional status allows the nurse to validate, monitor, and communicate clearly clinical impressions to other members of the interdisciplinary health-care team.

Activities of Daily Living

The Katz ADL scale (Fig. 15.4) is widely used to assess ADLs. It is a well-rounded tool that is appropriate for use in most settings, including home, hospital, and nursing home. ADLs are the activities performed in taking care of oneself. The following areas are considered ADLs: bathing, dressing, toileting, feeding, ambulating or transferring, and continence. Direct observation is the most valid indicator in assessing ADLs. Watch the older adult perform ADLs and check for abnormal body movements. Rate the older adult on each of the ADL items of the Katz scale. Using the scale supplies specific information on how the older adult performs in each of the ADL areas, and the composite score can give you and other members of the interdisciplinary health-care team an overall view of the person's level of ability. The score also gives an objective means to monitor progress over time. Goals in each of the ADL areas can be set on the basis of scores on the scale.

Instrumental Activities of Daily Living

IADLs include the ability to use the telephone, cook, shop, do laundry, manage finances, take medications, and prepare meals. These activities are needed to support independent living. Lawton's scale for IADLs is used widely (Fig. 15.5).

If possible, observe the older adult while he or she is performing IADLs. Look for abnormal body movements such as tremors or twitching, for lack of balance, or for poor vision. In addition to checking the person's ability to complete the IADL, it is important to assess the older adult with regard to safety. The older person may be able to cook a meal, but if the burner is left on, a serious safety concern exists.

In completing an IADL assessment, the nurse often must rely on reports from the older adult or family members. Keep in mind that individuals tend to overrate their abilities, and family members tend to underrate them.

Activities of Daily Living (ADL) Scale
Evaluation Form

Name _____ Day of evaluation _____

For each area of functioning listed below, check description that applies. (The word "assistance" means supervision, direction, or personal assistance.)

Bathing—either sponge bath, tub bath, or shower

☐	☐	☐
Receives no assistance (gets in and out of tub by self, if tub is usual means of bathing)	Receives assistance in bathing only one part of the body (such as back or a leg)	Receives assistance in bathing more than one part of the body (or not bathed)

Dressing—gets clothes from closets and drawers, including underclothes, outer garments, and using fasteners (including braces, if worn)

☐	☐	☐
Gets clothes and gets completely dressed without assistance	Gets clothes and gets dressed without assistance, except for assistance in tying shoes	Receives assistance in getting clothes or in getting dressed, or stays partly or completely undressed

Toileting—going to the "toilet room" for bowel and urine elimination; cleaning self after elimination and arranging clothes

☐	☐	☐
Goes to "toilet room," cleans self, and arranges clothes without assistance (may use object for support such as cane, walker, or wheelchair and may manage night bedpan or commode, emptying same in morning)	Receives assistance in going to "toilet room" or in cleansing self or in arranging clothes after elimination or in use of night bedpan or commode	Doesn't go to room termed "toilet" for the elimination process

Transfer

☐	☐	☐
Moves in and out of bed as well as in and out of chair without assistance (may be using object for support, such as cane or walker)	Moves in and out of bed or chair with assistance	Doesn't get out of bed

Continence

☐	☐	☐
Controls urination and bowel movement completely by self	Has occasional "accidents"	Supervision helps keep urine or bowel control; catheter is used or person is incontinent

Feeding

☐	☐	☐
Feeds self without assistance	Feeds self except for getting assistance in cutting meat or buttering bread	Receives assistance in feeding or is fed partly or completely by using tubes or intravenous fluids

SOURCE: Courtesy of Sidney Katz, MD. Reprinted with permission.

For additional information on administration and scoring refer to the followig references:
1. Katz S. Assessing self-maintenance: activities of daily living, mobility, and instrumental activities of daily living. *J Am Geriatr Soc.* 1983;31:721–727.
2. Katz S, Akpom CA. A measure of primary sociobiologic functions. *Int J Health Services.* 1976;6:493–508.
3. Katz S, Downs TD, Cash HR, et al. Progress in development of the index of ADL. *J Gerontol.* 1970;10(1):20–30.

FIGURE 15.4. Katz Activities of Daily Living Scale. (From Katz, S., Ford, A., & Moskowitz, R. [1963]. The index of ADL: A standardized measure of biological and psychosocial function. *Journal of the American Medical Association* 185, 914. Copyright 1963, American Medical Association, with permission.)

Instrumental Activities of Daily Living (IADL) Scale	
Self-Rated Version Extracted from the **Multilevel Assessment Instrument (MAI)**	
1. Can you use the telephone:	
without help,	3
with some help, or	2
are you completely unable to use the telephone?	1
2. Can you get to places out of walking distance:	
without help,	3
with some help, or	2
are you completely unable to travel unless special arrangements are made?	1
3. Can you go shopping for groceries:	
without help,	3
with some help, or	2
are you completely unable to do any shopping?	1
4. Can you prepare your own meals:	
without help,	3
with some help, or	2
are you completely unable to prepare any meals?	1
5. Can you do your own housework:	
without help,	3
with some help, or	2
are you completely unable to do any housework?	1
6. Can you do your own handyman work:	
without help,	3
with some help, or	2
are you completely unable to do any handyman work?	1
7. Can you do your own laundry:	
without help,	3
with some help, or	2
are you completely unable to do any laundry at all?	1
8a. Do you take medicines or use any medications?	
(If yes, answer Question 8b) Yes	1
(If no, answer Question 8c) No	2
8b. Do you take your own medicine:	
without help (in the right doses at the right time),	3
with some help (take medicine if someone prepares it for you and/or reminds you to take it), or	2
(are you/would you be) completely unable to take your own medicine?	1
8c. If you had to take medicine, can you do it:	
without help (in the right doses at the right time),	3
with some help (take medicine if someone prepares it for you and/or reminds you to take it), or	2
(are you/would you be) completely unable to take your own medicine?	1
9. Can you manage your own money:	
without help,	3
with some help, or	2
are you completely unable to handle money?	1

SOURCE: Lawton MP, Brody EM. Assessment of older people: self maintaining and instrumental activities of daily living. *Gerontologist.* 1969;9:179–185. Reprinted with permission.

For additional information on administration and scoring refer to the following references:

1. Lawton MP. Scales to measure competence in everyday activities. *Psychopharm Bull.* 1988;24(4):609–614.

2. Lawton MP, Moss M, Fulcomer M, et al. A research and service-oriented Multilevel Assessment Instrument. *J Gerontol.* 1982;37:91–99.

FIGURE 15.5. Instrumental Activities of Daily Living Scale. (From Lawton, M. P., & Brody, E. M. [1969]. Assessment of older people: Self maintaining and instrumental activities of daily living. *Gerontologist* 9, 179–185. Copyright © The Gerontological Society of America, with permission.)

Tools for assessing ADLs and IADLs are used to measure the older person's ability to do self-care and home-care tasks. They can be used to help identify needed services and to monitor the progress or deterioration of the older individual.

Social Function

Social function is how the older adult interacts with self, the environment, and others. It is the degree to which a person functions as a member of the community. Cultural and socioeconomic background and the older adult's environment define and limit social activities and relationships. Self-concept affects the older adult's ability to perform self-care activities. Psychological interventions may be necessary to enhance the older person's self-esteem before achieving independent functioning.

CONCLUSION

This chapter contains a great deal of information about performing a holistic physical assessment and a functional assessment. To be an effective gerontological nurse, you need to be very good at both of these skills. There is a great deal of information in this chapter. The only way you will learn it is to go over it several times, practice asking the questions, and practice the skills. Have the courage to use the skills (even with a cheat sheet) whenever you go to your student clinical assignments. This is not a chapter to read and then move on to the next one. This is the one you need to internalize through rereading and practice. Best wishes!

Miss S. is an 85-year-old woman who has been admitted to the medical unit where you work. She has been there for 2 days while being treated for CHF. You are assigned her care for the next 12 hours. In a report, you are told Miss S. is uncooperative and incontinent. Miss S. is responding well to her medication regimen for the CHF and will be discharged tomorrow.

Discussion

1. What is your priority in terms of assessing Miss S. today?
2. How will you meet the requirements of the priority assessment items?
3. What other points of concern should you address in your assessment?
4. How will you do that?

Solutions

In doing a holistic assessment, it is important that you determine the underlying cause of the "little" problems as well as the big ones. The big problem for Miss S. is the management of her CHF. According to the report, that is going well. You need to verify that her medical treatment is still managing her symptoms. This is the priority concern because it is life-threatening and the reason she was admitted to the hospital. How will you assess the CHF? Following are some suggestions:

1. Assess for edema by checking her ankles, abdomen, lumbosacral area, and hands for swelling, and listen to her lungs for adventitious breath sounds.
2. Is she able to perform ADLs without dyspnea?
3. Does she understand her medication administration?

Now let's consider her incontinence and lack of cooperation. Some nurses would not be concerned about these items, but because you are committed to holistic nursing care, these concerns are important to you. One idea should come to your mind right away. Assume Miss S. is on furosemide (Lasix) for the CHF. Lasix is associated with increased urination. At age 85, this probably is a major inconvenience for this person. Has she cut down on her fluid intake to decrease the stress urination and incontinence, which has resulted in an electrolyte imbalance and confusion? This is what I would investigate as I did my assessment. It will be a very serious problem if it is not resolved before Miss S. goes home.

Select the best answer to each question.

1. The following are normal aging changes except:

    a. Presbyopia, presbycusis

    b. Presbyopia, urinary incontinence

    c. Kyphosis, ptosis

    d. Osteoporosis, arteriosclerosis

2. Activities of daily living include:

    a. Shopping

    b. Managing finances

    c. Bathing

    d. Using the telephone

3. A common tool used for evaluating ADLs is:

    a. Lawton's scale

    b. The mini-mental status examination

    c. The Katz scale

    d. a and c

4. A common symptom of myocardial infarction in an older adult is:

    a. Chest pain

    b. Lethargy

    c. Confusion

    d. b and c

5. An important health problem that the nurse should help the older adult prevent is:

    a. Fecal impaction

    b. Dehydration

    c. Malnutrition

    d. All of the above

16 Common Clinical Problems: Physiological

Mary Ann Anderson

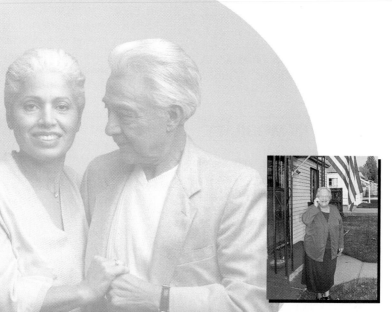

Learning Objectives

After completing this chapter, the student will be able to:

1. Identify the age-related factors that place the older adult at risk for impaired mobility and describe how the nurse can assist in maintaining mobility.
2. Define two categories of risk factors for falls in older people.
3. Identify two categories of incontinence.
4. Explain how prompted voiding and habit training schedules can be used by the nurse for prevention or reversal of incontinence.
5. Identify the mechanical and physiological risk factors for pressure ulcers.
6. Discuss the problems pertaining to adequate food intake in older people.
7. Describe two sleep disorders common to older adults.
8. Define iatrogenesis, and list common iatrogenic problems experienced by older persons.

INTRODUCTION

With aging, every body system undergoes some changes. These changes, although they do not result in illness or disease, cause health problems that are more prevalent in older people. As you learned in Chapter 14, most people who are older than 65 years of age have multiple chronic diseases. As a result of normal aging changes combined with underlying chronic diseases, the older person has less physical reserve than a younger person has to respond to the increased demand of an illness. With diminished physical reserve, the older adult is less capable of adapting to physical stressors and is at increased risk for clinical problems such as immobility, falls, incontinence, pressure ulcers, and alterations in nutrition and sleep. This chapter reviews the clinical problems that are common to older adults. In addition, effective management approaches, based on nursing diagnoses, are discussed.

ALTERATION IN MOBILITY

The process of aging, combined with the presence of chronic illness, places the older adult at risk for developing an alteration in mobility status. Immobility is a major medical disability for elderly adults and one that is frequently overlooked by health-care providers. Immobility often leads to numerous complications for older people in long-term care facilities, people in the hospital, and people in the community. Nursing management is essential to maintaining and improving one's ability to be mobile.

Musculoskeletal System

Normal aging changes that occur in the musculoskeletal system increase the risk of developing

---

> ### ▲ PRIORITY SETTING 16.1
>
> The priority for this chapter is easy to identify. After you understand the content of this chapter, you need to assist every older adult to whom you give care to achieve his or her maximum physical ability. Keep that thought in mind and do not stray from it. By doing so, you will enhance the lives of all of the older people in your care.

---

problems related to mobility. The bones of an older person are less dense and more brittle owing to changes in the formation of bone at the cellular level. As a result, older adults are likely to develop osteoporosis and subsequently be at risk for bone fractures.

With a fracture, mobility is restricted still further. Mechanical stresses, such as walking and standing, tend to stimulate the process of bone formation. When the body is immobilized, there is bone dissolution. This process is called *disuse osteoporosis*, and it makes the bones of the older person still more brittle.

Generalized muscle weakness is also a normal aging process. There is a noticeable decrease in muscle strength with aging. The antigravity muscles are most affected by this change so that standing up can be a difficult movement. In time, if muscles are not used, walking, balancing, and turning become severely impaired. At complete rest, muscle strength can decline at a rate of 5% a day. *The loss of muscle mass is not only a symptom of generalized deterioration, but it is also a factor in the risk of falling.*

The mobility of the joints is affected by the length and composition of the muscle fibers. When there is immobility, the muscles that bridge the joint shorten. With decreased muscle length and thickening of the joint cartilage (which is the connective tissue that surrounds the movable surfaces of the joint), the joints become stiff, which seriously impacts the ability of the person to move.

Osteoarthritis, or degenerative joint disease, occurs in 83% to 87% of people 55 to 64 years old. It is marked by deterioration of the cartilage and formulation of new bone at the joint surfaces. With aging, the cartilage is less elastic, thicker, and more easily stretched. As a result, the joint is stiff, and there is decreased range of motion (ROM) of the joint. Over time, an older adult can lose the ability to mobilize efficiently as a result of stiffness in the joints. As joints are immobilized, contractures (a permanent contraction of the muscles that bridge the joint) can develop and limit mobilization further.

Cardiovascular System

Many of the changes in the cardiovascular system that accompany aging are closely related to inactivity. Similarly, these aging changes can be exacerbated, or become more severe, when there are prolonged periods of immobility. One such aging change is in oxygen consumption, which is referred to as $\dot{V}O_2$. $\dot{V}O_2$ measures the body's ability to transport oxygen from the atmosphere to the various tissues of the body. In aging and during periods of immobilization, this ability decreases. $\dot{V}o_2$ is affected by cardiac output (the amount of blood pumped from the heart to the body), which is known to diminish in aging. Physical exercise causes the active tissue to use more oxygen and eliminate carbon dioxide, which increases cardiac output. With prolonged immobility, cardiac output during exercise does not increase as efficiently as in an active ambulatory person.

Oxygen consumption and cardiac output also are known to decrease with aging. This change is evident from the fact that the pulse rate of an older person does not increase in response to exercise as efficiently as in younger people. After physical exertion, the pulse takes longer to return to a normal level. The inefficient cardiac response to activity causes activity intolerance.

Respiratory System

As is true of all of the body systems, aging changes to the respiratory system put the older person at risk for complications when immobility is present. Normal anatomical changes in the aging body compromise lung function.

Increased rigidity of the rib cage, kyphosis, and osteoporosis reduce the compliance of the chest wall, making it more difficult to inflate the lungs fully. The reduced compliance of the chest wall makes it more challenging for the older adult to maintain activity, and it increases the potential for complications caused by immobility. The lungs of most older adults have diminished vital capacity (the amount of air that can be expelled from the lungs after inspiration). Other changes include less efficient gas exchange by the alveoli and less stretchability of the lung tissue. The result is impaired ventilation and decreased blood supply to the lungs. Such changes not only may hinder the older person's ability to move, but, more important, they also place the older person at increased risk for developing atelectasis (collapsed lung) and pneumonia when immobilized.

Response to Illness

Chronic health problems may cause older people to restrict their movement. Poor eyesight may cause someone of any age to avoid activity because of fear of falling over an obstacle. Pain in the joints owing to arthritis or pain in the lower extremities owing to impaired circulation

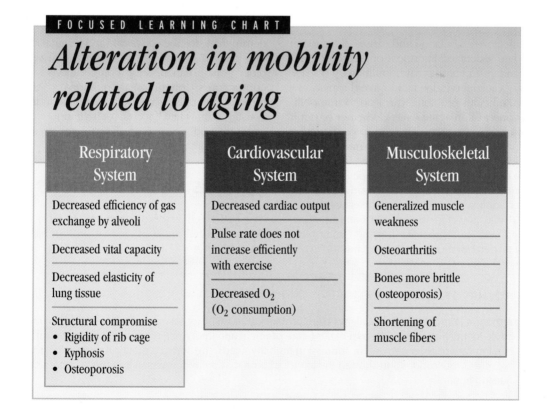

FOCUSED LEARNING CHART

Alteration in mobility related to aging

Respiratory System	Cardiovascular System	Musculoskeletal System
Decreased efficiency of gas exchange by alveoli	Decreased cardiac output	Generalized muscle weakness
Decreased vital capacity	Pulse rate does not increase efficiently with exercise	Osteoarthritis
Decreased elasticity of lung tissue		Bones more brittle (osteoporosis)
Structural compromise • Rigidity of rib cage • Kyphosis • Osteoporosis	Decreased O_2 (O_2 consumption)	Shortening of muscle fibers

Oxygen consumption in cardiovascular systems of older adults (V_{O2})

V_{O2} measures the body's ability to transport oxygen from the atmosphere to the tissues in the body; simply put, it is the amount of blood pumped from the heart.

Ability for O_2 consumption decreases (decreased V_{O2}) with:	Physical exercise causes:
Aging	More O_2 to be used
Immobility	More CO_2 to be eliminated
	Increased cardiac output, resulting in an increase in V_{O2}

generally limits ambulation and causes older adults to become sedentary. Shortness of breath or angina secondary to chronic cardiopulmonary disease also may cause the individual to avoid activity.

Acute health problems can lead to immobility. The onset of an acute illness, whether or not it requires hospitalization, may lead to confinement in bed. Often, well-meaning family members and health-care providers encourage immobility. Bedrest often is ordered during hospitalization for an acute illness. In contrast to a younger person, an older adult who is on bedrest deteriorates rapidly and may develop irreversible complications. Although rest can promote healing, immobility promotes deterioration. Prolonged immobility is detrimental to the physical and mental health of a person of any age. When immobilized, the older person can develop complications such as contractures, pneumonia, pulmonary emboli, thrombophlebitis, pressure ulcers, incontinence, constipation, renal stones, dehydration, loss of appetite, and psychological problems related to sensory deprivation and depression.

NURSING IMPLICATIONS

Nurses as well as the older people to whom they give care need to be aware that promoting physical activity not only prevents complications, but

POINT OF INTEREST

Although immobility is a prevalent health problem, it often is not addressed in the care of the older adult. Identifying immobility as a patient-care problem and intervening to prevent it are central to nursing care of older persons. In addressing mobility needs, the licensed practical nurse (LPN) may prevent complications and shorten the length of time that the older person is in the hospital or nursing home.

also slows the rate of the aging process. In the hospital setting, the time for enforced bedrest needs to be limited as much as possible. As soon as it is medically safe to do so, the nurse needs to ensure that the patient is up and out of bed. If orders for bedrest are in effect, it is the nurse's responsibility to inquire whether such orders can be changed. Even transferring the person from a supine to a sitting position has beneficial effects. While on bedrest, older adults can be taught isometric and active ROM exercises. If the person is incapable of performing these exercises independently, the nurse must assist the patient in meeting this need through passive ROM exercises.

As soon as it is medically indicated, the older patient should be ambulated with assistance. This intervention is as important to the patient's health as receiving the proper medication or a dressing change. Nursing staff should support physical therapy services by ensuring that appropriate sturdy footwear, eyeglasses, and any assistive devices such as canes or walkers are available. Because of reimbursement issues, hospital stays are becoming shorter. As soon as the person is physiologically able, attempts to restore functional ability should begin.

As in the hospital setting, promoting functional mobility is central to the care of the older person at home or in a nursing home. The nursing home environment offers different possibilities for fostering mobility. In contrast to the hospital setting, where the presence of an acute state may impede the nurse's attempts to restore function, the nursing home environment allows the nurse to monitor and promote mobility over an extended period. All residents should be considered for assisted walking unless the underlying chronic illness absolutely precludes such an activity. An older person who does not walk deteriorates even further and eventually loses all ability to walk. Family members and other caregivers for the older adult who lives at home need to be taught the importance of mobility.

⬤ POTENTIAL FOR INJURY FROM FALLS

As with alteration in mobility, the potential for falls is closely related to many of the bodily changes that occur with aging. The aging of the musculoskeletal system, which may cause deterioration in mobility, also may increase the older

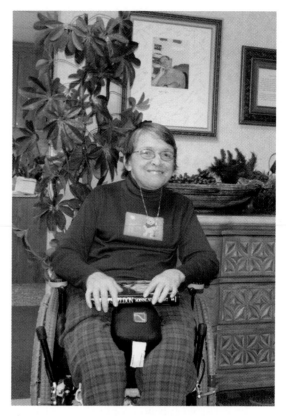

This woman has severe physical limitations, but she can get around because she is in the right type of wheelchair for her needs. She can see to read, as noted by the book she has in her lap. Observe that she is clean and neat, with matching clothes, jewelry, and a nice haircut and nails. What do these things say about her?

person's risk for falling. One-third of adults who are older than 65 years living in the community and one-half of adults older than 80 years living in the community fall each year. In nursing homes, a fall rate of two per resident per year has been reported. Most falls do not result in serious injury; however, 250,000 falls per year result in hip fractures, and 1500 persons 65 years old or older die each year as the result of a fall or fall-related injury. The presence of chronic illness accompanying the aging process places all older adults at increased risk for falls.

When an older person falls, the person often becomes fearful of falling again. The older adult may limit activities and become more withdrawn and dependent on others, less mobile, and more at risk for future falls. Caregivers also may place restrictions on the older person's mobility to prevent another fall. At home, the family may admonish the older person to restrict activities so that a fall does not occur again. In the health-care setting, restraints should never be used to prevent the risk of another fall. These options do not promote health for the person.

Factors that predispose to falling are typically divided into two categories: intrinsic and extrinsic. Intrinsic factors include factors inherent to the individual, such as normal aging changes, deficiencies in health status, changes in mental status, immobility, and changes in functional ability. Extrinsic factors refer to environmental conditions, which may include poor lighting, slippery floors, inappropriate or poorly placed furnishings, and inadequate footwear. Falls among older adults often stem from the presence of intrinsic factors that hinder the older person's ability to manage the environment or from environmental conditions (extrinsic factors).

Intrinsic Factors

Age-related changes in posture, balance, gait, and vision predispose an older person to falls. Postural changes are common in older people and are due to a decline in strength and flexibility. In older adults, the head tends to be carried forward, the shoulders may be rounded, and the upper back may have a slight curvature, or kyphosis. Changes in posture and spinal alignment can affect balance and increase the risk of falls.

Posture and Balance

The body's ability to maintain its coordination in a standing position and to react to prevent a fall depends on coordination among the musculoskeletal system, the neurological system, and the visual system. Postural sway occurs when one or more of these three systems are not functioning at an optimal level. Balance problems are associated with postural sway, which can cause falls. Prolonged bedrest, aging changes, medications, and the presence of some chronic diseases are contributors to postural sway.

Postural reflexes play a role in fall prevention by responding to disturbances in balance during standing or walking. With aging, these reflexes become slower; older people are less able to "catch" themselves when they trip or begin to fall. Inactivity may result in a slower response to disturbances in balance.

Gait

With aging, the gross motor movements necessary for maintaining posture and gait, or walking, are altered. The gait of older people often is marked by decreased speed and step height; small, hesitant steps; diminished arm swing; and stooped posture. These changes are almost universal in people older than 80 years. The alterations in speed of movement and maintenance of upright posture adversely affect balance and often lead to a higher incidence of falls by older adults.

Vision

All older people experience changes in vision as part of the normal aging process. With aging, there is a decline in visual acuity, peripheral vision, depth perception, night vision, and tolerance for glare. The loss of vision that accompanies aging is a risk factor for falls because there is a decreased ability to focus on objects at a distance and to judge distances correctly. The result is that an older person may miss a step or trip over a curb. The decline in peripheral vision may cause an individual to trip over objects at the edge of the visual field. Visual deficits can compound a gait disability because vision is necessary to maintain stability while walking.

These normal, age-related changes in posture, gait, and vision, when compounded by the presence of an underlying chronic or acute illness, make falls the leading cause of death from injury in people older than 65 years. Because of the presence of these intrinsic factors, many older people are less capable of coping with the extrinsic factors that may be in the environment.

Extrinsic Factors

At least 50% of falls affecting older adults result from environmental factors. Such factors include clutter in the halls, inadequate lighting or glare, and unsafe furniture or equipment in the person's immediate area. Attempting to function in an area that is not designed to accommodate the aging person's needs can diminish the older person's confidence. The individual may begin to fear falling and may eventually become more sedentary. Such behavior leads to an eventual loss of function and an increased need to depend on others for activities of daily living.

Nursing Implications

As health-care providers, it is important for nurses to understand the role that intrinsic and extrinsic factors play in falls. The individual's ability to maneuver safely in the immediate environment is best monitored by the nurse. In the home and the institutional setting, most falls occur in the bedroom and the bathroom. It is important to assess the older person walking about the bedroom, getting into and out of bed, and getting on and off the toilet. Only by assessing the individual's ability to manage these daily activities in his or her own environment can you, the nurse, begin to anticipate needs and take steps to prevent a fall before it occurs.

Having assessed the older person's safety, the nurse, along with members of the interdisciplinary health-care team (IDT), should plan care according to the observed need. The nurse may observe that the older person cannot safely get on and off the toilet independently and may advise the individual not to attempt this maneuver unassisted. If the person is not cognitively intact, you may use a toileting schedule to discourage the individual from attempting self-toileting when you, the LPN, or other caregivers are not present to assist. If the older person cannot safely ambulate alone, the IDT may decide that physical therapy is indicated or that a program of daily assisted ambulation should be initiated.

Older adults who cannot safely stand or walk unassisted, but who may still attempt these actions, should not be left alone for extended periods. One idea is to bring the person out of the room so that staff members can observe the older adult and in that way keep the individual safe. When someone who is not safe is left alone, mobility alarms would help the staff know when the individual is getting up unassisted. Mobility alarms can be attached to the bed and wheelchair. All members of the IDT need to remember to remove clutter and to maintain clear walking paths for older people, to adjust lighting to provide an optimal environment, and to wipe up spills from the floor as soon as they occur or are noticed.

⬤ ALTERATION IN ELIMINATION

Urinary Incontinence

Urinary incontinence, a problem that affects approximately 10 million Americans, is defined as an involuntary loss of urine that is sufficient to be a problem. It is a problem most often seen in the elderly population; 15% to 30% of noninstitutionalized people older than 60 years of age and half of all nursing home residents are affected. The cost of caring for individuals with urinary incontinence is approximately $7 billion annually for individuals living in the community

---

CRITICALLY EXAMINE THE FOLLOWING

You have been asked to present the educational section at the next staff meeting. Your nurse manager has requested that you develop a teaching plan for your colleagues regarding the importance of mobility in older adults. You have been asked to discuss two former patients who had mobility problems. As part of your lesson plan, write out the reasons an older person should be mobile. Identify ways mobility can be done successfully with the following patients:

1. An 87-year-old man with a fractured hip. He is deconditioned (a word from a previous chapter; do you remember it?), yet insists he can walk "by himself."
2. A 72-year-old woman who is "pleasantly confused" while recovering from a fractured femur. She is experiencing a great deal of pain and thinks you are her son.

   Address both patients' ambulation plans. Bring your best lesson plan to class to share with others.

---

and approximately $3.3 billion for nursing home residents.

Even greater than the economic cost are the psychological and social costs to the individual who is incontinent of urine. Incontinence is seen as a major reason older adults are placed in nursing homes. People who are incontinent may feel embarrassed and socially isolated. They may withdraw from participation in social activities and become depressed. Incontinence is associated with the development of other health problems, such as skin breakdown, behavioral disturbances, and urinary tract infections.

Age-Related Changes Affecting Incontinence

Although incontinence is more prevalent in older people, it is not a normal aspect of aging. There are, however, numerous age-related changes that make the older person susceptible to developing incontinence. In older adults, the bladder capacity diminishes to about half that of younger adults. The diminished ability of the kidneys to concentrate urine makes urinary frequency and nocturia (excessive urination at night) common problems for the older person. In addition, many older people experience sudden and unexpected contractions of the detrusor muscle (the smooth muscle that makes up the outside wall of the bladder), which cause an urgent need to void. Changes in the central and autonomic nervous systems of the older person cause a decreased ability to contract the external sphincter of the bladder, which exacerbates urinary urgency further. Many postmenopausal women experience thinning and weakening of the muscles of the pelvic floor and the urethra because of estrogen loss. In men, an enlarged prostate, often associated with aging, may lead to urinary retention, irritability of the detrusor muscle, and bladder spasms.

The urinary urgency that many older people experience often leads to incontinence in an institutional setting. When an older adult cannot go to the toilet independently or as often as needed, incontinence is likely to result. This situation is exacerbated further by the immobility that results from being ill or from needing medical interventions, such as intravenous therapy.

Types of Incontinence

For the nurse to intervene in the management of incontinence, it is important to understand the underlying causes of incontinence. Incontinence can be a result of a chronic problem, or it can be the result of an acute situation.

Acute Incontinence

Acute or transient incontinence is incontinence that occurs because of the presence of another medical problem, and it often resolves when the underlying illness is treated. The following mnemonic highlights the possible causes of acute incontinence:

D: Delirium
R: Restricted mobility, retention (acute)
I: Infection, inflammation, impaction
P: Pharmaceutical, polyuria, psychological

Delirium is an acute confusional state that is brought on by an acute illness and that disrupts the physiological homeostasis in the older person. In a delirious state, the person is unaware of the need to void, and the person does not have the capability to get to the toilet.

Restricted mobility, as already discussed, is a common cause of incontinence in elderly people. Acute urinary retention is often caused by anticholinergic and narcotic medications and may result in overflow incontinence.

Urinary tract infections cause frequency, urgency, and painful urination. This condition can lead to increased bladder contractions and incontinence. Many residents in long-term care have bacteria in their urine, a condition that is asymptomatic and does not require treatment. When bacteriuria is accompanied by urinary incontinence, however, the person should be treated, and the effect of the treatment on the incontinence should be noted.

Fecal impaction often obstructs the bladder outlet and may cause overflow urinary incontinence. In overflow urinary incontinence, the bladder retains urine, and when it reaches its capacity, the individual begins to drip or leak urine. In postmenopausal women, the changes that occur in the lining of the vagina and urethra because of lower levels of estrogen may cause inflammation and weakening of the pelvic floor, which can cause incontinence.

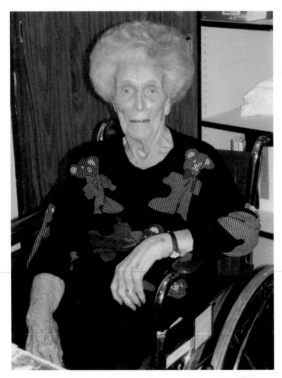

At age 83, this woman is incontinent. Many older adults admitted to nursing homes are put there because their family members cannot manage the problems associated with incontinence. This woman wears disposable briefs, which are changed by the nursing home staff on a regular basis, and quit dehydrating herself in an effort to control the incontinence. Her health has improved because of increased fluid intake, and the staff members keep her clean and free of urine odor.

Many drugs can cause urinary incontinence. Following is a list of drug groups that adversely affect an older person's ability to maintain continence:

- Sedatives/hypnotics
- Antipsychotics
- Narcotics
- Anticholinergics
- Alpha-adrenergic blockers
- Diuretics

Endocrine disorders that lead to hyperglycemia or hypercalcemia may cause urinary incontinence. Psychological causes that have been associated with urinary incontinence include depression and confusional states.

Nursing Implications

Most instances of bladder incontinence are transient and often reversible. In most cases, acute or transient incontinence can be resolved with treatment of the underlying illness or with discontinuation of a causative drug. Incontinence should never be accepted without first ascertaining that the older person has been assessed for underlying conditions and that treatment has been initiated.

Chronic Incontinence

There are four types of persistent or chronic incontinence. Incontinence is considered to be persistent if it continues after reversible causes have been ruled out or treated. In addition, persistent or chronic incontinence usually has a gradual onset, worsens over time, and occurs when there is a failure either to empty or to store urine. The four types of persistent or chronic incontinence are as follows:

Urge incontinence is the most common form of incontinence in long-term care facilities. It is closely associated with stroke and Alzheimer's disease. In this type of incontinence, the patient or resident feels the urge to go but does not have enough time to get to the toilet before the urine is released.

Stress incontinence occurs when a small amount of urine is released after there is a sudden increase in intra-abdominal pressure caused by coughing, sneezing, laughing, or lifting. This type of incontinence results when the bladder outlet sphincter is incompetent or weak. Stress incontinence is more common in women and is often a result of damage to the pelvic muscles during childbirth.

Overflow incontinence is present in approximately 15% of nursing home residents. It is caused by bladder outlet obstruction that results in impaired bladder emptying. When the bladder is not emptied sufficiently, the resident experiences frequent dribbling of urine.

Functional incontinence results when the individual is unable or unwilling to attend to toileting needs. In this situation, the bladder and urethra function normally, but cognitive, physical, psychological, or environmental impairments make it difficult for the older person to get to the toilet. Inaccessible toilets, unavailable caregivers, depression, and inability to find the toilet all are possible causes of functional incontinence.

Nursing Implications

Treatment of urinary incontinence is based on the underlying cause. Medication intervention may be used to treat infection or stop abnormal bladder muscle contractions and tighten sphincter muscles. Surgical intervention is used to correct anatomical anomalies and remove obstructions. Behavioral interventions require that the health-care professional provide education and positive reinforcement to the older adult and family members. Behavioral interventions sometimes may be used in combination with medical or surgical interventions.

Behavioral Interventions

Behavioral interventions, which are most often provided by nursing personnel, are also called training procedures and include the following:

- Bladder training (retraining)
- Habit training (timed voiding)
- Prompted voiding
- Pelvic muscle exercises

These techniques are most helpful with stress and urge incontinence.

Bladder retraining is used to restore the normal pattern of voiding by inhibiting or stimulating voiding. The goal is to lengthen the time between voidings. This is best done by instructing and assisting the individual to learn to suppress the urge to void in an attempt to increase the amount of urine the bladder can hold. This technique is used with individuals who are capable of understanding and remembering the instructions. Most bladder-retraining schedules begin with a schedule of toileting every 2 hours and gradually increase the amount of time between voidings.

Prompted voiding is different from bladder training in that the goal is not to increase bladder capacity, but rather to teach the incontinent person to be aware of toileting needs and to request assistance from the caregiver. In this technique, the person is asked to try to use the toilet at regular intervals and is praised for maintaining continence and using the toilet. The schedule that is followed usually involves toileting on awakening, after meals, at bedtime, and, if awake, at night. More voiding times can be added if the individual's voiding schedule indicates a need. This intervention works well with moderately confused people.

Habit training works best with cognitively impaired or confused people and requires the caregiver to take the patient to the toilet at regular intervals. The toileting schedule may be every 2 to 4 hours, or the caregiver may toilet the individual on awakening, after meals, at bedtime, and at night, if awake.

Kegel's exercises are used to alleviate stress incontinence. The goal of such exercises is to strengthen the pelvic floor muscles. Patients who are taught Kegel's exercises must be cognitively intact and willing to participate in this exercise regimen. The exercise consists of the person contracting the pelvic floor muscles and holding them for 3 to 4 seconds and then relaxing the muscle. This should be done 10 times in succession at least twice a day.

In dealing with incontinence, nurses play a key role in education and treatment. Incontinence is not a normal part of aging but is more prevalent in elderly people. Many forms of incontinence are reversible, and all attempts should be made to assess, treat, and resolve incontinence when it is present.

Constipation

Bowel functioning and the avoidance of constipation are common concerns for older adults. Many older people were raised during a time when anything but a daily bowel movement was considered abnormal. The concern regarding this problem is appropriate because numerous age-related changes in the gastrointestinal system make constipation more likely.

It is probable that an older person has an extended gastrointestinal transit time as a result of slower peristalsis. More water is removed from the stool when it is in the colon for longer periods. The stool becomes harder and more difficult to pass. Immobility, decreased exercise, and a lack of fiber and water in the diet are common problems in older people, and these factors tend to exacerbate the tendency to become constipated. Certain drugs also may lead to constipation, including the following:

- Aluminum-containing antacids
- Anticholinergics
- Calcium carbonate
- Iron salts
- Laxatives (when abused)
- Opiates
- Phenothiazines
- Sedatives
- Tricyclic antidepressants
- Diuretics
- Calcium channel blockers

Immobility is particularly problematic in the maintenance of regular bowel movements. Muscular atrophy, which is a loss of tone in the muscles of the intestine, and generalized weakness of the muscles necessary for the expulsive mechanism of evacuation occur during periods of immobilization. The overuse of laxatives also causes a loss of muscle tone in the bowel.

Immobility not only affects the physiological functioning of the gastrointestinal system, but it also prevents the individual from interacting efficiently with the environment to meet the needs of the body. Factors such as strange environments, disruption of the usual elimination patterns, being forced to defecate in an unnatural position in unnatural surroundings (as occurs with the use of a bedpan), and suppressing the urge to defecate because of the inability to get to the toilet inhibit normal defecation.

Nursing Interventions

Nursing interventions aimed at prevention of constipation should be focused on establishing a regular pattern of bowel elimination that is not associated with straining or discomfort. It is important for the older person's overall health to attempt to correct constipation without resorting to the use of laxatives. These interventions should include increasing physical activity, increasing water intake, increasing dietary fiber, and establishing a regular bowel routine. Regular exercise stimulates motility in the gut.

The older adult should be encouraged to drink 1500 to 2000 mL of fluids daily unless this is contraindicated by other health problems. Dietary fiber also plays an important role in the avoidance of constipation. Fiber holds water, making the stool softer and bulkier, which speeds the passage of stool through the intestine.

It can be difficult to increase fiber in the diet of the older person because of lifelong dietary preferences and poor dentition. It may be helpful to consult a dietitian. Although prunes and prune juice are often used to combat constipation, they may not be the best choice. Prunes have only 2 g of fiber per prune, and prune juice has none. Prunes mimic the action of cathartics, and there may be rebound constipation when the use of prunes is discontinued.

Assisting the patient to develop a regular bowel routine is an essential part of bowel maintenance and one in which the nurses play a pivotal role. In facilitating regular bowel routines, the nurse must assess how much, if any, assistance the person requires in getting safely to the toilet. The use of bedpans should be avoided whenever possible, but when they are used, the patient should be in an upright position unless this position is contraindicated. The nurse also needs to ensure that regular toileting times are maintained and that privacy is provided during toileting time.

● ALTERATION IN SKIN INTEGRITY: PRESSURE ULCERS

A pressure ulcer is defined as any lesion caused by unrelieved pressure that results in damage to the underlying tissue. Pressure ulcers are an extremely serious health problem that can lead to pain, extended hospital stays, and further complications from infection. In hospitals, the pressure ulcer rate has been estimated to be 29.5%, and in nursing homes it is estimated to be 23%. Older persons are particularly at risk, with persons older than 70 years accounting for 71% of all patients with pressure ulcers. Approximately 60,000 deaths per year are associated with pressure ulcers. In nursing homes, 66% of residents who develop a pressure ulcer die. It is estimated that patients with pressure ulcers require 50% more nursing care than patients without them. Because pressure ulcers are, for the most part, preventable, maintaining adequate skin integrity is a quality-of-care issue for all nurses. Even more important than knowing the various treatment modalities is knowing how pressure ulcers develop. You need to become an expert in prevention techniques.

Risk Factors

Mechanical Risk Factors

Four mechanical factors that contribute to the development of pressure ulcers are pressure, shearing, friction, and moisture.

- *Pressure* ulcers usually occur over bony prominences where normal tissue is squeezed between the internal pressure of the bone and an external source of pressure or friction, such as the chair or the bed. External pressure that lasts long enough and is sufficient enough to decrease blood flow results in inadequate oxygenation and nutrition to the area and the subsequent development of a pressure ulcer. Immobility is the most important risk factor in the development of pressure ulcers. Pressure of high intensity that is left unchecked for more than 2 hours can result in irreversible tissue damage.
- *Shearing* occurs when the head of the bed is elevated more than 30 degrees and the person slides toward the foot of the bed. In this situation, the skin over the sacrum does not move, whereas the subcutaneous tissue and gluteal vessels are stretched. Rupture of the blood vessels results. Subcutaneous fat, which lacks the ability to stretch, is particularly vulnerable to injury from shearing forces. Sores that develop on the sacrum, heels, and anterior tibial region are most probably a result of shearing. When shearing and pressure are both present, the amount of pressure necessary to cause tissue damage is half the amount that causes tissue damage when shearing is not present.
- *Friction* occurs when the skin is moved across the sheets, such as when the person is being pulled up rather than lifted up in the bed. The result of this motion is damage to the epidermis, which can lead to ulceration or a break in the skin. *Moisture* caused by perspiration or incontinence can increase the friction between the surface and the skin. Moisture also can cause maceration (softening of the skin), which weakens the skin and increases the risk of infection. In the presence of moisture resulting from urinary or fecal incontinence, the risk of pressure ulcer development on the sacrum and buttocks increases fivefold. Incontinence is a strong predictor of skin breakdown.

Physiological Risk Factors

In addition to mechanical forces, there are factors that are inherent to the individual that increase the risk of skin breakdown. Examples include aging skin, immobility, and malnutrition.

- *Aging skin* increases the likelihood of developing pressure ulcers because it is less resistant to the mechanical forces that can damage the skin. With advancing age, there is a decrease in the thickness of the cell layers of the epidermis, a flattening in the epidermal-dermal interface, and a loss of subcutaneous tissue. These changes cause impaired wound healing and decreased thermoregulation, causing the skin to become more fragile.
- *Immobility,* combined with the age-related changes of the skin, greatly increases the risk of pressure ulcer formation. Normally, spontaneous body movements that occur during sleep and throughout the day protect the skin from pressure. Many situations prevent the body from spontaneous movement, however, including physical disability, loss of sensation, presence of pain, or use of sedating drugs or anesthesia.
- *Malnutrition* is another physiological factor that can lead to pressure ulcer formation. Deficiencies in zinc, iron, vitamin C, and protein adversely affect the health of the skin. The more severe the malnutrition, the more severe the pressure ulcer. In older adults who have experienced weight loss or who are underweight, it is important to check the albumin level of the blood. A serum albumin level less than 3.5 g/dL indicates that nutritional intervention is necessary to prevent skin breakdown. Malnutrition and the subsequent weight loss lead to loss of muscle mass and subcutaneous tissue. This diminishes the body's protective padding and increases the pressure over the bony prominences.

Staging

Pressure ulcers are graded according to the degree of tissue damage. The staging of a pressure ulcer dictates the type of treatment to be implemented. Staging provides a means of describing an ulcer that allows for the ulcer to be monitored over time. Commonly used staging criteria are presented in the following list:

Stage I: Nonblanchable erythema of intact skin. (The skin is reddened, even in the absence of direct pressure.)

Stage II: Partial-thickness skin loss involving epidermis or dermis. The ulcer is superficial and manifests clinically as an abrasion, blister, or shallow crater.

Stage III: Full-thickness skin loss involving damage to or necrosis of subcutaneous tissue that may extend down to, but not through, the underlying fascia (fibrous membrane covering the muscles). The ulcer manifests clinically as a deep crater with or without undermining of adjacent tissue.

Stage IV: Full-thickness skin loss with extensive destruction, tissue necrosis, or damage to muscle, bone, or supporting structures (e.g., tendon or joint capsule). Undermining and sinus tracts also may be associated with stage IV pressure ulcers.

Prevention

Assessment of risk is a vital first step in prevention of pressure ulcers. If a person is found to be at risk for developing pressure ulcers, interventions to prevent skin breakdown can be initiated before an ulcer develops. Numerous assessment tools are available. Review the Braden Scale presented in Chapter 15.

Assessment should be done within the first 24 hours of admission to a hospital or nursing home and repeated 24 to 48 hours after admission. Ongoing assessment is necessary to prevent new skin breakdown. This should be done every 24 to 48 hours in the hospital, monthly in the nursing home, and whenever there is a change in the person's condition.

Inspection of the tissue of the feet requires special attention in elderly persons. They may neglect their feet because of the difficulty in bending over to see and manage any problems. Inspection of the feet is an important aspect of care. Hyperkeratosis of the nails (thick, hard nails, difficult to cut) may require a podiatrist visit to cut them. Cutting the nails of the feet should not be done by LPNs unless they are specifically asked to do so. Report all problems with the tissue or nails of the feet to the registered nurse (RN) so that appropriate referrals can be made for treatment.

When an older adult is found to be at risk for alteration in skin integrity, preventive measures should be aimed at reducing pressure on bony prominences, preventing shear or friction, keeping skin clean and dry, and providing adequate nutrition and hydration. To reduce pressure, the person should be repositioned at least every 2 hours. This regular repositioning decreases the amount of time that pressure is exerted on any one body part. The appearance of reddened areas indicates that more frequent turning or other interventions may be indicated. When placing an older adult on either side, a wedge should be placed behind the person to prevent the person from lying directly on the trochanter (which is the bony prominence located below the neck of the femur).

Although at one time it was common practice to massage reddened areas over bony prominences, this is no longer the practice. Massage may exert pressure on the area and may cause further breakdown of the small capillaries. In some cases, it may be necessary to use pressure-relieving devices, such as air-filled, water-filled, or gel-filled chair pads or mattresses, and foam heel protectors and mattresses. The use of egg-crate mattresses, although common, does not provide sufficient pressure relief to prevent pressure ulcers. Walking programs and passive and active ROM exercises not only improve muscle strength and joint flexibility but also are important in the prevention of skin breakdown.

CRITICALLY EXAMINE THE FOLLOWING

You are a home-health nurse for a 79-year-old woman who is cared for by her husband with drop-in visits from three daughters. Sarah, the patient, is home bound because of general fatigue and postoperative total hip replacement. She can ambulate with a cane but is fearful and will not leave the house except on rare occasions. She says she is happy to be at home with her husband and not to have the arthritic hip pain. The problem is she is either in bed or a recliner chair most of the day and night. Her husband lifts her to and from the chair and bed when Sarah is "too tired to move herself."

You have noticed that Sarah's buttocks are reddened, as are her heels. What should you do about your assessment? Focus on a teaching plan for this couple. (I know this is the second teaching plan you have been asked to do in this chapter. My hope is that after doing the first one and sharing it with your fellow students, this one will be easier to write.) What do they need to know about pressure ulcers? What is the best way for you to share the hazards of immobility with Sarah? What can you do to prevent the stage I pressure ulcers from developing into something worse? Do your best thinking and be prepared to share it with the class.

To reduce friction, persons should be lifted and not pulled when repositioned. The use of a lift sheet or a turn sheet is essential to distribute the person's weight evenly and avoid undue friction and stress on the skin. Shear can be reduced by decreasing the amount of time and frequency that the person's head is elevated in the bed. When out of bed and in a chair, the person should be repositioned at least every 2 hours, and long-term sitting should be discouraged. While in the chair, the individual needs to be examined for appropriate posture and alignment because an inappropriate sitting posture can lead to pressure ulcers and increased shearing forces.

Although skin should be kept clean and dry to prevent pressure ulcers, older adults do not need to be bathed daily. Excessive bathing and rubbing can be drying and damaging to the skin. Using a mild cleansing agent that does not promote dryness and patting the skin dry are essentials of good skin care for the older person.

Treatment

Despite vigilant nursing care, a pressure ulcer sometimes develops. Often an underlying disease state can defeat attempts to prevent skin breakdown. The treatment of pressure ulcers is extremely individualized, and there is much controversy as to which treatments and skin care products to use. The technology and products for treatment of pressure ulcers are changing every day. Treatment is aimed at promoting a healing environment by providing adequate circulation and oxygenation to the impaired tissue and maintaining a clean and dry wound area. Exudate should be removed as much as possible, and infection should be treated with the appropriate antibiotic. Any necrotic tissue needs to be débrided or removed before treatment of the ulcer can proceed; this should be done only under the supervision of the RN.

● ALTERED NUTRITIONAL STATUS

Adequate nutrition is essential to the maintenance of health, prevention of disease, treatment of chronic illness, and recovery from acute illness. When the body is inadequately nourished, the individual is more likely to develop an illness and is less able to recover from illness. Caloric or protein malnutrition is present in 12% to 50% of older people.

To be adequately nourished, the body must have a sufficient intake of carbohydrates, fats, proteins, vitamins, minerals, and water. Difficulty obtaining appropriate nutrition can be a result of lack of knowledge about good nutrition, inadequate income or means of obtaining the appropriate foods, lack of socialization (which may lead to disinterest or overindulgence in food), or housing that is inadequate for storing and preparing nutritionally sound meals. The older person's diet is often lacking in calcium, vitamin C, riboflavin, niacin, and iron. A deficiency of any essential nutrient can cause changes to the body that, if left unchecked, can lead to illness.

Risk Factors

Anorexia (loss of appetite) is a major cause of inadequate nutritional intake in older people. Poor dentition, poorly fitting dentures, or lack of dentures may make it difficult for the individual to chew, and a soft or puree diet may be unappetizing. Not only may diminished mobility make it difficult for the older person to obtain and prepare food, but a sedentary lifestyle also may lead to a decreased appetite. Polypharmacy, a common situation with elderly patients, can adversely affect appetite by altering taste sensation, impairing cognition and mood, or interfering with the absorption of nutrients. Other causes of anorexia in older adults may include the increased incidence of chronic illness, social isolation, depression, and unappetizing institutional foods.

Changes in the metabolism of older people translate into changes in nutritional requirements of the body. With aging, there is a decreased metabolic rate, and the body requires fewer calories for maintenance. Decreased mobility and the loss of muscle mass associated with aging also suggest that older people may need to decrease their caloric consumption. Older adults use more energy, however, than younger people to do the same activities. If the individual is active, there may be a need to increase the caloric intake. With aging, the body does not metabolize protein as efficiently, so older people may need more protein in their diet.

Maintaining adequate nutrition in older persons who have a disease process poses a particular challenge to the nurse. People with advanced dementia may have weight loss even when there is an adequate intake of nutritional requirements. It is suspected that this weight loss may be due in part to the increased use of antibiotics in a population that tends to have a higher rate of infection. Neuroleptics, another commonly used class of drugs in demented patients, also may cause a loss of appetite. It has been postulated that there may be a disturbance in the metabolism of patients with advanced Alzheimer's disease, and this, too, may account for the unexplained weight loss in these patients. The term "failure to thrive" has been used to describe another entity associated with weight loss. Failure to thrive occurs when some elderly nursing home residents experience a gradual decline in physical and cognitive functioning associated with weight loss, withdrawing from food, withdrawing from human contact, and exhibiting signs of depression.

A significant problem for many older adults who have had a stroke or generalized weakness is aspiration, the inhalation of solids or liquids into the upper respiratory tract. This is a critical problem because of the serious consequences of an aspiration. It can cause pneumonia or death by choking. The symptoms of aspiration include a sudden severe cough or cyanosis while eating or drinking, voice changes, and increased respiratory rate after eating or drinking. The possibility of aspiration is increased with dysphagia (difficulty swallowing) and gastroesophageal reflux problems.

Assessment

Assessing the nutritional status of the older person can be a difficult task for the nurse. The recommended daily allowance (RDA) that is established by the National Academy of Science Research Council is one way of monitoring how well an individual is meeting nutritional requirements. The RDA does not consider the specific needs of the population older than 65 years of age, however. Additional nutrients that may be needed as a result of infection or chronic illness are not addressed by the RDA.

Complicating the assessment for malnutrition further are the changes of the aging body itself. Many physical manifestations of malnutrition are similar to changes that are associated with aging. These changes include dry, thin hair; dry, flaky skin; sunken eyes; dry oral mucosa; weight loss; and muscle weakness. Using skinfold measures to estimate percentage of body fat may not yield accurate information because mean body mass (muscle tissue) decreases with age. Probably the most reliable indicator of adequate nutritional intake is a normal serum albumin level (3.5 to 5.5 g/dL). Monitoring an individual's weight over time is also an appropriate means of recognizing alteration in nutritional status.

Nursing Implications

To reestablish adequate nutritional intake, health-care providers should strive to maintain oral feedings, possibly with appropriate modifications. The diet may need to be made more palatable with foods that have different textures and flavors. Providing the individual's food favorites whenever possible is also a good approach. Family members can be asked to provide favorite foods for the older person. Ensuring that the older person has dentures and that they fit well and providing a diet that is appropriate for the person's dental status are imperative.

Everyone responds well to meals that are served in an attractive manner and in an environment that is relaxed and pleasant. Nursing staff should strive for this kind of atmosphere during mealtime by not raising their voices and trying to keep noisy dietary carts out of the eating area. Eyeglasses help the resident to see the food on the tray, and hearing aids allow the resident to socialize with tablemates during mealtime. It is important that the nurse ensure that the individual has whatever assistive devices are needed to make the eating experience a more pleasant one.

If the person's nutritional status does not improve despite these efforts, the nurse needs to consider other interventions. It may be necessary to offer more assistance with meals. The individual may need to be fed or have containers opened, or he or she may just need ongoing gentle encouragement throughout the meal to continue eating. Often, gently touching the arm or shoulder while encouraging feeding helps the older adult to attend to the task of eating. Touch is a caring behavior that indicates value and respect for the person being touched. Older people often are not touched or hugged frequently and generally respond positively to the act of being touched. A nutritional supplement also may be needed.

The dietitian should assist in deciding what, if any, supplements are needed. Liquid dietary supplements are best offered between meals so that the supplement is not substituted for the meal itself. The supplement can provide a large percentage of the RDA requirements but does not completely meet all dietary requirements.

Tube feedings and parenteral feedings can be used when all other attempts at oral feedings have failed. These methods have numerous complications, however. Striving to maintain adequate oral intake should be the goal of all

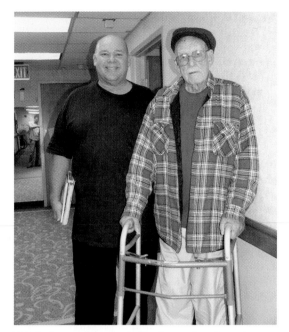

This father and son have lived together since the father's discharge from a nursing home. He was admitted for falling and for generalized weakness; he was malnourished. The son enjoys cooking and caters to his father's wishes, which has improved the older man's health remarkably. Now, the two of them go to the nursing home to visit the father's friends there.

nursing personnel. Adequate nutrition affects every aspect of the individual's health and well-being.

● SLEEP PATTERN DISTURBANCES

Older people often complain of not getting enough sleep or not feeling well rested after sleeping. Sleep disturbances increase with age. It is estimated that sleep pattern disturbances affect half of people older than 65 years who live at home and two-thirds of older people living in institutions.

Normal Sleep Patterns

A review of normal sleep patterns is necessary to understand the changes in sleep patterns that tend to occur with aging. There are five stages to normal sleep. Refer to Chapter 9 if you need to review this material.

Age-Related Changes in Sleep Patterns

In the course of aging, people tend to sleep less than 8 hours per night. Older people have an impaired capacity to maintain sleep; sleep tends to be marked by more frequent and prolonged awakenings during the night. In addition, stage IV and REM sleep diminish. In extreme old age, changes in cerebral blood flow and organic brain syndrome also are associated with a shortening of the REM stage of sleep.

The sleep patterns of older people can be disturbed by factors such as needing to void frequently during the night (nocturia) and changes in vision and hearing that cause incorrect perceptions of their immediate environment. These changes can lead to ineffective sleep or sleep deprivation. Sleep deprivation is marked by fatigue, tiredness, eye problems, muscle tremor, muscle weakness, diminished coordination and attention span, apathy, and depression.

Sleep Disorders

In addition to age-related changes in sleep patterns, some sleep disorders are common to older adults. Sleep apnea, a medical condition in which breathing stops for 10 seconds or longer numerous times throughout the night, affects 20% of older people. Sleep apnea is associated with high blood pressure, obesity, heart disease, and stroke. Death can result because of the effect on the cardiovascular and respiratory systems. The affected person complains of excessive daytime sleepiness and constant interruption of sleep. Cessation of breathing for 10 or more seconds, followed by very loud snoring or choking, is the primary objective symptom of sleep apnea.

Night-shift personnel are often the first people to discover the symptoms of sleep apnea when a patient or resident is admitted to the hospital or nursing home. The treatment for sleep apnea is usually weight reduction, continuous positive airway pressure (CPAP), oxygen, and occasionally surgery. CPAP is a technique that forces air down the nose, through the throat, and into the lungs; it is used during sleep for persons who have been diagnosed with sleep apnea.

Sundown Syndrome

Sundown syndrome is another disorder that affects many older people. Sundown syndrome is defined as the appearance or exacerbation of symptoms of confusion associated with the late afternoon or evening hours. This syndrome is marked by behaviors such as agitation, restlessness, confusion, wandering, and screaming that occur usually in the evening hours (sundown). Little is known about this disorder, which is a tremendous management problem for caregivers. Risk factors for sundown syndrome seem to be impaired mental status, dehydration, being awakened frequently during the night for nursing care, and recent relocation either to a new room or to the institution.

Nursing Interventions

Sleeping medications, tranquilizers, and sedatives are commonly used to promote sleep but should be avoided at all costs in older persons. Sedatives and barbiturates that depress the central nervous system may lead to other problems by depressing vital body functions, lowering basal metabolic rate, decreasing blood pressure, and causing mental confusion. Sleeping medications decrease spontaneous body movements that may lead to skin breakdown. Most of the medications used to promote sleep are not efficiently metabolized by the aging body, and the person may experience a hangover effect the next day. In addition, these drugs tend to cause blurred vision, dry mouth, and urinary retention. Because it is known that an elderly person cannot sleep as long as a younger person can, it is unreasonable to put an individual to bed at 8 p.m. and expect that person to stay in bed until 7 a.m. the next day.

There is much the nurse can do to promote sleep without resorting to the use of medications. Meeting the individual's comfort needs by offering back rubs or snacks such as warm milk, assisting with toileting needs, providing socks or an extra blanket to increase body temperature (which may be diminished in an older person), repositioning, and alleviating pain are just a few of the nursing interventions that may reduce insomnia. If these interventions do not promote sleep, it is prudent to allow the older person to come out of the bed and perhaps sit for a while in a comfortable chair near the nurses' station. This may reassure the individual of the surroundings and prevent attempts to get out of bed unassisted, perhaps risking a fall. During the daytime, increased motor activities and time outdoors, if possible, have been found to promote sleep.

IATROGENESIS

Iatrogenic disorders can be defined as disorders that a person acquires as a result of receiving treatment by a physician, nurse, or other member of the IDT. Iatrogenesis also can occur if the person does not receive treatment when it is indicated or receives incorrect treatment. An older person often presents with numerous chronic conditions that require complex interventions, numerous medications, and increased exposure to the health-care system; this puts older adults at increased risk of experiencing untoward effects of medical treatment. Iatrogenic disorders include the disorders previously discussed in this chapter: immobility, falls, incontinence, malnutrition, pressure ulcers, and disturbances in the sleep-wake cycle.

Studies have found that 30% to 40% of people older than 65 years have iatrogenic complications. Common causes of iatrogenesis in the hospital are misuse or overuse of drugs, prolonged immobilization, nosocomial (hospital-acquired) infections, and malnutrition and dehydration secondary to preparation for diagnostic tests. In the nursing home, common iatrogenic disorders include immobilization, adverse drug reactions, falls, pressure ulcers, and nosocomial infections.

Iatrogenic disorders often cause a vicious circle in which one disorder quickly leads to another. Consider the older person who is admitted to the hospital for abdominal discomfort. This person is unable to sleep and is prescribed a sleeping pill. Having taken this medication, the person is groggy when getting out of bed and sustains a fall. The staff, not wanting the patient to be hurt again, assigns a volunteer to sit with the person to remind him or her not to get up. The older person is now unable to get up and suffers from some of the adverse sequelae of immobility, such as incontinence, disorientation, and pressure ulcer formation. In time, the person's muscles become deconditioned, and the next time the patient is assisted out of bed, there is another fall, the person sustains a hip fracture, and the cycle continues. One can see what a high price is paid for the effects of negative medical and nursing interventions.

CONCLUSION

The health-care needs of older adults are multiple and complex. Health-care providers often are not educated in the normal aging process or in the older person's response to illness and health-care interventions. As a result, the layperson and the health-care provider may believe that there is little that can be done to improve the health status of older adults. Not only is this not true, but also this attitude can lead to a self-fulfilling prophecy in which older people are expected to be ill and to experience functional decline. Assessment and interventions aimed at correcting the illness, promoting function, and averting a subsequent decline may not be initiated, and the older person is likely to become more ill and more dependent on others.

LPNs can and should play a pivotal role in ensuring that the health-care needs of older persons are being met. They also need to be aware of the problems that besiege the older person as a result of medical interventions. Iatrogenesis can be prevented. Many of the clinical problems that the older person faces in health and in illness can be averted or alleviated with nursing interventions that are focused on improving and maintaining wellness and promoting function.

Mrs. S. is an 84-year-old widow who was admitted to the hospital after a right-hemisphere cerebrovascular accident (CVA). Her medical history includes hypertension, atrial fibrillation, and bilateral total hip replacements because of degenerative joint disease. Before the CVA and this hospitalization, she was living in her own apartment, where she was social and able to meet her own needs except for shopping and heavy housecleaning. Her family did those things for her. When admitted to the hospital, she was found to have left-sided weakness and some speech problems, although she could be understood.

The family is planning to admit her to the nursing home; they do not know if she will be able to return to her apartment, but they are hopeful that she will be able to go to an assisted-living apartment. The report given to the nursing home from the hospital includes the following facts:

- During her hospitalization, she became incontinent. A Foley catheter was placed to control the urinary incontinence, but she subsequently developed a urinary tract infection, so the catheter was removed.
- She developed aspiration pneumonia, which the physician assumed was due to aspirating food because of a swallowing deficit from her stroke. Her diet was changed to puree, and she has had no further episodes of aspiration, although she is taking only about 30% of her diet.
- She has started physical therapy and has progressed from the parallel bars to short distances with a walker. She does not own a walker, so she has not walked on the unit; she has only walked in the therapy department.
- Mrs. S. has not spoken much during her hospitalization, although she follows simple directions. The nurse thinks that she "might be a little confused at times."
- Her blood pressure is well controlled with diuretics.
- The family is very concerned that if she falls, she may damage the hip replacements, and they have requested that she be restrained.

Discussion

Examine the list of facts in the case study for iatrogenic problems. How would you prevent such problems? How would you deal with them?

Solution

In this case study, there are numerous potential iatrogenic problems that the nursing staff should address. The report from the hospital notes that Mrs. S. had a Foley catheter inserted because she was incontinent. The question the nurse should be asking here is, "Why is Mrs. S. incontinent?" True, the incontinence can be a result of damage from the stroke, but until attempts are made to take the patient to the bathroom, one cannot be certain. It may be that Mrs. S., having had a stroke that affected her speech, could not tell the staff that she needed to go. She may have to go to the bathroom as soon as the urge presents itself. A prompted voiding schedule would be helpful in beginning to assess whether this incontinence is reversible. A Foley catheter should not be the first intervention used in the presence of incontinence. In this case, the use of the catheter prolonged the hospitalization by causing a urinary tract infection.

Another possible iatrogenic problem may be aspiration pneumonia. In this case, iatrogenesis may be a result of something that should have been done that was not done. In a person who has had a stroke and who has difficulty talking, one should consider the possibility of a swallowing deficit. A patient such as Mrs. S. should never be left alone to eat. In addition, the nursing staff should be assessing her during mealtime for any difficulty swallowing. If a difficulty is noted, a speech and swallowing consultation is warranted. When the diet was changed to puree, Mrs. S. apparently had no further problems with swallowing but had a decreased nutritional intake. The nurse needs to assess the person to understand why the diet is not being taken. There may be many reasons. The patient may not like her diet, she may still be having difficulty swallowing and is afraid of choking again, or she may be depressed and without an appetite.

It is a positive step that Mrs. S. has been started on physical therapy and is walking, but there is more that the nursing and physical therapy staffs can do to promote functional ambulation. Walking does not have to be done just in the therapy department. The therapist needs to lend a walker to Mrs. S. or to instruct the family to buy one for her so that ambulation can be done on the nursing unit. Therapy takes place for only about 1 hour a day. Walking the person on the unit augments therapy, improves the person's gait, helps her to regain her confidence in her functional ability, and prevents the negative effects of immobility.

The nurse reports that Mrs. S. might be confused; however, there is little evidence here to support that conclusion or to suggest that confusion should be expected. From the report, Mrs. S. was not confused before her hospitalization. If she is confused, it may be related to the urinary tract infection, the pneumonia, the relocation to the hospital, or the depression from the stroke. The possibility of confusion should not deter the nurse in any way from pursuing a plan of care that focuses on promoting the highest level of functional ability for this patient.

The family requests that Mrs. S. be restrained to prevent injury to her hip replacements. Instead of a restraint, the staff needs to consider ways of preventing a fall so that the family will understand that a restraint is not needed. Possible interventions to prevent a fall might include helping Mrs. S. to understand her limitations, toileting her at regular intervals, promoting lower extremity strengthening through exercise, keeping her out of her room and within sight of the staff, and perhaps using an alarm if she is unpredictable in her attempts to get up. Because Mrs. S. is taking diuretics, one would want to assess her for orthostatic hypotension as a possible fall risk factor. Honoring the family's request for a restraint may serve only to cause contractures, skin breakdown, a worsening of her urinary incontinence, depression, and general deconditioning related to immobility. The family needs to be educated to the dangers of using restraints. The use of restraints would not promote a positive outcome for this patient.

Select the best answer to each question.

1. An example of an intrinsic risk factor for falls in the older person is:

   a. The use of diuretics

   b. Weakened muscles in the lower extremities

   c. Glaring lights in the hallway

   d. The use of a cane

2. To promote mobility in the older adult, the nurse would:

   a. Turn the patient every 2 hours

   b. Encourage the patient to cough and take deep breaths

   c. Ask the family to bring in the patient's walker from home

   d. Assume that the physical therapist is helping the patient to walk

3. The best way to promote urinary continence in the older person is to:

   a. Stop giving the diuretic because it causes the patient to have urinary urgency

   b. Obtain a urine specimen for culture and sensitivity

   c. Offer the bedpan every 2 hours

   d. Assist the patient to the toilet in the morning, after meals, and at bedtime

4. When seeing a reddened area on the patient's coccyx, the nurse would do all but one of the following interventions:

   a. Turn the patient every 2 hours

   b. Ask the physician to order a medication to treat the skin

   c. Help the patient to the toilet more frequently

   d. Measure how much of the diet the patient is taking every day

5. Which of the following is not an example of an iatrogenic disorder?

   a. Falling because of dizziness after receiving medication for pain relief

   b. Depression because of a stroke

   c. Incontinence because the patient could not find the bathroom

   d. Loss of weight because the patient cannot chew the food that is provided

17

Psychological Assessment

Mary Ann Anderson

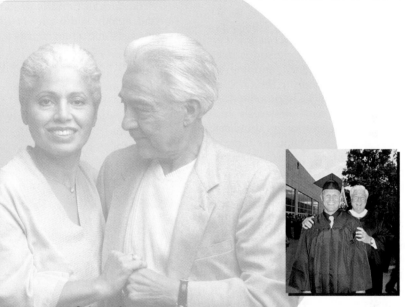

Learning Objectives

After completing this chapter, the student will be able to:

1. Identify three cognitive functions.
2. Describe two benefits of using a standardized examination to screen for cognitive functioning.
3. Identify four uses of psychological assessments.
4. Describe the impact of depression on the mental status score.

INTRODUCTION

Psychological assessments are essential tools in identifying the mental health of older adults in all health-care settings. Such assessments provide the basis for determining the psychological illness or wellness of a person as well as determining how much of a return to normal an individual can expect to achieve. Psychological assessments are important in any health-care setting, but especially when the focus is restorative care.

Restorative care, in its truest application, requires a body-mind-spirit connection. Relate this concept to Jean Watson's theory of caring—the two theories are conceptually the same, and it is hoped that they are beginning to have meaning for you in your practice. Nurses practicing within this framework are concerned with the physical indications that a person is declining, such as falling, incontinence, and immobility. Even though behavioral or psychological indicators have received less prominence in terms of restorative care, they are equally important. Some examples of psychological indicators are failure to eat and a decline in functional level, such as severe memory loss or confusion without a physiological basis.

Although one can expect a certain amount of decline in older people who have vascular and central nervous system disease, it is important to identify the psychological areas of decline and recognize when interventions are essential. Maintenance of mental health and cognitive functioning is as important to restorative care as the maintenance of physiological processes. Nurses working with elderly people need to understand basic concepts of mental health and cognitive function so that they can participate in the care of the older adult more effectively. Assessment tools provide a brief, methodical approach to noting changes commonly found in individuals with cerebrovascular diseases, delirium, and dementia disorders.

MENTAL HEALTH

Over the years, clinicians in the field of mental health have tried to diagnose symptoms, traits, and patterns of behavior that identify disease. The view that identification and treatment of disease result in optimum health is known as the medical model. The simplest definition of mental health would be the absence of identifiable disease. Most people have short-term or long-term psychological disorders at intervals throughout their lives; examples include grief over the death of someone close, post-traumatic stress disorder, or an eating disorder. A more comprehensive approach to mental health is to define the traits of the mentally healthy personality.

Practitioners use terms that have been formulated by theorists to describe and discuss psychological problems. Words such as *id, ego*, and *superego* are used by therapists who base their practice on Freud's theory. *Enmeshment* is a term used by some family therapists to describe interactions among family members that keep them dependent on each other. A therapist practicing within a Gestalt framework may focus on the feeling experiences of an individual.

The current trend is to identify wellness in mental health. Although it is difficult to define wellness, some characteristics have been described by psychologists, nurses, and physicians and are included in the following list:

- A clear meaning and purpose in life
- A strong reality orientation
- An ability to cope creatively with life's situations
- A capability for open, creative relationships

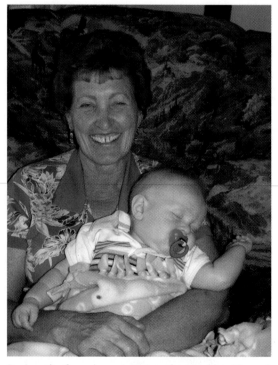

Review the four characteristics of mental health, and then look at this woman's face. You would need to interview her to determine whether or not it is true, but she does have the appearance of someone with purpose and meaning in her life.

Notice how these statements complement the concept of gerotranscendence? If an individual has achieved gerotranscendence, that person has increased personal life satisfaction, made a redefinition of self and relationships with others, and become open to new and creative possibilities. Gerotranscendence is psychological well-being.

Mental health is not a product of good nurturing or of a life of positive experiences. There are individuals who function well in life—for example, they maintain a satisfying job and career, have a family, and make a contribution to their community—despite poor nurturing and environmental handicaps. Most views of mental health now embody a continuum of health and illness. This continuum is dynamic rather than static. Many situations have an impact on the functioning of an individual, including the following:

- The death of someone close
- Unemployment
- The birth of a child
- Relocation

Any individual, if sufficiently stressed, can show some signs of impairment. One concept refers to the continuum of functioning as a scale of the differences in people. Individuals who are higher on this scale require more stressors to impair their functioning than individuals who are lower on this scale, and they choose a life course based on thought and conviction rather than on impulse; they also show an ability to stand by a belief that is different from that of their peer group.

It is important for nurses working in gerontology to identify and promote positive mental health traits. Nurses can reinforce healthy traits and interactions in older persons. This is nursing care being given in the nursing model (Watson's theory) rather than the medical model. Because it is nursing model care, it is caring and holistic, which are strong traits of the profession of nursing and characteristics that you want to work to develop as a licensed practical nurse (LPN).

Cognition

Cognition is a mental activity concerned with processing information. It refers to a broad range of mental behaviors, including awareness, thinking, reasoning, and judgment. This process is very complex and involves many abilities or functions. Because it cannot be directly observed, many psychologists define cognition in terms of cognitive functions. The cognitive functions can be conceptualized in numerous ways. One scientist's definition is perceiving, thinking, remembering, communicating, orienting, calculating, and problem-solving.

Memory

Generally, the more active people have been, the better their overall memory is as they age. A dysfunction in memory occurs in almost all of the cognitive disorders common in older adults. Psychologists generally refer to two categories of memory: short-term memory (STM) and long-term memory. The time interval for measuring STM is seconds, whereas for long-term memory it is minutes and beyond. More recently, there has been an interest in the study of remote memory. Many elderly persons demonstrate excellent long-term recall, although this recall may be rooted more in a belief than in fact; this is the nature of remote memory. It means that the stories older persons tell of their childhood or young adulthood are stories based on their belief systems rather than on what actually happened. This skill may be enchanting to staff and can be used effectively as a tool for reminiscence to strengthen a person's self-esteem.

Memory functions are extremely important to a person's ability to think. A deficit in STM means that a person is unable to recall some of today's events. An older adult with severe impairment of STM experiences the routine of each day as a new experience. Such a person is trapped in an endless cycle of requesting basic information about the environment from strangers, such as "Where is my room?" or "When do we eat?"

Memory impairment limits the ability of a person to form a new idea or relate one fact with another. It is nearly impossible for memory-impaired individuals to organize new information into categories. A place where one can put something (a pair of glasses) for safe keeping may change several times a day. This makes a never-ending search for an important item an everyday event.

Screening for memory impairment is the most important part of any assessment for an elderly patient. The loss of STM is the first symptom of Alzheimer's disease. A stroke also may impair memory function, but in this case, the type and extent of impairment depend on the location of the damage. Other STM deficits may be due to depression. Individuals with depression are inattentive to their environment. They often are preoccupied or self-absorbed. A decline in STM is an important finding on assessment and should prompt further investigation.

Perception

Psychologists believe that all behavior depends on how one sees oneself, the situation one is in, and the interaction between the two. Behavior changes as individuals become aware of details in their surroundings. Learning, problem-solving, remembering, and forgetting all are part of one's awareness of the environment. Effective communication with an older person depends on the nurse's ability to understand the perceptual world of that person. With such an understanding, the most bizarre behavior often becomes comprehensible.

The first phase of forming a perception is the ability to use the five senses to collect

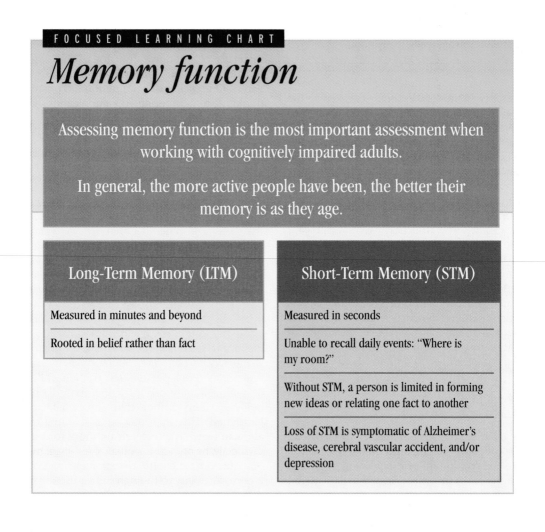

FOCUSED LEARNING CHART

Memory function

Assessing memory function is the most important assessment when working with cognitively impaired adults.

In general, the more active people have been, the better their memory is as they age.

Long-Term Memory (LTM)	Short-Term Memory (STM)
Measured in minutes and beyond	Measured in seconds
Rooted in belief rather than fact	Unable to recall daily events: "Where is my room?"
	Without STM, a person is limited in forming new ideas or relating one fact to another
	Loss of STM is symptomatic of Alzheimer's disease, cerebral vascular accident, and/or depression

information about the environment. Frequently, older adults have impairments in the sense organs. In Chapter 2, you learned about the deficits in vision, hearing, touch, taste, and smell that may occur in older persons.

There is an emotional or feeling component to perception as well. Individuals take in information from the environment and form opinions about such information. Perceptions are normally evaluated against past experiences. An older adult may compare a meal eaten within the institutional setting with recollections of meals eaten with the person's own family. These recollections of past experiences are a part of forming perceptions.

Perceptual distortions also are known as hallucinations and delusional thinking. Although both may indicate a psychiatric illness in younger individuals, perceptual distortions are common in illnesses with dementia. Impaired memory and a natural distrust of a strange environment exaggerate this tendency in an institutionalized older person.

Orientation

Orientation refers to a person's awareness of self in the context of a particular time and place. Tests for orientation determine whether the persons being tested know their names, where they are, and the approximate time of day. Sometimes the expression "oriented times three" is used to indicate that an individual's orientation to time, place, and person is correct. Assessment of orientation is covered on every mental status examination. This is important information because a disturbance in orientation is one of the most frequent symptoms of brain disease. Awareness of time and place requires that individuals know where they are and can remember it. In this way, individuals keep in touch with ongoing history. Orientation depends on a person's ability to link each minute with the previous minute. Disorientation with respect to time is the first major confusion to occur as a result of dementia. Loss of a sense of place is likely to follow. Finally, the person loses the ability to

---

CRITICALLY EXAMINE THE FOLLOWING

You are caring for an 81-year-old woman who was just admitted to the medical unit where you work. The charge nurse asked you to do something about the woman because she is screaming, "Don't hurt me! Don't hurt me!" and thrashing out at the staff. Because you are experienced in gerontological nursing, you assess the woman to determine the problem rather than restrain or confine her because her behavior is inconvenient. Think in terms of first-stage dementia and list three reasons why this woman would legitimately be fearful. Then, list what you can do about it. The first clue is in the section you just read on perception. The next clue is that the woman was just admitted and might be experiencing transitional stress. You think of a third reason and list all three with an appropriate intervention. Be prepared to share your thinking in class.

---

recognize other people and, eventually, cannot remember who he or she is.

Thinking

Every area of the brain is involved in the mental operation of thinking. The ancient Greeks believed there were "higher" levels and "lower" levels of thinking, a distinction that is still relevant. Higher level thinking includes the ability to form concepts and think in an abstract manner. Asking a person to interpret a proverb tests the person's ability to think abstractly. If a person interprets the proverb "a stitch in time saves nine" in a way that conveys that prompt attention to a problem prevents trouble in the future, the person's ability to think abstractly is considered intact. A concrete interpretation adheres closely to the exact meaning of the phrase. Concrete thinking is a "lower" mental ability. Someone with concrete thinking may answer the question about the proverb with something like, "If I make nine stitches, the cloth will hold."

POINT OF INTEREST

Orientation is easily determined by asking the older adult to state his or her name, the date, and the location. If the patient answers all three questions correctly, he or she is oriented times three; two questions, the patient is oriented times two; one question, the patient is oriented times one; and if he or she is unable to answer any of the three questions, the person is disoriented.

Thinking processes have a hierarchical order. The lower mental abilities are more enduring and less affected by brain injuries and disease processes. The higher levels of thinking tend to be more fragile. At first glance, interpreting proverbs may seem a bit removed from a person's ability to function in the real world. The use of good judgment, the ability to think abstractly, and the capacity to reason are higher level abilities, however, that indicate the difference between independent and supervised living. To some extent, these abilities can be determined by proverb interpretation. In general, tests for abstract thinking are not included as part of the short tests of mental function.

Communicating

The only vehicle for assessing thinking processes in an individual is communication. People understand human thought when it is reflected in language. It is important to assess language problems because they are common in cerebrovascular and dementia disorders. Assessment of communication patterns, word order, and the general sense of a sentence provides a window into the dementia process. This is especially true with a person who has experienced a stroke. Sometimes persons who have had a stroke have severe problems with communication. Small connecting words such as "if," "and," and "but" are missing. There are also several types of aphasia that impair an individual's ability to communicate.

CRITICALLY EXAMINE THE FOLLOWING

Whenever you are asked to complete this type of exercise, you are asked to think on a higher level. Has it seemed that way to you? Think back to your reactions in doing the critical thinking assignments. Did you avoid doing some? Were you irritated or upset at any of the assignments? Did you enjoy the challenge of doing them? Were you bored with them or saw them as not being a challenge? Take some time and consider your reactions to these assignments. Consider how you felt when certain items were discussed in class. Did you benefit from the thinking of your classmates? Were your ideas and thinking valued by others? Take the time to write your reactions regarding the higher level thinking experiences. Be prepared to share them in class.

Calculating

Calculating is a cognitive function that must be assessed carefully in terms of the person's intelligence and educational level. Poor performance may indicate dementia or delirium, anxiety, or depression. Serial 7s is one test that can determine a person's ability to calculate. The person is asked to subtract 7 from 100 and then to subtract 7 from that remainder, continuing five times. A nurse interviewed a moderately to severely impaired patient with Alzheimer's disease. Although the patient was completely disoriented with regard to time and place and could not recall the names of three objects seconds after they were told to him, he performed magnificently with the serial 7 calculations. In seconds, he completed the operation and then turned to the nurse, announcing proudly that mathematics was always his favorite subject. The patient had been a judge.

Problem-Solving

Problem-solving skills are essential to an individual's ability to function in any environment. Even some very demented people can exhibit aspects of problem-solving ability. Individuals in the early stages of Alzheimer's disease frequently make lists. Lists are coping devices that enable the recall of event sequences. When asked questions of orientation, some elders search for familiar cues in the environment. Examples of this behavior include the patient who was asked the date, spied a newspaper, and then winked and, smiling broadly, gave the correct answer. Another patient called to a nursing assistant passing by the door. When the nursing assistant entered the room, the patient asked him for the date and promptly relayed this information to the nurse interviewer.

An individual's environment is filled with a multitude of clues that facilitate orientation, aid a failing memory, and maintain a stable perceptual field. Use of these clues enables older adults to maintain communication with nurses, other patients, and family members. Because a patient's environment is rich with problem-solving clues, room changes and unit changes should be made infrequently and only after the most careful thought.

ASSESSMENT TOOLS AND HOW TO USE THEM

Mental status examinations are the most frequently used psychological assessments. Mental status assessment includes probing of the cognitive functions and level of consciousness (LOC). In selecting a tool, it is important to remember that examinations with brief instruments are generally better tolerated by an elderly person. A short examination is much less tiring for an older person to sit through than a lengthy one. No brief instrument is a perfect detector of cognitive impairment, however.

Screening tools initially may seem intimidating or cumbersome to use in clinical practice. Most tools are short and can be easily committed to memory after using them a few times. All of the following tests are easy to learn and administer: Pfeiffer's Short Portable Mental Status Questionnaire (SPMSQ) (Pfeiffer, 1975), Folstein's Mini-Mental Status Exam (MMSE) (Folstein, Folstein, & McHugh, 1975), Kahn's Mental Status Questionnaire (MSQ) (Kahn, Goldfarb, Pollock, & Peck, 1960), Jacobs' Cognitive Capacity Screening Exam (CCSE) (Jacobs, Bernhard, Delgado, & Strain, 1977), and Kiernan's Neurobehavioral Cognitive Status Examination (NCSE) (Kiernan, Mueller, Langston, & Vandyke, 1987). These scales are compared in Table 17.1 and are listed with a brief description in Box 17.1.

An important factor to consider in the scoring of all tests is that the educational level of the person being tested influences test results. An older adult with a lack of a formal education can score several points lower than an older person with greater deficits but more education. Some mental status tests have a method of scoring to correct for education.

There are important reasons for an LPN to gain skills in using assessment tools. A standardized test allows you, as the caregiver, to collect pertinent information in a short time. The collection of this information is organized and methodical. The initial test establishes a baseline and allows for comparison of changes over time.

Memory

Assessing memory function is the most important assessment in working with cognitively impaired older adults. There are three steps in the memory process. Each step needs accurate assessment. The steps are reception (encoding), storage (retention), and retrieval (recall). Folstein's MMSE tests memory by asking the older adult to repeat three words after the nurse three times—for example, apple, ball, and lamp. The number of trials it takes for the older person to recall the three items is noted. Immediate repetition enables the nurse to determine whether the person has heard the three words correctly. After the older adult repeats the words accurately, the nurse requests that the person remember them. In 5 minutes, the nurse asks again for the older adult to recall the three words. Each word recalled is given a score of 1.

Orientation

All short mental status examinations include questions about orientation. Time orientation is tested by asking for the date (day, month, year, and day of the week) and the time of day. Because older adults often become quite skilled in using clues from the environment, it is important to remove newspapers or calendars that may help them find the answer. An older adult can sometimes have an accurate sense of time passing yet may not remember the exact date. The nurse may ask questions such as "How long has it been since you last saw me?" or "What was your last meal?"

Assessment of orientation in place generally begins with questions about the name or location

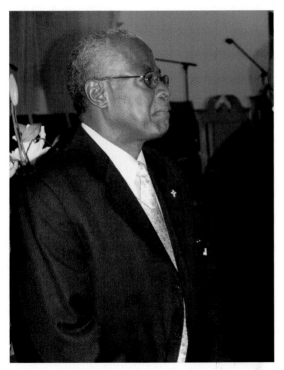

This man is a deacon in his church. This responsibility requires that he communicate, calculate, and problem solve. He also needs a good memory to do his job well. Interviewing people about their activities gives you important information for a psychological assessment.

TABLE 17.1 **Mental Status Examinations**

	NCSE	MSQ	SPMSQ	MMSE	CCSE
Level of consciousness (LOC)	X			X	X
Cognitive functions					
Remembering	X	X	X	X	X
Communicating	X				
Problem-solving					
Perceiving					
Thinking	X				X
Orienting	X	X	X	X	X
Calculating	X	X	X	X	X
Corrects for education and culture	X	X	X		
Number of questions	2 PG	10	10	30	30
Time required (minutes)	5–20	5	5	10	10

Source: Gurland, B. J. (1987). The assessment of cognitive function in the elderly. *Clinical Geriatric Medicine 3*, 53–63.

NCSE = Neurobehavioral Cognitive Status Exam; MSQ = Mental Status Questionnaire; SPMSQ = Short Portable Mental Status Questionnaire; MMSE = Mini-Mental Status Exam; CCSE = Cognitive Capacity Screening Exam.

of the place in which the person is being examined. You, as the LPN, need to determine whether patients know the kind of place they are in—a nursing home or hospital. Short mental status examinations ask questions about the state, county, or country of residence. Many people with moderate to severe dementia are unable to recall places. It may be more functional to question an older adult regarding the location of the bedroom or the dining room, for example, "Can you tell me where your room is?"

Level of Consciousness

The determination of a person's LOC is an important assessment to make in the event of delirium or a head injury. Folstein's MMSE is one tool that screens for LOC. It is important for the nurse to know the four levels of consciousness and to be able to define each in behavioral terms. The first level is *alert,* which means that the person is awake and responding in an appropriate manner. The next level is *lethargic.*

BOX 17.1 **Brief Description of Common Screening Tools**

The MMSE was developed by Folstein to be used with medical and psychiatric patients. Scores in the range of 9 to 12 indicate a high likelihood of dementia. Scores of 25 and higher are considered normal.

The *SPMSQ* was developed by Pfeiffer. This test is a little quicker to administer than Folstein's MMSE. Questions of orientation and memory are addressed, and there is one question concerning calculation. LOC is not assessed. An advantage over the MMSE is that there are specific directions for scoring this test to correct for education and race. A test score of 8 to 10 indicates severe intellectual impairment; 5 to 7, moderate impairment; 3 to 4, mild impairment; 0 to 2, intact status.

The *MSQ* was developed by Kahn. This questionnaire has two versions: one for institutionalized elderly patients and the other for use with adults in the community. Five or more errors indicate severe impairment, three to five errors indicate some impairment, and fewer than two errors indicate no impairment.

The *CCSE* was developed by Jacobs. This mental status questionnaire was adapted specifically to diagnose diffuse organic mental syndromes on busy medical wards. A score of less than 20 indicates diminished cognitive capacity.

The *NCSE* was developed by Kiernan for use with behaviorally disturbed adults in acute diagnostic units. This test differs from the others in that it has two separate scores. One score is given for LOC, orientation, and attention. Another score is given for language, construction, memory, calculations, and reasoning. The two separate scores enable clinicians to differentiate areas of impairment more clearly. This examination is 2 pages long, with directions to the clinician on how to administer it. It can be completed in 5 minutes by nonimpaired patients and by most patients with impairments in 20 minutes.

A person is lethargic when the individual can be aroused and, when aroused, responds in an appropriate manner and with an orientation that is consistent. The third LOC is *stuporous*. If a person can be aroused but responds inappropriately when aroused and then returns to sleep when the stimulus is stopped, the person is stuporous. This response may be the initial phase of a delirium. *Comatose* is the fourth level. A person who is comatose does not respond to any stimulus except deep pain.

Delirium and the Mental Status Examination

Nurses sometimes have a difficult time recognizing delirium. Sudden onset is the most significant feature described by experts. Older individuals may develop a delirium gradually, however, over the course of 2 or 3 days. One sign is a fluctuating LOC. This can vary from mild confusion to stupor in an active delirium, which is frequently characterized by visual hallucinations. A nursing home resident was being assessed for delirium by the nurse. The resident, who was talking about snakes in her bed, suddenly stopped and turned to the nurse. "Your hands are very chapped," she said. "You should use gloves to do your housework. I always did." Then the resident returned to her delirious state.

Another feature of delirium is disorientation. One person may be mistaken for another. Sometimes an older adult imagines being at home or in another location. Other cognitive functions may become impaired. There also may be a disturbance in the sleep cycle. Many delirious elders are awake all night and then sleep during the day.

Validity and Reliability of Assessment Scales

Whenever a questionnaire is used in any clinical setting, psychologists are concerned about two questions: validity and reliability. Is the test question a valid question? For example, does the question really measure memory, or orientation, or thinking? *Validity* is determined by the agreement reached by a panel of individuals who are experts in the content of the particular test questions used. The more experts that are involved in designing the process, the greater the validity of the test questions. *Reliability* is concerned with consistency. Would two nurses, each asking the same person the same questions, get the same

answers? When the answer to this question is "yes," the test questions are reliable. All standard mental status questionnaires considered in this chapter are valid and reliable instruments. They have been used by a variety of experts for many years with consistent results.

Because rating scales are designed to collect standard information about older persons in a methodical way, nurses should review the methods of using the rating scales together. This practice ensures that information is gathered in the same way. One nurse can interview an older adult while another nurse observes. Then they can reverse roles and compare the answers they received. Some experts recommend continuing this technique with 10 patients or until 80% of the ratings are the same.

WHEN TO ASSESS

Many hospitals and nursing homes use some sort of standard mental status examination to screen for gross impairments on admission. This is an excellent practice. Although some initial confusion, agitation, or depression is often seen in older adults who are newly admitted because of transitional stress, this practice, if consistently done, helps staff to get a baseline of the person's overall cognitive function. The assessment can be repeated if the older adult exhibits acute changes in behavior, mental status, or functional level—for example, if there is a decline in activities of daily living (ADLs). Although screening tools are not diagnostic—that is, they do not point out the exact nature of the problem—they do show, in a factual way, specific areas that have changed.

ASSESSMENT TECHNIQUES

Older adults generally remain cooperative unless they perceive the questions asked as challenging their mental competence. Catastrophic reactions such as screaming or leaving the room angry can be precipitated when a person is pushed to perform beyond the person's competency. An older adult's refusal to answer questions should be accepted. This information in itself is significant. Older persons, aware of their cognitive impairments, may become defensive when their vulnerabilities are exposed. Attention to the following factors promotes the success of the psychological assessment.

Timing

The timing of an interview is an important factor in determining success. Regular staff members, especially nursing assistants in the nursing home setting, are especially skilled in knowing the best time to interview a resident. Allowing an older person to select a time may be the most effective way to gain cooperation.

Privacy

Privacy is very important. Questions that to caregivers may seem routine are often considered deeply revealing and very personal to older persons. All interviews should be conducted in the person's room or in a location that ensures confidentiality.

Elimination of Interruptions

Interruptions undermine the importance of psychological assessments. They negatively affect a person's attention span, and they distract the nurse from focusing on the person being interviewed. Some interruptions are beyond your control as the nurse and occur regardless of the precautions taken. Reasonable efforts should be made to eliminate as many interruptions as possible because they have an impact on the reliability and validity of the assessment.

Positive Introduction of the Assessment

Introducing the psychological assessment in a positive and respectful manner is useful. Describing the test as "a lot of silly questions" may prompt the response that "If they are so silly, why should I answer them?" Let the older adult know that the information gained from this assessment will help the nurses in planning and giving care.

WHAT TO DO WITH THE ASSESSMENT INFORMATION

All information obtained from the older person must be used on the individual's behalf. This information should be dated and appear in an accessible place on the chart with a notation that this document must remain on the chart. Assessment information generally is not updated unless a person exhibits a behavioral problem or has a marked decline in functional level.

Applications in Clinical Practice

In the hospital or nursing home, psychological assessments may be used as one of the factors determining the unit assignment of a new resident on admission. They contribute to the identification of the person's strengths and potentials. When used in conjunction with the person's ability to perform ADLs, psychological assessments may point out the need for psychiatric evaluation. When a person's mental functioning seems much lower than the score of a psychological assessment might indicate, a mental illness is suspected.

Psychological assessments can be used as a basis for care planning. This assessment is especially important when an older adult's social graces lead staff members to conclude that the person is functioning at a higher level than is the case. Many individuals with dementia learn strategies to cover for losses in cognition. They may rely on list making, props in the environment, and social cues from others. Staff members sometimes can make excessive demands on older persons if they are unaware of cognitive deficits.

Psychological assessments can allow a broad determination of the effects of an intervention. For example, a person with sadness, who wishes to die, may be treated with an antidepressant. Effective treatment may enhance the abilities of depressed older persons to attend to their environment, improving memory and perception. On the mental status examination, such people

---

POINT OF INTEREST

As an LPN, you should develop polished skills with one of the assessment tools. Learn it well, practice it on people many times, and then be prepared to share your skill and knowledge with the interdisciplinary team. This will make you a strong, positive asset to the place where you work.

may achieve higher scores in the area of recall. This information is useful to a consultant when a more extensive evaluation is considered necessary. It is helpful to be able to tell a consultant that an older adult has dropped 4 points on Folstein's MMSE because the examination was conducted 6 months earlier. It also is useful to note the specific area of decline—for instance, the area of decline is in orientation to time and place or in immediate recall.

Older adults vary greatly in symptom severity and the rate of progression. Although older persons in the later stages of dementia present similarly regardless of disease process, the initial symptoms may clearly indicate one disease over another. The initial symptom of Alzheimer's disease is the gradual progressive decline in the ability to learn new information. The most significant early symptom of Pick's disease is a change in personality. This is an important distinction.

Symptoms of dementia are a moving target that must be tracked. The tracking is done by frequent, well-recorded assessments. If an assessment tool has been used to establish a baseline in the early stages of the disease process, it may contribute to the diagnostic process.

⬤ OTHER ASSESSMENTS

Assessing Depression

Although research indicates that depression is no more prevalent in older people than it is in younger people, its manifestation is different and difficult to identify. It is important for you, as the nurse, to gain skill in the assessment of depression because of your focus on the quality of life for all people. There is a heavy emotional cost to depression that ultimately affects the immune system, which can lead to cancer and other physical illnesses and infections.

Depression predicts the onset of disability almost as powerfully as disability predicts depression. Older individuals who are depressed are in a high-risk category for institutionalization because they are less motivated to care for their personal hygiene and nutrition. This lack of self-care increases their vulnerability to disease. In addition, depressed individuals are frequently withdrawn and socially isolated, and so they have weak support systems. The path to a nursing home for these individuals is apt to be very short and direct.

It is a fact that people older than 65 years of age are beginning to face some significant losses: economic, vocational, family supports, and friendships. Physical disabilities are frequently viewed as the beginning of the end. "If you have your health, you have everything," one grandmother reports. The loss of health signals a life of dependency for most older adults.

Generally, the most impressive feature of depression is an unpleasant mood. To psychiatrists, the term *clinical depression* refers to a cluster of specific symptoms. These symptoms are clearly defined in a diagnostic manual called the *Diagnostic and Statistical Manual of Mental Disorders (DSM)*. Depression may be chronic or acute, and the symptoms may vary in intensity. Severe depression is thought to impair cognitive functioning at any age. Memory seems to be the

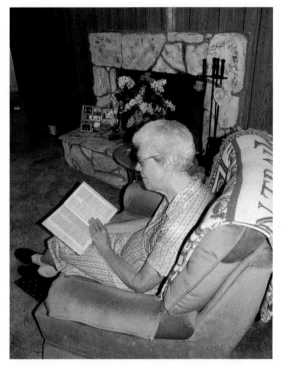

Older people experience significant losses. This woman has lost her husband, can no longer drive a car, lives alone, and has experienced the deaths of friends and family members. A concerned neighbor reported that the woman is "very" depressed. As a volunteer mental health nurse, you are asked to talk to her to determine if she is depressed and needs an intervention. What you find is a delightful woman who serves in her church and has friends and activities in her life. She is quiet and reserved, however, which you suspect is the reason someone mistook her for a person with depression. Nothing is more important in a psychological assessment than your physical presence with your knowledge and life skills.

function most influenced by a depressed mood, but there are many ways that memory can be affected. Information committed to memory when a person is depressed is likely to be biased. Other clinicians focus on the ability or lack of ability of older adults to attend to their environment as the indicator of a depression. Methods for the identification of depression in elderly adults are controversial. Use your own skills and life experience to process the responses of the older adult you are interviewing to try to identify expressions or behaviors of depression. Report your results to the registered nurse (RN).

Assessing Pain

Chronic pain may leave a person totally fatigued and unable to participate properly in a restorative care program. In addition, some behavioral problems in institutionalized older adults stem from ineffective pain management. A psychiatric evaluation may be requested for screaming or abusive behavior on the part of a resident of a nursing home who in fact is experiencing physical pain. A failure to identify pain as a factor affecting behavior and function may result in poor medical management.

Pain in older people is frequently either overtreated or undertreated simply because it is difficult to assess. Some older adults want every ache treated with a drug, whereas others maintain a stoic attitude: "Why bother? There is nothing that can be done, anyway." Older people often perceive pain differently. Some pain receptors may not be as acute as they were in the past. Medical journals document clinical cases describing "silent" myocardial infarctions or "painless" intra-abdominal emergencies. These cases may not be silent or painless but may reflect an older person's normal aging situation.

Cognitive impairments, delirium, and dementia are some barriers to pain assessment. People who have a dementia process or a stroke and become aphasic may be unable to give an accurate pain history. They may be unable to describe when the pain started or at what point in the day the pain becomes most severe. Most people describe the pain in the here and now.

A person in pain is often self-absorbed and inattentive to activities in the environment. Because pain frequently leads to depression, the mental status examination score may show a decline in recall.

Delirium may be one manifestation of an attempt to treat a person's pain. An assessment for delirium should be made whenever there is a change in the LOC after the start of any new drug, particularly a pain medication. A sensitivity to medications that results in delirium makes pain management difficult for older people.

Multiple chronic disease processes and acute processes compound the difficulty. There may even be an acute exacerbation of a chronic problem. These multiple sources of pain make diagnosis difficult, and pain management becomes a challenge.

Myths of Pain

One myth regarding pain in older adults is that pain is normal. As body systems begin to wear out, one might expect an increase in pain. At any age, pain is the most common symptom of a disease process, however, and should be investigated and treated.

Another myth is that pain and sleep are incompatible. Nurses often disbelieve a patient's complaint of pain when they bring a pain pill and find the person asleep. The wrong conclusion is drawn. It is believed that an individual really in pain could not possibly sleep. The exhaustive feature of pain is seldom considered in the assessment process.

The last myth is that narcotic drugs are not safe for older people. Narcotics provide effective pain relief for some chronic conditions and terminal illnesses. These drugs should be used on a scheduled basis, such as every 4 hours or every 6 hours. Use of a narcotic on an "as needed" basis does not provide effective pain management. Some nurses believe that narcotics dull an older person's LOC. They fear that an older adult would be unable to benefit from the support of family or friends in the time remaining before death. Effective relief of pain actually promotes interaction, and the initial drowsiness soon wears off.

Methods of Assessment

Although pain is a highly subjective experience, there are two methods for assessing it. *Simple observation* from a nurse who knows the person well can be very effective. A grimace or clutch of the chest provides a vivid picture of pain. *Assessment questions* may follow these observations. Clinical practice guidelines for acute pain management identify the quantifiable measures of pain that should be considered in an assessment, including the intensity of the pain, the duration of the pain, the quality of the pain, and the personal meaning this pain has to the older adult. The impact on the person's functioning is also included.

Assessment tools are available. A good tool addresses the older person's pain history and coping strategies for dealing with pain and medications in the past that have been effective. It is important to ask questions that help to describe or define the pain. Noting the intensity and duration assists in providing an objective measure to a highly subjective experience. Simply asking "How is your pain today?" may prompt the response, "Well, it is there."

The simplest method of pain assessment is the use of a pain intensity scale. You, as the nurse, can draw a line indicating that the far left (L) end of the line defines no pain and the right (R) end represents the most pain the person has ever experienced. The person can point to the place on the line that reflects current pain level. Another commonly used method is to ask the older adult to rate the pain on a scale from 1 to 10, with 10 being the worst pain imaginable.

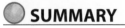

SUMMARY

Observations of a person's behavior and functional status are subjective and often inconsistently reported. It is difficult to get a clear idea of decline or progression over time without objective measures. Psychological assessments and other assessment tools provide the means for collecting factual information about older adults.

Brief mental status examinations universally identify assessments of memory and orientation as the two features that provide the most information about an individual's cognitive functions. Assessments help establish a person's baseline functioning. They can be used to establish a diagnosis, plan care, and evaluate treatment efforts. Psychological assessments also enable the nurse to define problem areas in a more specific manner to consultants. Older adults cooperate well with assessments if the nurse is sensitive to timing, respects the person's privacy, limits interruptions, and presents the assessment tool in a positive manner. Other assessments that can provide important information in planning care are those that address depression and pain.

CONCLUSION

Many institutionalized elderly people are well aware of their declining abilities. These losses have a dynamic impact on their self-concept. A life once vital and central to a young family now does not seem worth the effort to maintain. A lowered self-concept and diminished self-esteem complete the picture of physical decline. The process can become circular without the intervention of a caring and knowledgeable staff.

The performance level of most individuals improves in a supportive environment. Recognition and reinforcement of cognitive skills and abilities and of attributes of mental health can positively affect restorative care efforts. Nurses who consistently identify strengths in a factual way are instrumental in improving the quality of life for older adults in their care.

Ms. F. is 81 years old. She had a long career with the government that involved traveling all over the world. Although she never married, she is a devoted aunt and a vital member of her extended family. She is the youngest of three siblings. Her two older brothers live in New York and California. Despite the distance, the three communicate regularly through letters and telephone calls. Nieces and nephews are always attentive to Ms. F. She never spends a holiday alone.

The retirement years for Ms. F. became the highlight of her life. She continued her travels, sometimes with friends and at other times with a niece or nephew.

Only one problem seemed to dampen Ms. F.'s life. In her middle years, every once in a while (3 to 5 years), she became depressed, or "blue," as she describes it. Two episodes she "toughed out" on her own. Although she continued to function in her job, her appetite diminished. She woke up at 3:00 a.m. on most days and had no energy to do much of anything. In a couple of months, the depression lifted, and she returned to the good life. These periods seemed to have no precipitating event. She saw a psychiatrist for the first time when she was 54 years old. He prescribed an antidepressant, nortriptyline (Pamelor). This medication was successful in treating the depression. After 6 months, the medication and brief therapy were stopped. She did quite well in the following years.

When she was 78 years old, Ms. F. made the decision to come to a nursing home. Her family thought she was having some minor problems with memory. Although she denied feeling depressed, she noticed a real decline in her energy level and ability to do for herself. She was placed on a unit with other residents who functioned independently. A niece came to help her decorate her room. Whatnots displayed unique treasures from a life of travel.

Based on this information, answer the following question:

1. With respect to the administration of the mental status examination, the charge nurse decided:
   a. Not to give the examination. It would be insulting to Ms. F. to be questioned in such a way.

   b. To check with Ms. F. regarding a good time to conduct some routine admission assessments, which would include the MMSE.
   c. That Ms. F. was doing so well that there was no need for such a test.
   d. To ask the social worker to conduct this examination in a few weeks after the resident had adjusted better.

Ms. F. was a trim woman, and her clothing was exquisite. From the start, the other residents seemed to respect her. Although she did not become a member of one of the unit cliques, there was no one who did not accept her and welcome her company when she sat down. Her admission MMSE score was 29/30. She was unable to recall one object after 5 minutes.

A few months after admission, some of the residents began to remark to the staff that Ms. F. was ignoring some of their efforts to engage her in a conversation. She started retreating to her room a little more. She seemed more withdrawn in general. She favored a chair off to herself rather than an available seat in a group of other residents.

Based on this information, answer the following question:

2. The charge nurse was concerned. She went to visit Ms. F. in her room. The two problems the charge nurse was assessing in this interview were:
   a. Delirium and dementia.
   b. Depression and dementia.
   c. Depression and hearing loss.
   d. Depression and possible delirium.

Ms. F. was a little vain and disclosed to the charge nurse during this interview that her hearing was not what it used to be. "I don't want to wear a hearing aid," she said. The charge nurse convinced Ms. F. that a routine audiology appointment might be useful.

She was scheduled for a clinic appointment the following week. She had a great deal of wax buildup that was interfering with her hearing. When the wax was removed, her hearing improved, but the audiologist convinced her that a hearing aid would be most beneficial and told her, "It's an attractive device and can be made to fit your glasses." The persuading force was Ms. F.'s love for classical music. She had been unable to enjoy her music with the hearing loss. She ordered a hearing aid.

The bad weather set in, holidays came and went, and Ms. F. holed up in her room "reading the paper." As spring approached and there were a few days of good weather, Ms. F. could not be dissuaded from staying in her room. When Ms. F. was weighed routinely, staff members noted a disturbing 10-lb weight loss. In reviewing the minimum data set (MDS), it was noted that she had lost a total of 15 lb in 3 months.

Based on this information, answer the following question:

3. The charge nurse decided to conduct a mental status examination. Ms. F. agreed to being tested. The nurse noted that it took four repetitions of the objects for her to recall them. In 5 minutes she could not recall a single object. Because Ms. F. was well oriented, the nurses believed that:
   a. There was some dementia.
   b. She needed a battery for her hearing aid.
   c. She was depressed.
   d. A combination of a, b, and c.

The psychiatrist was called to assess Ms. F. He determined that she was depressed and recommended nortriptyline (Pamelor), an antidepressant. The primary physician prescribed Pamelor 25 mg every evening. After 3 weeks, the nurses reported that Ms. F. was smiling and seemed to be out of her room more. Her appetite was a little better; at least she ate a good breakfast. The primary physician conferred with the psychiatrist and increased the Pamelor to 50 mg daily. Six weeks later, Ms. F. was on the porch enjoying lovely June days. She had been in the facility for a year. The charge nurse decided to repeat the mental status examination to determine whether there was marked improvement in her depression. Ms. F. was able to recall two out of the three objects. Her recall had improved. She was a little vague about the date; however, she knew the season, month, and year.

Based on this information, answer the following question:

4. The charge nurse wondered if:
   a. Ms. F. was just a little confused.
   b. Ms. F. might have a disturbance in orientation related to a dementia process.
   c. An adjustment in the antidepressant might be appropriate.

   d. She should discourage Ms. F. from subscribing to a daily newspaper because it might be too tiring for her declining abilities.

Toward the end of November, Ms. F. slipped. Although she did not fall, she injured her back when she grabbed onto the support rail in her bathroom. The nurses noticed that she held on to the furniture and walls as she walked. She had radiographs, which revealed osteoporosis. The staff and primary physician discussed with her the idea of using a walker to get around. She agreed to try this and went to physical therapy (PT) for an evaluation and a walker. Two weeks later, Ms. F. was still complaining of pain. She stayed in her bed more and did not come out for meals. Aspirin was ordered for her pain. Staff members came by to visit. A few more weeks passed. Answer the following questions about this situation:

5. Some of the staff members believed that:
   a. Ms. F. was exaggerating her problem to get more attention.
   b. Ms. F. was depressed because of the pain and decline in function.
   c. Ms. F. had more extensive physical problems than they realized.
   d. Further assessment was needed to determine the factors behind Ms. F.'s decline.

6. The charge nurse decided that the following assessment or assessments would help staff members understand Ms. F.'s decline:
   a. Pain history and physical assessment per physician
   b. Nurse interaction focused on identifying depression, if it existed
   c. MMSE
   d. All of the above

Ms. F. described the pain as severe, the worst she had ever experienced. The physician decided to hospitalize her for more tests. Hospital laboratory work showed dehydration. Magnetic resonance imaging (MRI) revealed that there was a disk pushing in on the spinal cord. The physician ordered intravenous fluids and meperidine (Demerol) to manage the pain. When the charge nurse stopped by the hospital to see Ms. F. on the way home from work, she was shocked to find that Ms. F. did not remember her and believed it was nighttime. She had no idea where she was and had no recall from

Continued on page 306

one moment to the next. It was January, and she believed it was June.

Answer the following question regarding this situation:

7. The charge nurse realized that Ms. F.:
   a. Was depressed.
   b. Was in extensive pain.
   c. Had not heard a word she had said.
   d. Was delirious.

During her hospital stay, Ms. F. was treated for gastrointestinal problems related to aspirin use and had back surgery that resulted in some postoperative complications. When Ms. F. returned to the nursing home, it was spring. She had a marked decline in her functional ability. She was now in a wheelchair and had been assigned to another unit. The staff members from her original unit visited her to help her get adjusted. They focused on her abilities and her life of travel. They invited her to visit them and attend groups on the first floor. Ms. F. seemed very vague to them. The nurses felt sad and wondered whether Ms. F. would ever again be as bright and interested in her surroundings as she had been on their floor.

The MMSE was repeated. The nurses realized from the MMSE that Ms. F.'s cognitive status had changed significantly. There were deficits in orientation and memory. Her ability to perform calculations had not declined, however.

In a postadmission care conference, the staff members identified Ms. F.'s resident care needs. Answer the following question about this determination:

8. The staff members believed that they must implement all of the following except:
   a. To assist the resident to accept her decline
   b. To assess her ability to move about and participate in a walking program
   c. To request a psychiatric evaluation
   d. To encourage her to participate in all unit activities

Ms. F. slowly began to respond to the staff's plan of care. She was restarted on an antidepressant that had been stopped while she was in the hospital. She responded well to a walking program. Although she had lost some of her agility, she achieved some independence with a walker. Her dementia had advanced slightly, but she could and did participate in activities. It was decided that staff would continue to do an MMSE annually to monitor her progress.

Solutions

1. b
2. c
3. c
4. b

5. d
6. d
7. d
8. a

Select the best answer to each question.

1. The health-care providers who are best qualified to conduct psychological assessments, such as Folstein's MMSE, are:

a. Psychologists

b. Nurses

c. Social workers

d. Psychiatrists

2. The social worker of a unit annually conducts an MMSE on all the residents. She informs you that Mrs. H.'s score in the area of orientation has dropped 2 points from last year. You suspect that the drop is due to:

a. Delirium

b. Arthritis

c. Progression of dementia

d. Depression

3. The activities department has alerted you to the fact that recently Mr. J. has not been interested in attending programs sponsored by their department. This morning, he complained to you that he believes that he is having problems with his memory. He did not eat breakfast and only picked at his lunch. He denies feeling depressed. You conduct an MMSE. There is a change in score from the admission MMSE conducted 3 months ago. His immediate recall of three objects on Folstein's MMSE has declined. You suspect:

a. Delirium

b. Progression of dementia

c. A urinary tract infection

d. Depression

4. Mrs. C. does not come out of her room for breakfast. The night shift staff members report that she was up all night and that she has a fever. You go to Mrs. C. to determine whether you can assist her. She seems to be asleep. When you touch her arm, she opens her eyes. She does not quite recognize you, her favorite nurse. She believes that it is bedtime and her main concern is that her husband (who has been dead for 20 years) is late coming home from work. When you leave the room, she returns to "sleep." Yesterday her MMSE score was 30/30. You know immediately that she is:

a. Depressed

b. Having a massive stroke

c. Delirious

d. Confused, owing to dementia

5. Important considerations when conducting psychological assessments are:

a. Timing

b. Privacy and elimination of interruptions

c. Positive introduction of the assessment

d. All of the above

18

Common Clinical Problems: Psychological

Mary Ann Anderson

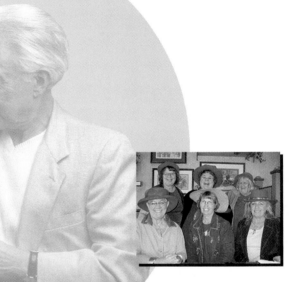

Learning Objectives

After completing this chapter, the student will be able to:

1. Recognize three behaviors that may signal the presence of a psychological problem in an older adult.
2. Explain how to use nursing interventions for older adults with common psychological problems.
3. Discuss how to manage difficult behaviors of older adults.
4. Compare reality orientation, reminiscence, remotivation, resocialization, and validation techniques.
5. Select important information about psychological medications to include in teaching.

INTRODUCTION

Psychological problems are disturbances in mental or emotional health that occur as a result of external or internal stimuli. These problems are usually assessed by examining thought patterns, behaviors, and emotions. Because psychological difficulties are not as obvious as some physical problems that can be diagnosed by laboratory tests, it may be difficult to diagnose and treat older adults with these problems correctly.

Almost any psychological problem that can occur with other age groups also can occur with older adults. A few common psychological problems found in clinical situations are described in this chapter. A glossary of terms used in this chapter is presented in Box 18.1.

BOX 18.1 Glossary of Psychological Terms

Anxiety: Generalized unpleasant feeling of apprehension.

Behavior modification: Treatment method of changing behavior.

Bipolar affective disorder: Psychological disease involving mood swings from mania to depression.

Delirium: Sudden, reversible state of confusion.

Delusion: False, fixed idea or belief.

Disorientation: State of not knowing what day or time it is, or not knowing where one is.

Hallucination: False sensory impression, often seeing or hearing something that is not there.

Illusion: Misperception of a real event or object.

Neurolinguistic programming: A way of communicating using neurological, behavioral, and speech patterns.

Neurotransmitter: A chemical in the brain that carries electrical impulses to neurons.

Paranoia: A way of thinking that systematically interprets others as being intentionally harmful.

Phobia: Exaggerated fear of a particular object or group of objects.

Schizophrenia: Psychological disease involving severe thought and perception disturbances.

Sensory deprivation: Condition of decreased stimulation that can cause hallucinations, illusions, and disorientation.

Social support: Emotional and physical assistance given by loved ones.

Somatization: Extreme preoccupation with physical problems.

GENERAL GUIDELINES FOR COMMUNICATING WITH OLDER ADULTS

It is helpful to review some basic principles for good communication, particularly as they relate to communicating with an older person with a psychological disorder. It is important to practice the skills outlined throughout this chapter to develop your own style for working in an individualized way with each person in your care.

Forming Relationships With People Who Have Psychological Problems

Generally, relationships have three stages. During each stage, there are concepts with which you should be familiar. At the beginning of a relationship, people sometimes are uncomfortable. After all, they are sick, and you are new to them. As time goes on and trust is established, people enter a stage of the relationship that allows for more open communication that can be therapeutic in its purpose. The last stage of a relationship involves termination or saying goodbye. Problems in relationship-building can be prevented by understanding these normal stages.

Beginning a Relationship

People who have psychological problems may not be easy to get to know initially. They may have had problems starting relationships all of their lives, and forming a relationship with a new nurse might be difficult. Some people with mental illnesses have trouble trusting others and find it difficult to trust a new nurse or a new roommate in a hospital or long-term care facility. There are some things that can be done to help make the beginning of a relationship more comfortable.

If the person with a psychological problem does not talk or becomes upset at first, do not take it personally. The person may be feeling uncomfortable and unsure of how you will react. You, as the nurse, can be creative in dealing with problems such as this and need to respond in a natural way. Some approaches to consider are using humor to diffuse tension or finding an interest of the person's, such as fly tying or crocheting, and asking him or her about it.

Important points to keep in mind are the need to establish trust and not to reject the person. You may need to say to the individual, "It seems like you'd rather not talk right now. I'll come back in an hour and sit here (or at the desk, or at a table) just in case you want to talk to me then."

Developing a Relationship

Once you have developed a trusting relationship with an older adult, you are ready to be an instrument in the work of healing for a person with psychological problems. With the development of trust, the older person is able to share with you emotions such as fear and anger and the symptoms of more serious illnesses such as delusions or hallucinations. Your responsibility is to listen and guide the discussion.

If the older person has a serious disease, most of the verbal therapy is done in group or private sessions with nurse practitioners or psychologists. Your responsibility is to listen, be genuine, and report anything unusual to the registered nurse (RN).

Ending a Relationship

Nurses begin and end relationships with many people every day. Sometimes this happens in small ways, such as taking a weekend off or going away for a conference or vacation. Sometimes it is more permanent, such as discharging a person to another facility or to the home, changing jobs, or saying goodbye to a person who is dying. During this phase of a relationship, people generally try to avoid the termination process. This often is exhibited when the patient ignores you and other staff members or acts out.

If a nurse is going away for a short time, the older adult may start demanding more attention by ringing the call light more frequently, becoming angry or irritated by small things, or not responding or talking. To prevent this from happening, it is best if the person knows as soon as possible when to expect the separation. Provide opportunities for the older adult to talk about it openly with you. If a permanent separation is approaching, some kind of formal farewell, such as a goodbye party, might be helpful. Taking pictures with patients and staff also can help ease the difficulty of a separation. If an older person is being discharged home, do not always assume it is a joyous occasion. Sometimes the situation at home is worse than being in the nursing home or hospital. Even if a person is looking forward to going home, mixed feelings may exist about having to adjust to another new situation. Remember the difficulty of transitional stress.

It is not unusual for a patient who is ready to go home suddenly to become worse. If this happens, it may be a clue to you that the person is having problems with ending his or her present relationships. If you, as the nurse, talk about this openly by sharing feelings, such as "Things just aren't going to be the same around here without you, Mr. M.," the person may be more willing to discuss personal feelings.

Verbal Communication

Communication skills described in general nursing books also can be used successfully with older adults. Some skills are important to emphasize when working with elderly people who have psychological problems. The following discussion includes validation techniques, which are especially useful with disoriented individuals. Validation therapy is discussed in more detail later in the chapter.

Open Questions

Verbal communication can be helpful by using open questions instead of closed questions. A closed question is a question that can be answered with a simple "yes" or "no." An open question tends to encourage the person to talk more. Open questions are asked using such words as "who," "what," "where," "when," and "how." "Why" questions usually are not helpful, especially with someone who is disoriented. Some people with psychological problems may be unable to answer a "why" question logically or rationally. If a resident in a nursing home says she is looking for her mother, you may validate her by asking open questions, such as "What did your mother look like?" "What did you like to talk about with your mother?" "What did you and your mother do together?" If you were to ask, "Why do you want your mother?" the resident likely would be unable to tell you.

Giving Instructions

When giving directions, it is best to do so slowly, one step at a time. Individuals who are disoriented may be unable to perform any self-care activities unless they are prompted by very simple cues. Telling someone who is disoriented to brush his or her teeth may not get any results. If you tell the person to pick up the toothbrush, then pick up the toothpaste, then put the toothpaste on the brush, then put the brush in the mouth, and then brush up and down, the person may be able to do more than you originally thought.

Guided Choices

Some people may not respond to open questions as well as they do to guided choices. When asked, "What would you like to do today?" someone with a psychological problem may not know how to respond. When given a choice between two activities, with choices given one at a time, however, the person may be able to make a choice. An example of guided choices is: "Would you like to go to singing time today, or would you rather go for a walk outside?"

Empathy and Genuineness

When a nurse shows the desire to understand someone, it promotes more meaningful communication. Empathy can be expressed by maintaining eye contact, using a caring tone of voice, listening closely to what someone says, and making statements such as "This must be difficult for you," or "It sounds like you are having a rough time right now."

The opposite of empathy is patronizing a person. Using a tone of voice as if talking to a child is an example of being patronizing. This type of communication keeps the nurse from using empathy and is not helpful in communicating with older adults. Referring to an older person as "honey" or "dearie" is also patronizing and a hindrance to effective communication. Another example of patronizing behavior is referring to an older person in a report to another nurse as a "real cutie" or a "sweetheart."

It is important that the nurse be genuine when showing empathy. Being genuine means that nurses must truly represent themselves. Finding things you sincerely want to say to a person is more important than saying the right thing from a book.

Listening

Listening to someone includes listening to feelings, words, and behaviors. Sometimes people with emotional problems may forget or confuse the facts or use words that do not make sense. When this happens, it is especially important to listen to feelings instead of trying to get the facts straight. If a resident is incomprehensible but is speaking loudly and has tearful eyes, you might respond by saying, "This is extremely frustrating for you."

Another aspect of listening is to ensure the older adult can hear you. A review of the basic principles may help you. Start by placing yourself directly in front of the person. Stand so that there is not a bright light (e.g., a window on a sunny day) behind you so the person can read your lips as well as listen to you. Speak in a normal tone; do not shout even if the person cannot hear you. If you suspect the person is having difficulty hearing you, move closer to the person. Ask permission to move close to one of the person's ears and repeat what you were saying, in a normal tone. If the person seems comfortable with touch, place your hand on a shoulder and express nonverbal acceptance and caring with touch. Remember to smile and do not act rushed even if you are. You may find other successful methods for promoting the older adult's way of listening. If so, use them and share them with others.

Values and Culture

There are many different motivations for behavior during a conversation. Two that can enhance or interfere with effective communication are the values and culture of the nurse and the older adult. What one person sees as normal may be seen as unacceptable or offensive by a person who has different values or comes from a different cultural background. For example, a nurse who has been educated to value touch as a way of communicating concern and an older adult who perceives touch without permission as an invasion of privacy would have problems with the communication process.

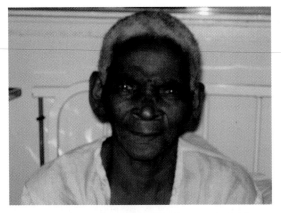

Do you recognize the cultural background of this man by looking at him? It is important to gather information quickly on cultures unfamiliar to you so that you can give caring, holistic health care. This man is from Sudan and has suffered horrific family deaths and persecution from the terrorists there.

Nurses know that older adults, as with other age groups, come from a wide variety of backgrounds. A Hispanic resident may stand very close while talking to staff members. A staff member who is unaware of this cultural difference may interpret such behavior as being intrusive. An older Japanese person who values modesty may have difficulty talking openly about bowel and bladder problems. Some Native Americans want their Shaman, or medicine man, to perform a sacred "sing" to help them heal. This ritual involves music, dance, and numerous family members and friends. To have meaningful communication with older adults, all caregivers need to understand and respect the various differences that can occur because of personal values and cultural behaviors. Review Chapter 8 if you feel you need more information on cultural awareness.

Being patient also is very important. Some nurses have to be available to the older person to whom they are assigned for several days before seeing a positive response. When the results do come and the nurse is able to communicate successfully with the older person, it is a very rewarding experience.

Nonverbal Communication

Psychologists say that nonverbal communication, such as tears or the inability to smile, is the most honest communication a person can make. To be an effective listener, you need to watch and listen to what is being said. Using direct eye contact and a caring tone of voice can help the communication process. Positioning the body at eye level also helps.

Touch

Touching is an important part of communicating with people. Many older people miss human contact and enjoy being touched. A person with psychological problems, however, may become frightened, withdrawn, or agitated if touched. When the nurse touches someone who has an emotional problem, it is a good idea to ask the person first if it would be all right. Saying "Would it be okay if I gave you a hug?" might be a way of asking for permission. Carefully note the response of the person to the question and the actual touch. Some people who are very withdrawn may respond only to touch.

Touch can be used to stimulate sensory memories as well. Different people respond to touch in different ways. Table 18.1 lists common responses to touch. A person who talks about his mother or says "Ma, ma, ma" repeatedly may respond well to stroking on the upper cheek. This stimulates the rooting reflex and can bring back memories of a loving mother. Stroking the upper arm from the shoulder to the elbow is perceived by many people as a universal symbol of friendship. It feels comforting and safe to have someone touch in that way. If a patient is agitated, you can try stroking his or her upper arm while you talk quietly and gently to the patient.

Matching and Mirroring

Research has determined that it helps the communication process if a person can match or mirror another's behavior. Mirroring is doing exactly what the person is doing as if the person were looking into a mirror. Matching is using the same pattern or intensity of tone the person is using. This technique must be done in a respectful way and not as a way of making fun of the individual.

TABLE 18.1 **Common Responses of Disoriented Older Adults to Touch**

Remind Client of	Touch Technique
Mother	Palm of hand in a light circular motion on the upper cheek
Father	Fingertips, in a circular motion, medium pressure, on the back of the head
Spouse/lover	Hand under the earlobe, curving along the chin, with both hands, a soft stroking motion downward along the jaw
Child	Cupped fingers on the back of the neck, with both hands, in a small circular motion
Brother or sister or good friend	Full hand on the shoulders and upper back by the shoulder blades; use full pressure in a rubbing movement
Animals or pets	Fingertips on the inside of the calf

Source: Feil, N. (1989). *Validation: The Feil Method.* Cleveland, OH: Edward Feil Productions, pp. 47–48, with permission.

If the nurse feels uncomfortable doing this, it is not genuine and does not help communication.

Matching and mirroring are nonverbal ways of helping someone know that you hear what he or she is saying. Matching of emotions can be done by labeling the emotion out loud and using the same intensity used by the older person. Mrs. C. may pound her fist on the arm of her wheelchair and say, "I hate them, I hate them, I hate them." Using matching and mirroring, the nurse would pound on the table with the same rhythm she is using and say, "You're angry, you're angry, you're angry," using the same intensity of emotion.

Universal Symbols

A universal symbol is an object in the present that represents something important from the past. Sometimes these symbols increase in importance for people who develop disorientation as they grow older. The symbol can be something that has meaning to the older person, such as a reminder of a hobby or life's work, or it can be a different type of symbol. Some typical symbols are listed in Table 18.2. An apron can be made with a large pocket in the front that can contain significant symbols. A farmer may touch farm tools placed in the pocket of an apron and by doing this revive a memory of a time in life he enjoyed. As the farmer touches the tools, the nurse can encourage communication using these symbols of his previous life.

Problem Behaviors

If a person with a psychological problem begins to display any unusual behaviors, it may be due to numerous different causes. Recent changes in relationships may contribute to increased wandering, shouting, and aggressive or withdrawn behaviors. These behaviors are common after a room or roommate change or when the person is becoming accustomed to new staff members. These behavioral changes also may indicate that a medication change needs close monitoring or that symptoms of the person's illness are becoming more acute.

When you are caring for a person who is exhibiting difficult behavior, you need to take special precautions. Be alert to any situation that would place you, the older adult, or other patients in danger. Report anything suspicious to the RN, and stay calm.

All persons with psychological problems do not act in a dangerous way. Some sit quietly and never talk or move. This person needs your attention and expertise as well. Talk gently and kindly to the person. Sit with this quiet individual even if there is no conversation. Touch the person if it seems acceptable. All of these simple acts indicate acceptance of the person and are important for healing.

What should you do if an older adult is "yelling" at you? First, do not respond with anger. Stay calm. Be empathetic and kind. Listen to what is being said to identify what the problem really is. Get help if you need it. Be alert to what is going on throughout the unit and with the individuals in your care.

Some older adults with psychological disorders have hallucinations, delusions, and illusions.

TABLE 18.2 Universal Symbols and What They Can Mean

Symbol	Possible Meaning
Jewelry, clothing	Worth, identity
Shoe	Container, womb, male or female sex symbol
Purse	Female sex symbol, vagina, identity
Cane or fist	Penis, potency, power
Soft furniture	Safety, mother, home
Hard furniture	Father, God
Napkin, tissue	Earth, belonging, baby
Flat object	Identity
Food	Love, mother
Drink from a glass	Male power, potency
Any receptacle	Womb
Picking the nose	Sexual pleasure
Playing with feces	Early childhood pleasures

Source: Feil, N. (1989). *Validation: The Feil Method.* Cleveland, OH: Edward Feil Productions, p. 73, with permission.

These are symptoms of serious mental illness. People exhibiting these symptoms may think that they are Jesus Christ, or they may see bugs crawling all over their arms, or they may think you are a princess and want to wait on you. When dealing with such problems, the first rule is to stay calm. The next most important thing is to tell the truth. Do not play into the symptom by saying, "Yes, I am Princess Laura," or something of that nature. Be caring, honest, and genuine with the person. If you feel uncomfortable or in danger, get help; this is never a wrong response.

AGITATION

Agitation can occur as a result of physiological or psychological problems. Some people become agitated because of physical causes that result in delirium. Common psychological problems that can cause agitation are the manic phase of bipolar affective disorder, stress or anxiety, flashbacks from traumatic experiences, reactions following abuse, or dementia. When people become agitated, they also may become violent. Such violence can be directed toward themselves or others. Preventing agitation and managing it when it occurs can be accomplished by following a few simple principles, as follows:

- Watch for signs of agitation. Some people show signs of increasing irritability before a severe problem occurs. Others may have sudden, explosive outbursts. Notice if someone is talking very loudly, pacing more or faster, or making threatening comments to staff or others. Before an actual outburst occurs, try to keep the person talking to you by using some of the communication skills discussed in this chapter. With many people who are agitated, simply matching their breathing patterns or tone of voice is calming.

With most people who are agitated, it is best to step back about 4 to 6 feet while talking with them. With disoriented elderly people, the reverse may be true, especially if a sensory deficit is present. It may be more calming to move closer to maintain sustained eye contact and touch. This movement must be done cautiously to protect your own safety and that of others. If there is the possibility that other patients or visitors may be harmed, move them out of the way.

- If a person becomes physically aggressive, it is important to remember that the thumb is the weakest point of the hand. If a person has a hold on you, the way to remove yourself is by rotating away from the thumb of the person's hand. Most psychiatric facilities provide training sessions that allow you to practice dealing with these behaviors in a way that minimizes harm to yourself and protects the agitated person.

Dealing With Psychological Problems Caused by Stress

This section provides some general guidelines for dealing with older adults with psychological problems who are experiencing stressful situations. Making an extra effort to assign the same staff members to an older person in the hospital and in the nursing home may help to prevent emotional distress. A hospitalized patient may be assigned nine different nurses during a 3-day stay. The sheer number of names to remember is difficult, but it is especially challenging for an older adult with emotional problems.

In addition to the "normal" stress of being admitted to a hospital or nursing home, an older person with psychological problems has to deal with whatever illness caused the admission and the symptoms of the psychological illness. An example is a person who has hallucinations. Hallucinations are real to the person experiencing them, and they add a tremendous level of confusion to the daily life of the person. Hallucinations interfere with one's ability to perceive information accurately. The nurse's instructions or even a greeting may be misinterpreted; medications may look like spiders; walls and doorways may keep moving. The approach to such problems includes keeping the same caregiver with the patient throughout his or her stay. The nurse will begin to understand the behaviors of the older adult and be able to work within the limitations of the mental illness of the person.

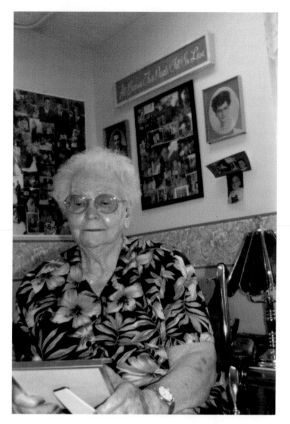

Reminiscence is an excellent tool to use to strengthen an older person's self-esteem.

It also helps when an older person's familiar belongings can be kept in the room; this promotes self-worth and helps to prevent disorientation. Small objects and pictures can be placed near the older person during a hospitalization to prevent the disorientation that can accompany stressful changes during an illness. Playing taped music of familiar songs generally is better than television viewing in preventing

CRITICALLY EXAMINE THE FOLLOWING

A 78-year-old woman, who is legally blind, attempts to hit a staff member when she is being returned to bed.

Possible Solutions

1. Call resident by name.
2. Move close to her face and touch her if acceptable.
3. Match her voice tone and breathing while talking to her.

sensory overload. These are just a few examples of simple nursing interventions that can be used to prevent psychological problems caused by stress in older adults.

Violent Behavior

If older adults start to act violently, the nurse must remember to protect these individuals from their own behavior at all times. The nurse needs to call for help and, as a member of a team, decide what the intervention should be. Do not raise your voice; stay calm. These are the basic rules for handling someone who is violent.

Some violent behavior can be life-threatening. If you are in that type of situation, slowly gather any endangered patients and take them to safety. There is no formula for what to do in every possible situation. Simply stay calm and safeguard the patients and yourself.

CRITICALLY EXAMINE THE FOLLOWING

Mrs. C. starts yelling and shouting, "Call the police, call the police," while she is throwing items at her roommate.

Possible Solutions

1. Maintain eye contact, speak in a calm voice, and call Mrs. C. by name.
2. Tell her to talk to you and ask, "Are you frightened of something?"
3. Have another employee remove the roommate to safety.

CRITICALLY EXAMINE THE FOLLOWING

Mr. J. walks into the visitor's area, unzips his trousers, and begins to masturbate.

Possible Solutions

1. Gently approach him and get his attention by moving in close and speaking to him. Say his name.
2. Quietly lead him to his room; make sure that he is safe and then give him privacy to do whatever he wishes sexually. Ask his roommate to go to the dayroom with you if necessary.
3. Give affection and attention when he is not sexually acting out.

Sexual Acting Out

Acting out feelings of anxiety may take many forms. Sometimes older adults with dementia lose social controls and express sexual feelings openly. Some people, such as individuals in the early stages of Alzheimer's disease, have an increased desire for sexual activity. People with other types of psychological problems, such as bipolar affective disorder, show sexual feelings in ways that are socially inappropriate. Dealing with these behaviors is almost always difficult, no matter how experienced the nurse is. Always consider if the acting out is an expression of the need for affection and touch. Notice any factors that seem to trigger the behavior to intervene before the behavior occurs.

● SPECIALIZED COMMUNICATING SKILLS

The hallmark of nursing care for persons with psychological problems is the ability to communicate effectively. In addition to the skills just described in this chapter, there are other communication skills that can be used to make it easier to talk to older people with psychological problems. Some standard communication skills and concepts from neurolinguistic programming (Bandler, 1985) and validation (Feil, 1993) are described in this section.

Neurolinguistic programming uses observation of a person's words and behaviors to help establish the best way of relating to that person. Validation, a communication approach for relating to disoriented older adults, helps disoriented persons express themselves. Sometimes communication with someone who is disoriented is blocked by the listener's need to have the disoriented person think or talk in a "logical" way. When the listener is able to put aside the need to communicate in a normal way, it becomes possible to communicate in other, more effective ways. The listener becomes able to understand and validate the disoriented person's experiences.

Preferred Sense Words

All people relate to their surroundings through their senses. Most people respond more through one sense than through others. How a person talks can give an idea of that person's preferred sense. If Mrs. J. says, "I see what you mean. Look at this," she probably is a person who responds best to sight or visual words. Some people respond best to hearing or auditory words, and others respond best to words about feelings or movement (kinesthetic words). Table 18.3 lists commonly used visual, auditory, and kinesthetic words. The nurse can use the person's preferred sense to establish rapport. If an older adult says, "No one listens to me anymore," a response such as "What would you like for me to listen to, Mr. J.?" would receive a better response than "What would you like me to see, Mr. J.?"

Vague Pronouns

If a person is unable to fill in the details with enough facts to be understood, try using vague or ambiguous pronouns to help foster communication. Sometimes people refer to all women as "she" and all men as "he." If the nurse becomes too concerned about accurate details, the opportunity to communicate may be lost. Instead of worrying about the facts, such as who "he" or "she" is, try to focus on the feelings. If an older person says, "She's all alone. She can't stay there," you can respond, "You're worried about her. She's important to you." That type of sensitive response generally elicits more communication.

Speaking Slowly

Many people who have emotional problems have slowed thought processes. When this problem is combined with normal aging changes, it is very important for the nurse to use slightly slower speech and wait a little longer for the person to respond. Asking questions one at a time, instead of running several questions together, can also make it easier to talk to an older person with an emotional problem.

TABLE 18.3 **Commonly Used Preferred Sense Words**

Visual	Auditory	Kinesthetic
See	Listen	Feel
View	Hear	Grasp
Picture	Sound	Move
Look	Loud	Touch

Asking the Extreme

When someone who is disoriented is upset about something he or she thinks happened, ask questions about the extremes of the situation. What is the worst? What is the best? Imagine the opposite. When is it better? When does it not happen? Suppose every night an elderly woman thinks some men are coming to attack her. The nurse might ask, "When do they usually come? When are they not there? What helps you feel safe? What doesn't help you very much?" Often by looking at the extreme of a situation, the person can recognize what is happening in the "here and now."

● GRIEVING AND DEPRESSION

Surviving losses is part of the aging process. An older person may lose relationships with people through death, retirement, or relocation, or he or she may lose the ability to maintain contacts with friends and family because of physical problems. An older adult also may experience the loss of valued social roles, a home, financial security, vision, hearing, or other body functions. The loss of a loved one is one of the most powerful losses a person can experience.

Dealing With Grief

It is helpful to keep in mind the stages of the grieving process—denial, anger, bargaining, depression, and acceptance—when dealing with losses (see Chapter 10). These stages do not always occur with every person. Some people who experience losses may become angry but not go through the other stages. As a nurse, it is important to accept each person's response to grief and not have a preconceived idea of how a person should respond.

If an older adult is grieving over the loss of a job, the nurse can help him or her to talk about the grief by asking open-ended questions, such as "What did you do at your former job?" "When did you start working there?" "How did you get started working there?" Asking open-ended questions about feelings also can help another to express grief. Sometimes it can be uncomfortable to hear a person talk about negative emotions such as anger and sadness. Encouraging someone to express feelings and allowing expressions of anger or crying can help that person deal with feelings effectively. Saying something like, "How did you feel about that?" or "What upset you the most about that?" can encourage someone to talk about feelings. Telling someone who is sad and grieving "Don't cry now, it will be all right" only gives false reassurance and tells the person to keep such powerful emotions inside. If emotions are not expressed, they tend to be expressed later in dysfunctional ways, such as extreme anger, agitation, or withdrawal.

Depression

Because depression is a part of grieving and loss, it is a serious problem among elderly people. Other factors may contribute to depression as well. Most current theories about depression have a strong emphasis on neurobiological causes and take into account the fact that depression tends to run in families. Most researchers conclude that depression is linked to the amount of the neurotransmitters serotonin and norepinephrine present in the nerve synapses. Lower serotonin and norepinephrine levels seem to be associated with depression. Factors within the body can deplete these substances, but external factors such as stress or decreased exposure to light also can influence the amounts of neurotransmitters available to a person.

As health-care providers, nurses also know that regular exercise can help maintain a higher level of endorphins in a person's body. Endorphins are naturally produced morphine-like substances that help people feel better. If the ability to exercise is impaired, the body and mind are affected, and depression may result. Getting exposure to sunlight also can affect some people by changing their mood. For a homebound elderly person, this may be a problem. A poor diet also may contribute to the development of depression. Many older people have poor nutritional intake because of various psychological and physical factors, such as poor denture fit, cost of nutritious foods, changes in taste sensations, and eating alone. When the effects of the losses of aging are combined with the effects of physical risk factors, it is clear why many elderly people are depressed. The good news is that most people who have depression can be helped by treatment. Medications that are used to treat depression are generally effective.

Tricyclic antidepressants were widely prescribed in the past and are still effective for many people. Major problems with using tricyclic antidepressants are side effects related to the cardiovascular system and urinary retention. Many elderly persons have problems with heart disease and hypertension, and men may have prostatic hypertrophy. These problems can be contraindications for the use of tricyclic drugs. With the advent of serotonin-selective reuptake inhibitors such as fluoxetine (Prozac), sertraline (Zoloft), and paroxetine (Paxil), safer treatment options are available for people who have depression and other physical problems. Another antidepressant used very effectively with many elderly people is bupropion (Wellbutrin). Wellbutrin must be monitored closely if there are any eating disturbances or if there is a concern over weight loss.

Medications are an important part of treating depression but are most successful when used in conjunction with other types of therapy. Individual therapy with a counselor educated to work with older adults can help the person develop coping skills for dealing with depression.

Depression and Confusion in the Elderly Person

Assessing someone who is depressed is complicated by factors that occur as a result of normal aging. Chapter 17 describes how to assess someone with depression and how to use standard measures of depression. Some of the behaviors seen in people with depression may be very similar to behaviors seen with other problems that are common in older people. Individuals who are depressed may not care about their surroundings and begin to be disoriented and confused as they draw inward. It can be very difficult to know whether the mental slowing and memory loss attributed to depression are actually caused by the depression or represent changes commonly found in the early stages of

---

CRITICALLY EXAMINE THE FOLLOWING

Mr. N. usually walks well, but since starting on an antidepressant, he has fallen three times in the past week.

Possible Solutions

1. Check lying, sitting, and standing blood pressure.
2. If he has orthostatic hypotension, teach him to sit on the side of the bed for a few minutes before standing up slowly.
3. Talk to his physician to determine whether another drug could be used.

dementia. Many elderly people who have depression are thought to have dementia and are not treated for their depression (see Table 18.4).

Depression and Suicide

Assessing for the risk of suicide is essential for someone who is depressed. The suicide rate among older adults is high. It may not seem likely that an older person would have thoughts about suicide, but it happens too frequently. If an older person says something like "I just don't want to live anymore," the tendency may be to discount the person and say, "Oh, you don't mean that," or "You'll feel better tomorrow, you're just having a bad day." If a person expresses a wish to die, makes funeral plans, has a major change in life, or begins to give away cherished possessions, these can be signs that the person may be planning suicide.

Asking people whether they are having thoughts about killing themselves is not "putting the thought into their heads." Many people are relieved to talk to someone about suicide if asked in a calm, matter-of-fact manner. Finding out whether the person has a plan and what it is are essential pieces of information. If a homebound older adult describes a hoard of potassium supplements or cardiac medications that are readily available, and if the person's conversation indicates a plan to take the medication after the nurse leaves, the situation requires immediate action. Persons who say they do not want to live but have not thought about how they would end their lives are at a much lower risk for an immediate suicide attempt than persons who

have a plan. Many incidents of so-called noncompliance with medications are actually intentional attempts to overdose. If an older adult is having thoughts about suicide, listen carefully, intervene immediately if necessary, and refer the person for treatment.

Failure to Thrive

The term *failure to thrive* is most often applied to young children who do not grow and develop as expected. Some elders who are depressed also may have a failure to thrive or a giving-up complex. This may be the case when the older person no longer makes an effort to continue with life, such as by refusing to eat, refusing medications, or choosing to resist or refuse treatment for

TABLE 18.4 Differences Between Delirium, Dementia, and Depression

	Delirium	Dementia	Depression
Onset	Rapid	Slow	Rapid
Duration	Short	Long	Short or long
Night symptom	May worsen	Frequently worsen	Usually do not worsen
Cognitive functions	Variable	Stable	Variable
Physical causes	Common	None	Possible
Recent changes	Common	None or minimal	Common
Suicidal ideation	Rare	Rare	Common
Low self-esteem	Rare	Rare	Common
History of psychiatric symptoms	Not usually	Rare	Common
Mood	Labile	Labile	Depressed
Behavior	Labile	Labile	Slowed thought and motor processes

health problems. If there is not an intervention that involves the interdisciplinary team and the family, the older adult may die in this situation.

DELIRIUM AND DEMENTIA

Because depression can cause some confusion and disorientation, it can be difficult to determine whether the older person has a problem with delirium, dementia, or depression (Table 18.4). Many factors influence a person's ability to think clearly.

Emotional stress and change can cause anyone to have difficulty remembering scheduled appointments or to be distracted easily from activities of daily living, such as turning off the burner when cooking. Sometimes physical factors such as illness, insufficient oxygen, or high or low blood glucose levels may cause a person to behave in a bizarre way. A person who has a problem with disorientation can be found in any setting. When a person becomes disoriented, the caregivers may become resigned to the problem and consider this to be a normal part of the aging process. That is not a correct assumption. Clarification of the differences between delirium and dementia can provide guidance for effective intervention in both situations.

Delirium

Delirium refers to a situation in which an older person has a rapid change in behavior and thinking ability. Mental status changes that occur with this acute problem usually affect an individual's ability to recall where he or she is, what day or time it is, or even the individual's own name. Delirium may cause agitation or rapidly changing moods. Someone who is delirious commonly has an anxious facial expression. Short-term memory may or may not be intact. With delirium, the older adult pays little attention to surroundings or may respond slowly to new surroundings.

A person with delirium usually talks in a rambling way that does not make sense. The individual may have difficulty staying awake, or the individual could have increased activity and be awake all the time. Sensory and perceptual disorders, such as hallucinations and delusions, may be present. A person with delirium may perceive that a nurse holding a syringe has a knife or that a baby is crying when no baby is there. Changes in thought content and process also may be present. Fixed ideas or beliefs as

---

CRITICALLY EXAMINE THE FOLLOWING

A 75-year-old man who has just had surgery develops delirium, is agitated, and tries to pull out his nasogastric tube.

Possible Solutions

1. Check for physical causes.
2. Ask a family member or a volunteer to sit with him to prevent removal of the tube.

An 82-year-old woman, who has just received oxycodone, thinks the nurse who enters the room with a stethoscope is going to hang her with a rope.

Possible Solutions

1. Stop oxycodone use and notify the physician.
2. If possible, remove the stethoscope and return later when she is less agitated to take her apical pulse.
3. If she is not too agitated and is able to listen, speak to her in a quiet and caring way. Do all you can to help her overcome her agitation.

---

well as disjointed or flighty thoughts may be evident.

Delirium can result from various physiological causes and can be reversed. Malnutrition, electrolyte imbalance, infection, acid-base imbalance, change in blood glucose, hypoxia, drug reactions, dehydration, and head trauma are common causes of delirium. It is important to determine what is causing the delirium because the sooner the problem can be treated, the sooner the delirium resolves.

When an older adult has a period of delirium, it can be very upsetting for the family and nursing staff. Explaining what is happening to all involved can help reduce stress and make it easier for everyone to handle the problem behaviors that occur.

Dementia

The symptom of dementia is usually defined as the loss of intellectual abilities to the extent that it interferes with normal activities of daily living. Dementia is characterized by problems with cognitive ability, personality changes, memory impairment, decreased intellectual functioning, and changed judgment and mood.

Dementia usually occurs gradually, over months or years, and is the result of deterioration of the brain. Neurological diseases such as Pick's disease or Huntington's disease can cause this damage, or the damage can be the result of vascular problems such as multi-infarct dementia. Advanced AIDS also has an associated dementia. The most common type of dementia is associated with Alzheimer's disease (AD). It is estimated that in the future dementia will outweigh heart disease and cancer as a major health problem. This estimate is based on the growing number of elderly people in the population and the strong correlation between aging and AD.

Because dementia is such a significant concern, new approaches to dealing with this problem are being examined. Validation therapy is a way of communicating with people who have dementia (Feil, 1993). Validation means respecting the feelings of the person and confirming that, from the individual's perspective, the experience is true.

Validation therapy is being used in many countries for people who are disoriented to decrease stress, to promote self-esteem and communication, to reduce use of chemical and physical restraint, and to make it possible to sustain independent living for a longer time.

A brief introduction to validation therapy follows. More information on communication strategies is given later in this chapter. For those with a special interest in validation, additional information is available by doing a topic search on the Internet.

Stages of Disorientation

Naomi Feil (1993) has described four stages of disorientation that occur with people who are "old-old" (older than 80 years of age). These changes occur in people who have had fairly normal lives until they reach their 80s, when they begin to show signs of disorientation. The stages are malorientation, time confusion, repetitive motion, and vegetation.

Malorientation
Malorientation is the first stage of disorientation. People who are maloriented may initially appear as if nothing is wrong with them. These people may be oriented as to where they are and who the president of the United States is, but they are beginning to forget information important for maintaining normal activities of daily living. They may try to cover up their memory loss by making up excuses. They do not like to be around people who are disoriented because they are threatened by their own memory loss. They deny their feelings and blame other people for their problems.

People who are maloriented respond best to open questions about facts, not feelings. It is important to hold on to acceptable social roles and rules for people who are maloriented. Encouraging someone who has been a teacher to lead the Pledge of Allegiance may be a way of helping maintain dignity and promote self-esteem. Often, the technique of using commonly preferred sense words assists this person to relate to the caregiver. It is best to listen to a maloriented person until you identify what the person's preferred sense is and then address the person with words that represent that sense. For example, someone who often says, "Oh, yes, I see what you mean," probably is a visual person and may respond to visual words better than to other choices (see Table 18.3).

Time Confusion
As people become more disoriented, they withdraw more from the real world and retreat into their own inner world. During this stage, people lose a sense of real time and respond to an inner sense of time.

A person may think about his or her mother (who is dead) and because past time has fused with present time talk about her as if she was present. Because the nurse feels a need to orient the time-confused person, he or she might say something like, "Your mother is dead; you can't go to see her." This only agitates and distresses the individual, who has no real need to stay in a painful present reality. Using the validation approach, the nurse would move close, use touch, and say, "You miss your mother. What color eyes did she have? Blue or brown?" This is an effort to stimulate pleasant thoughts and memories for the person. There are several different methods of touching a person with dementia that are designed to evoke feelings about a loved one. See Table 18.1 to review common forms of touch.

Repetitive Motion
If people with dementia continue to retreat from present reality, they may enter the stage of repetitive motion. During this stage, movements or sounds are repeated constantly. Usually, speech is limited to single-syllable words, and eye contact is made only after someone touches and talks to the person. The use of touch with these people is very important. Individuals with repetitive motion are often ignored emotionally, with caregivers providing physical care only. Validation techniques of sustained eye contact, stroking, and touching can help reach people in this stage of disorientation and prevent the final

stage, which is that of vegetation. When persons are in the repetitive motion stage, they often communicate through universal symbols. These people use objects to represent thoughts. A common example is carefully folding and holding or caressing a napkin, which could represent a baby. Other examples are given in Table 18.2.

Vegetation

The final stage of disorientation and withdrawal is vegetation. In this stage, very little movement or sound is noted. Eye contact is very rare. Using touch and familiar music can help reach a person in this stage.

Alzheimer's Disease

The most common type of dementia is AD. The disease was first described in 1906 by a neurologist, who observed neurofibrillary tangles in an autopsy sample of the brain. Although there have been many advances regarding AD over the years, the only way to diagnose AD conclusively is at autopsy. This means that AD is usually diagnosed clinically by first ruling out any other causes of delirium or dementia. When symptoms of dementia are present and no other organic disease causing behavioral and mental changes can be found, a diagnosis of AD can be made.

AD is commonly found in persons older than 80 years of age, but it can occur in persons as young as 30 years. Research findings indicate a strong correlation for increased incidence of AD as people age. There also seems to be a significant correlation between Down's syndrome and head trauma in relation to AD.

At least half a dozen drugs are being investigated for use in the management of dementia. At present, the medication tacrine (Cognex) is being used with mixed success in the treatment of mild-to-moderate AD. Because of the effects of this drug on the liver, it is necessary to make frequent checks of liver enzymes.

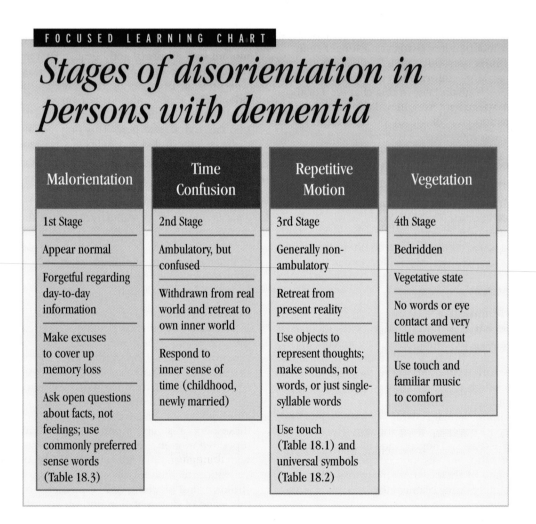

FOCUSED LEARNING CHART

Stages of disorientation in persons with dementia

Malorientation	Time Confusion	Repetitive Motion	Vegetation
1st Stage	2nd Stage	3rd Stage	4th Stage
Appear normal	Ambulatory, but confused	Generally non-ambulatory	Bedridden
Forgetful regarding day-to-day information	Withdrawn from real world and retreat to own inner world	Retreat from present reality	Vegetative state
Make excuses to cover up memory loss	Respond to inner sense of time (childhood, newly married)	Use objects to represent thoughts; make sounds, not words, or just single-syllable words	No words or eye contact and very little movement
Ask open questions about facts, not feelings; use commonly preferred sense words (Table 18.3)		Use touch (Table 18.1) and universal symbols (Table 18.2)	Use touch and familiar music to comfort

PARANOIA

Some people with emotional problems fear that other people are trying to hurt them. Such paranoid ideas are an indication of problems the person may have with trusting others. This paranoia can occur with dementia, schizophrenia, or other psychological problems. People who are paranoid often seem very convincing and logical. Developing trust is the priority with someone who is paranoid. Being consistent and reliable in all that you do with the person can be the best way to develop trust. Do not make promises you cannot keep. If you say you will do something, following up with the paranoid person is especially important. It is particularly important to avoid putting medicines in food or drink without the paranoid person's knowledge.

DEVELOPMENTAL DISABILITIES

Historically, people who had developmental disabilities did not live to an old age. With advances in health care, more individuals who have developmental disabilities, such as Down's syndrome, are living longer. There is evidence that as individuals with Down's syndrome grow older, they are at high risk of developing AD.

Individuals with developmental disabilities may have some of the problem behaviors that have been identified in this chapter. Principles for setting limits on behavior include the following:

- Recognize the person's feelings and encourage expression of them.
- State the limit clearly.

- Point out ways that behavior can be expressed within the limits and what is outside the limits.
- Allow the person to express anger at having limits placed on him or her.

SUBSTANCE ABUSE

Health care workers who are working with people who have chemical dependency problems recognize that there are a growing number of older adults with substance abuse problems. Because many older people are treated for a wide variety of physical problems, sometimes they receive prescription drugs from several different sources. The availability of prescription drugs contributes to the problem of drug abuse among older persons.

Alcoholism is another problem for many elderly adults. Many of the same reasons that people use substances to self-medicate (e.g., depression, losses, loneliness) in other stages of life are even more of a problem for elderly people. Because many memory lapses found with substance abuse are similar to the memory lapses in the early stages of dementia, substance abuse may not be discovered until it is advanced. Sometimes families have difficulty confronting older family members about substance abuse problems. The denial of a problem, which is characteristic of most substance abuse problems, is especially difficult to deal with when working with older adults. This situation creates a problem with the treatment process. If a substance abuse problem is suspected, it is best to contact trained professionals to assist with interventions.

EATING DISORDERS

Often, the reason for seeking health care is a problem with eating. Problems with eating can be due to physical factors, such as loss of taste sensation or poor denture fit, but eating difficulties often are due to psychological problems. Anorexia can be a symptom of a psychological problem, such as depression, or it can be a problem in itself.

Compulsive resistance to eating or anorexia historically has been most commonly found in young women. Clinicians are increasingly describing similar symptoms in elderly people. Eating or not eating can be used as a way of exhibiting controlling or resisting behaviors, especially in stressful situations. Compulsive overeating also can occur in elderly people, as can the bingeing and purging found in bulimia. Some elderly patients with psychological problems have phobias related to certain foods. Others may become paranoid about food that they believe is poisoned or contaminated.

Regardless of the specific problem, treating someone who has an eating disorder may require tremendous creativity. Sometimes, the only effective treatment is using a feeding tube until adequate weight gain is achieved. Behavior modification techniques, such as giving privileges for weight gain and withdrawing privileges for weight loss, may need to be planned by the health-care team or a psychiatric nurse specialist.

GROUPS FOR THE ELDERLY

Many older adults with psychological problems can benefit from group interactions. Some types of group therapy that have been used successfully with older persons are discussed next.

Reminiscence

Based on memories of similar events or experiences, many older adults form bonds in groups. Stimulating memories of childhood or early adulthood can serve to improve feelings of self-worth and provide an opportunity to review their lives. Memories may stimulate laughter and happiness or other emotions and serve as a way of coping with present circumstances. Groups can be conducted around an important event, such as Pearl Harbor Day. Common, shared experiences, such as early school days, can be recalled to promote socialization and provide mental stimulation. Reminiscence also can be used individually as a means of helping people process any unfinished business in their lives.

A very structured form of reminiscence is the life review process. This process provides an opportunity for evaluation and integration of life experiences. People in more advanced stages of disorientation are unable to benefit from this type of therapy.

Remotivation

To improve interest in and quality of life, remotivation techniques can be used. The emphasis with remotivation is the use of real objects to stimulate senses and provide new motivation in life and the surrounding world. Pictures, plants, animals, or sounds can be used to encourage group interaction. Holidays, birthdays, or hobbies can be used to focus on participating in the here and now. The focus is on factual information as opposed to exploration of feelings. These groups work best with people who have depression or early stages of disorientation.

Resocialization

Encouraging residents to assume social roles can stimulate feelings of increased self-esteem. The focus for this group is on social roles and not on problem-solving. Discussion may occur about previous social gatherings and how people behaved during these events. The emphasis is on the present and on the discussion of factual information.

Many older adults with psychological problems can benefit from group interactions. Group members are assigned roles, such as the greeter, or to serve each other refreshments. Feelings are not the focus of resocialization groups, which can be helpful for mildly disoriented individuals.

Reality Orientation

The goal of reality orientation is to help residents become oriented to present reality. Constant reminders about the present—that is, where they are and what day it is—are given. Current events on the television or in the newspaper can be used as topics to stimulate discussions. The season of the year, holidays, and the weather are other topics to promote orientation to reality. These groups are focused on keeping people oriented to present reality and are not usually very effective with people who have more than mild disorientation.

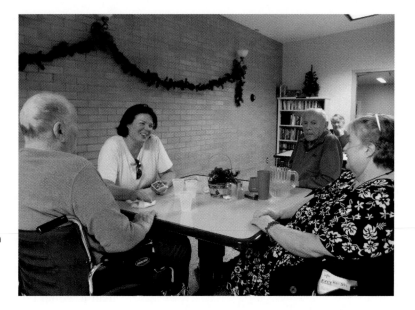

This group of older adults is being led in a resocialization group. Many older adults with psychological problems benefit from group interaction.

Validation

Validation groups combine some of the other types of techniques with group problem-solving and a focus on support. Members are assigned roles, sing familiar songs, serve each other refreshments, and reminisce about the past. Movement is encouraged during group activities. The group is presented with a problem to solve. Resolving losses and expressing feelings are emphasized. Validation groups are most effective for people who have moderate disorientation.

PSYCHOTROPIC MEDICATIONS

As with all medications, adaptation is necessary when using psychotropic medications with an older adult. Teaching the older person and his or her family about the reason for the medication, side effects, toxic effects, and what to do if a dose is missed are very important when psychotropic drugs are used.

Many psychotropic drugs require time—sometimes several weeks—before a therapeutic effect is achieved. This waiting period may be longer for some older people. Older people may show more signs of toxicity at lower-than-usual doses because their ability to excrete the drug is impaired, resulting in a buildup of the drug in the bloodstream. Older people could also be more difficult to treat because of side effects that occur secondary to the difference in distribution and excretion of drugs in the aging body.

Psychotropic medications work in the brain in various ways. Most medications work by helping to change the level of neurotransmitters or chemicals in the brain. It is hoped that reestablishing a more normal balance will help the person have fewer psychological problems. Because these drugs work on the brain, it is important to use them only for psychological problems and not just because the resident has behaviors that irritate other people. Before any drugs are used to sedate a person with problem behaviors, all other types of nursing interventions must be used along with documentation of the interventions.

Because of physical health problems, some medications used to treat mental health problems may be contraindicated or may require careful administration in the older patient. For example, an elderly man who has prostate disease may have extreme difficulty voiding if given a tricyclic antidepressant.

A common side effect of many psychotropic drugs is constipation. When combined with normal aging changes, the constipation resulting from psychotropic medications can become a problem for the elderly person.

Orthostatic hypotension results from many psychotropic drugs. Simple teaching techniques can help manage some of the postural blood pressure changes; however, these changes often are severe enough to require that the medication be discontinued.

PHYSICAL AND MENTAL HEALTH

Because there is such a strong relationship between physical and mental health, many professionals believe that all diseases have physical and emotional aspects. Some older people grew up in a time when it was frowned on to admit that mental illness existed, but it was more socially acceptable to have a physical problem. One grandmother described a time early in her marriage when she became so upset with her husband that she became "sick" and took to her bed for a week.

This expression of emotional problems through physical complaints is called somatization. If a stressful situation is encountered, the person who uses somatization may develop a backache, headache, or stomach ache to avoid dealing with problems. This does not mean the ache is "all in the head," but it may mean that the person finds it easier or more acceptable to have a physical pain than an emotional one. For someone who has done this for 80 or 90 years of life, it may be difficult or impossible to change this way of coping. The nurse can help the patient learn to meet needs more directly by encouraging the person to talk about feelings openly.

PATIENT RIGHTS AND LEGAL RESPONSIBILITIES

The current standard of care in nursing homes and in mental health centers is that the older person has the right to the least restrictive form of treatment. Federal and state regulating agencies such as the Health Care Financing Administration have specific regulations protecting these rights. In most states, treatment can be administered involuntarily only if a danger exists to the individual or to others. The length of time allowed for this type of treatment varies from state to state but is usually only a few days. If a longer treatment schedule is required and the older person is unwilling to consent, an application for guardianship may be made; the person's rights to make personal decisions are taken away and assigned to a guardian. This procedure may be necessary for people with some types of mental illness, including dementia.

When agitated behaviors become severe, the nurse has to make a decision about how to handle the problem. Points that must be considered are the patient's right to the least restrictive treatment environment and the legal issues related to the use of chemical and physical restraints. If an older adult has an episode in which increased symptoms of bipolar affective disorder or schizophrenia are exhibited, an antipsychotic drug is likely to be more effective than it would be for someone with dementia or delirium. Before giving a chemical restraint, it is necessary to try talking to the person as well as using behavioral interventions. When all else fails, physical restraints may be necessary on rare occasions. If using physical restraints, remember the following safety precautions:

1. Use the least restrictive device.
2. Check on the person often.
3. Remove the restraints every 2 hours for a brief period.

CONCLUSION

The care of elderly people in all arenas of nursing is an opportunity to practice the art of nursing at its highest level. The skills and understanding that are needed to give meaningful care to the elderly patient with psychological problems are complex, and they require a personal and professional commitment to the needs of people as they age.

Mr. A. is an 80-year-old retired farmer. He lived with his wife on the farm until 1 year ago, when he became too ill for his wife to manage his care alone. At that time, he became a resident of a nursing home in a nearby town. He has been forgetful for several years and now wanders the halls looking for his pickup truck. During the winter, he walked away from the nursing home and wandered for several hours. This resulted in frostbite on several fingers and toes. He becomes agitated when he is told that he cannot go back to his home. What actions can be taken to assist Mr. A.?

Solution

Working with the entire nursing staff, a plan is developed for using validation therapy with Mr. A. When he asks about his truck or home, the staff ask him questions such as, "What color is your truck?" "What did you do with your truck?" "Where did you go?" "With whom?" Coveralls with a front pocket are obtained, and a small hammer and screwdriver are placed in his pocket. His toolbox is brought into his room. The staff has put him in charge of a small garden outside the nursing home. Individual sessions of validation are scheduled 20 minutes a day, three times a week, by the activities staff.

Over a 6-week period, the staff notices that Mr. A. spends quiet, productive time in the garden area. He carries his toolbox with him most of the time but does not use its contents. He no longer leaves the building except to work in his garden. He is still forgetful.

Select the best answer to each question.

1. The best intervention for an elderly resident of a nursing home who has paranoia is:

   a. To encourage him to lead a large group singing

   b. To plan one-on-one activities with staff and other residents

   c. To invite the resident to sit on the residents' council of the nursing home

   d. To have the resident join a weekly bingo group

2. An elderly homebound person taking medication for a psychological problem needs to know which of the following?

   a. If dizziness occurs, notify the nurse.

   b. It may take several weeks to get the desired effect.

   c. Report any changes in vision.

   d. All of the above.

3. Validation techniques are best described as:

   a. A way of helping someone resolve past experiences

   b. Helping someone find new meaning in growing older

   c. A reminder of a painful present reality

   d. Bringing someone from the past into the present world

4. When a hospitalized older adult suddenly becomes disoriented, the best intervention is which of the following?

   a. Ignore the person's feelings because they are a normal part of aging.

   b. Tell the person to cheer up because things are not so bad.

   c. Do not allow the person to talk about being sad because that makes it worse.

   d. Encourage the person to discuss feelings openly because it helps to talk about problems.

5. When teaching older adults or their families about the use of psychotropic drugs, one of the most important concepts to teach is:

   a. The meaning of the different colors of the medications

   b. The stress psychotropic drugs put on the kidneys

   c. To anticipate the chronic light-headedness that most people experience

   d. Not to expect the full effect of the drug for several weeks

19 Rehabilitation and Restorative Care

Kathleen R. Culliton

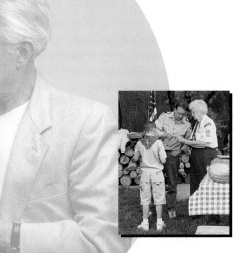

Learning Objectives

After completing this chapter, the student will be able to:

1. Define rehabilitation and restorative nursing in a holistic framework.
2. Identify the clinical implications of restorative care in walking programs, continence training, and feeding and self-help programs.

INTRODUCTION

Nurses strive to promote the health of older adults. Generally, nursing care involves assisting older persons in overcoming the symptoms of an acute health problem or the worsening of a chronic condition. Nurses use medications, treatments, and referrals to help the individual overcome physical, psychological, social, and spiritual illness. In the acute-care setting, nurses assist older adults through the crisis of illness and discharge them back into the community to their homes or a supportive living environment. The goal of nursing care is to assist older adults back to the highest level of health possible and to allow them to live in their homes or whatever environment provides them with optimal safety. Assessment of their general health and ability to meet their personal needs are considerations during the discharge process. Sometimes older adults are no longer physically or emotionally able to return safely to their homes. You, as the licensed practical nurse (LPN), play a significant role for institutionalized older adults who need restorative care.

This chapter presents an overview of gerontological nursing concepts based on rehabilitative and restorative care. Rehabilitative and restorative nursing care surpasses the traditional custodial approach that prevailed in the care of older adults before the initiation of the 1990 Omnibus Budget Reconciliation Act (OBRA) regulations. Data collection for residents in nursing homes is done on the minimum data set (MDS) (see Chapter 3) and emphasizes restorative care of older adults as a major priority of care.

With the aging process comes increased disability for many older persons. It has been projected statistically that 40% of all disabled people in the United States presently are 65 years old or older. With the elderly population increasing, nurses are called on to provide rehabilitative and restorative care to more and more older people as they enter health-care facilities.

UNDERSTANDING REHABILITATION AND RESTORATIVE CONCEPTS

Rehabilitation is the process of teaching and training individuals to achieve their highest level of independent function. People are most familiar with rehabilitation programs for spinal cord injuries. For older adults, rehabilitation

---

PRIORITY SETTING 19.1

When dealing with rehabilitation and restorative care, there are three priorities for you:

1. Get to know the person admitted to the unit and the person's family and significant others. To make the rehabilitation and restorative program meaningful for the person receiving treatment, you need to know the person's personal goals and dreams. Because people are not brought to a rehabilitation and restorative care unit in a life-and-death crisis, you have time to meet this priority. Take the time to identify the person's goals and share them with the rest of the IDT team.

2. Use your knowledge and skills as a nurse to prevent disabling consequences (i.e., footdrop, contractures, pressure ulcers, depression) while carrying out rehabilitative and restorative programs.

3. It is assumed that you will carefully follow all physicians' orders. The third priority goes beyond doing what is legally and morally required of you, such as following orders. It is to support the people in your care as they go through the challenges of a rehabilitative or restoration program. It is difficult and demanding. Your support can make a significant difference in the outcome for each individual.

---

often is prescribed for a cerebrovascular accident (or stroke) or deformity from arthritis and after surgery for severe arthritis. Rehabilitative care is a multidisciplinary care model. Physical therapists, occupational therapists, speech therapists, dietitians, respiratory therapists, recreation therapists, social workers, psychologists, nurses, and rehabilitation physicians all are members of rehabilitation care teams.

Rehabilitation is initiated after an extensive assessment of an individual's physical, emotional, spiritual, and functional assets and liabilities. To develop a rehabilitative plan, assessment information and the resources available to assist the individual are reviewed. Often, an individual does not need all available services. The team is restructured to include the necessary health-care team members. This team works with individuals and their families to develop rehabilitative goals and to decide the best way to work toward the goals.

Selecting a short-term or long-term living environment is one of the first choices that a rehabilitation team must make. Every care environment has the potential to be a place for rehabilitation. Limiting factors often are insufficient family support, environmental safety, insurance reimbursement, and access to the rehabilitation team. An older adult with a total hip replacement may want to go home, but home has an upstairs bathroom, and there is no one available to prepare meals. These factors present a problem. A man may be recovering well from knee surgery and wants to have intensive inpatient therapy, but his insurance company does not approve the cost. An elderly woman may want to go to her rural community hospital for rehabilitation after a stroke, but the services she needs are unavailable in that community. The rehabilitation team works to help the person access support services and find the most appropriate environment for the rehabilitation process.

Restorative nursing care is related to rehabilitation. It has the same goal—to assist older people with reaching their highest functional ability. The major difference is the intense involvement of the entire health-care team. Because of the direct involvement of therapists and other health-care professionals, rehabilitation is an expensive service. Restorative care is initiated after an older person has reached the rehabilitative goal or has not shown any further improvement. The whole health-care team is involved in designing restorative care plans but is not directly involved in the implementation. An older person who is in a rehabilitation program after a stroke would have the benefit of a physical therapist to learn exercise, safe walking, and transferring techniques. The older adult continues to need assistance with exercises and walking, but a nurse or a nursing assistant encourages the person to do as much as possible independently and assists him or her only if necessary.

Rehabilitation provides individuals with intensive short-term strengthening and retraining, whereas restorative care continues the process over time. Older adults often have a major health crisis and go through intensive therapy and training only to move to an environment where everything is done for them, and the benefits of the therapy are lost. Examples of restorative programs are ambulation, personal care, feeding, and toileting. The challenge for the nursing team is to continue to promote high levels of independent function. It is faster to transfer a person into a wheelchair and push the person to the dining room for breakfast, but that is not promoting independence.

This same concept of needing to hurry is associated with high incidences of incontinence. It is often perceived as faster to change an older adult's briefs and bedclothes than to anticipate the need for voiding and walking the person to the bathroom. With rehabilitative and restorative nursing care, "faster" is not the goal.

The same principle applies to eating and personal care. Have you ever watched someone struggle to put a shirt on a paralyzed arm? Watching that struggle is uncomfortable because nurses know they could help that person get the shirt on faster and without as much stress and strain. It is very difficult to watch someone try to eat independently when they have a disability and to see the stress and frustration that can occur. Yet that older person deserves the right to feel the satisfaction of accomplishing a task or meeting a personal goal.

The concepts of rehabilitation and restorative care are crucial to promoting an older adult's optimal level of function. The focus of rehabilitative and restorative care is to maximize the abilities and functions of older adults to ensure the highest level of independence and quality of life. Rehabilitation and restorative care are not isolated treatments with limited application. They embody a broad set of principles to incorporate into every facet of nursing care in all settings.

Within the context of the interdisciplinary team (IDT) effort and after clinical conferences with the team to determine what plan is to be designed, LPNs, working cooperatively with the registered nurse (RN), prepare the goals and the nursing care plan. In this capacity, the LPN's role becomes one of practitioner, educator, counselor, case manager, researcher, and consultant.

● NURSING ROLES

Bedside Caregiver

As caregivers, LPNs provide direct care to older adults until the skills necessary for self-care have been developed by the individual. Nurses need to give older adults positive reinforcement, encouragement, hope, and an opportunity to develop and use their physical and social skills.

Educator

When serving in the role of educator, nurses provide older people and their families with information related to the disability and its treatment and management. Included in the education plan should be health measures to obtain and retain function and to prevent further disability. Effective outcomes are more likely to occur when older adults and their families are included in the process of determining the goals of rehabilitation and restoration of function and treatment. It is important for older adults and the family or other caregivers to recognize that they are responsible for the decisions made and actions that result from those decisions. That is a predominant principle of rehabilitative and restorative care.

Counselor

As counselors, nurses assist elderly people with describing, analyzing, and responding to the current situation that makes rehabilitation or restorative care necessary. Counseling is the process of helping people solve and cope effectively with their problems. Counseling disabled people and their families is an ongoing process that requires supportive behaviors from the entire IDT. LPNs, after establishing trust and rapport with the older adult and the family, need to focus on assisting them in dealing with their grief over the losses imposed by the older person's current disability. The opportunity to express personal feelings assists the elderly person in developing coping skills related to the event of trauma that made rehabilitation and restorative therapy necessary. The LPN should counsel disabled elderly persons and their families to respond to the feelings of loss, frustration, and anger that they generally feel. It is important to express and deal with such feelings as a family.

Advocate

When assuming the role of advocate, LPNs use their influence and power as health-care professionals to bring about necessary changes for the older person and the family's well-being. That advocacy allows the rehabilitation and restorative care to have maximum effect. The LPN's interventions aid the older adult and the family members in obtaining necessary community-based services; the community-based services assist older disabled adults in maintaining their status as fully functioning, independent individuals within the constraints of the limitations imposed by the disability. Such interventions may include the use of assistive or adaptive devices such as crutches, a walker, a plate guard, and a padded spoon.

Case Manager

Generally, an RN is the case manager for disabled persons. In some situations, the LPN is asked to serve in that role. The case manager role places the LPN as a central figure working with the total health-care team throughout the entire episode of illness. The major focus for a case manager is to resolve actual problems and prevent potential problems for the aging person. The treatment plan, once agreed on by the IDT, is under the supervision of the licensed nurses (RNs and LPNs) working in conjunction with each older adult and family. When the plan is agreed on, a contract is entered into by the individual, family members, and nurse. This contract allows the plan to be implemented with clear communication with each person involved. This management may take place in a hospital or nursing home and continue into the community where home-based care is provided.

Researcher

Many LPNs work in conjunction with RNs and a qualified nurse researcher to gather data on the rehabilitation and restorative care of older adults. Many questions remain unanswered regarding rehabilitative and restorative care of older adults in numerous areas. Each area provides a rich arena for research. Some research interests are the following:

- Management of behavioral symptoms
- Feelings about placing disabled family members outside the home and into an institution for care on a permanent basis

---

POINT OF INTEREST

Refer back to the chapter on end-of-life issues (Chapter 10). Review Kübler-Ross's five stages of grief. The older adult and the family will be going through these stages because of the loss that has brought them to the IDT for rehabilitation and restorative care.

- Barriers that prevent the use of respite and day-care services
- Accurate measures of caregiver burden
- Effective coping strategies used by caregivers
- Types of educational and support programs needed to assist caregivers
- Services needed to individualize care at different stages of an illness or injury

All of these clinical questions need to be raised when older individuals experience a traumatic episode and require nursing care. The nurse is responsible for raising questions regarding the specific needs of the older individuals and seeking systematic answers through research. A research approach helps build a body of knowledge regarding rehabilitation and restorative care.

GOALS OF REHABILITATION AND RESTORATIVE CARE

A goal is defined as a written statement of desired behavioral outcomes from which steps or strategies may be designed to achieve that desired end. Goals provide direction. They are the measuring tool for an effective plan of care. For example, "I will buy a car today" is a statement of the desired outcome. A defined series of steps needs to be taken before the accomplishment of that goal. Some of the steps are establishing a means to pay for the car, deciding what type of car to buy, finding out the selling price of cars at various car dealers, checking on insurance, and buying the car.

From the time of injury or disability, the efforts of all health-care professionals involved in care of the older adult are to be focused on the ultimate goal: the highest level of personal independence possible within the limitations imposed by the injury. In setting goals, LPNs assess the older person to determine what assets of mind, body, and spirit are present that would aid in the accomplishment of the goal. For instance, can the person ambulate sufficiently to make trips to the bathroom, dining room, and physical therapy department? The LPN might ask the following questions:

- Is the person able to communicate needs verbally?
- Can the person feed himself or herself?
- What are the goals of the older adult?

The information derived from the assessment is important in determining realistic and achievable goals for each individual. For lifelong quality of living, the components of a successful rehabilitation and restorative program must include the following goals, which should be individualized toward increasing the function and performance of the individual:

- Independence and self-care
- Mobility
- Involvement in activities—social, civic, family, church, and recreation
- Fulfillment of life's goals
- Holistic approach to living with a disability

You must be knowledgeable in evaluating the current holistic status of the older adult. For older adults, major changes in three areas are crucial to the success of a rehabilitation and restorative care program. Changes must be noted in physical, functional, and psychological status. Each of these areas can greatly affect the ability of the older adult to carry out the goals identified in the plan of care.

Physical Changes Affecting Restorative Care

Numerous physical changes may be present when an older adult sustains an injury or trauma necessitating rehabilitation. Existing health problems must be considered in planning rehabilitative and restorative care, as follows:

- Musculoskeletal changes secondary to old fractures, osteoporosis, arthritis, osteoarthritis, muscular dystrophy, or loss of strength in arms and legs can create mobility difficulties. Such situations can occur because of muscle atrophy, decreased bone mass, loss of subcutaneous fat, and decreased flexibility of the joints and limbs.
- Cardiovascular changes secondary to diminished cardiac output, irregular heart rate, and increased blood pressure readings can result in diminished circulation that does not bring sufficient oxygen to the body. Such conditions often cause a lack of activity because of fatigue. Cardiac changes may be the result of thickening of heart valves, thickening of blood vessels, or delayed response to stress.
- Respiratory changes related to diminished respiratory rates can create ventilation challenges for the older person and may be caused by long-standing asthma, obstructive lung disease, emphysema, tuberculosis, upper respiratory illnesses, limited rib cage expansion, atrophy of respiratory muscles,

Holistic functional assessment

Psychological	Physiological	Sociological
Memory	ADLs	Interaction with others
Judgment	IADLs	Family support
Thinking ability	Current health status	Involvement in the community

decreased arterial oxygen tension, decreased vital capacity, and diminished cough.

- Renal and digestive tract changes create elimination difficulties that may impair the proper implementation of a restorative program. These changes may include decreased peristalsis of the intestinal tract that results in constipation or diarrhea, decreased intestinal enzyme levels that reduce the ability to digest foods properly, diminished glomerular filtration in the kidney, and decreased bladder capacity resulting in incontinence or retention of residual urine. The last-mentioned may create edematous lower limbs that make it difficult for the older person to ambulate comfortably.
- Consciousness and mental status changes may result in short-term memory loss, slower thought processing, and decreased pain threshold.
- Perceptual changes may be exhibited by loss of visual acuity, diminished hearing, decreased sense of taste, lower sensitivity to touch, and decreased proprioception (spatial sensitivity or awareness of where things are in the available space).

Functional Changes Affecting Rehabilitative and Restorative Care

Changes in function in older adults may result from the impact of social and environmental situations and can include the following:

- Inability to negotiate stairs in the home
- Functional implications of acute or chronic disease processes
- Physical factors, such as limited range of motion (ROM), strength, and endurance
- Inability to consume sufficient nutrients to maintain optimal health
- Inability to cook food, clean a home, or complete the laundry and other crucial chores

These functional changes need to be assessed by a nurse so that realistic goals can be established.

POINT OF INTEREST

When LPNs are asked to be involved in research, they are asked to gather data for the principal investigator. This is an opportunity you should take. You will learn from the principal investigator, will be able to spend time with older adults while gathering data, and will have pride in the finished research project.

Psychological Changes Affecting Rehabilitative and Restorative Care

The psychological status of an older adult is a crucial component of any rehabilitation and restorative care program. When the older person possesses psychological well-being, there is a strong motivation to work toward the highest possible level of function. When older people feel needed and wanted by family, friends, and associates, they generally possess self-esteem and a positive self-image—two critical factors in developing a high degree of motivation to proceed with the restorative care program.

● DEVELOPING GOALS FOR REHABILITATIVE AND RESTORATIVE CARE

When developing goals for rehabilitative and restorative care, LPNs need to complete a full nursing assessment under the guidance of the RN. The nursing assessment should include a database with the following elements:

- Nursing history that includes the older adult's past medical conditions, psychological impairments, hospitalizations, and previous injuries (see Chapter 15)
- Physical assessment of all bodily systems (see Chapter 15)
- Functional assessment to check for functional ability and mobility (see Chapter 15)
- Mental status and psychological parameters that may be present, such as depression or anxiety (see Chapter 17)
- A spiritual assessment to determine any spiritual needs or deficits that may be a deterrent to good rehabilitation progress

Following the assessment, the LPN and RN work together as a team to analyze the data and prioritize rehabilitative and restorative goals for the older person. The following principles of holistic nursing care should be the guidelines for identifying goals:

- When the older adult enters the hospital or nursing facility, rehabilitation must begin immediately.
- Proper body alignment is to be maintained at all times.
- Pressure ulcers are to be prevented on all body parts.
- Rehabilitation is to be implemented concurrently with the illness, whether chronic or acute, temporary or permanent, or disabling or nondisabling.
- All joints must be kept free through proper exercise and ROM.
- Convalescence is a gradual process and may extend over a considerable period of time for the older person.
- Nurses must understand the person's self-concept and feelings of dependency and isolation, if they exist.
- The time period for rehabilitation depends on the person's psychological acceptance of the condition and his or her physical condition.
- People born with disabilities usually have less difficulty accepting their condition than persons who acquire disabilities later in life.
- More severe emotional reactions are produced when accidents are traumatic.
- Loss and its meaning vary with every person.
- Any personality problems that may be exhibited are generally the result of the person's personality characteristics before disability.
- The usual initial reactions to physical injury are shock, fear, disbelief, and anxiety.
- Periods of grief occur when loss of any physical ability is experienced.
- Depression, anger, and denial may be present.
- Values are examined and limitations are put in perspective over time.
- Time is essential for acceptance.
- The family needs emotional support and comfort during the acute phase of the trauma or illness.
- All information should be given to the family and older adult, including information about resources for rehabilitation services and economic assistance.
- The nurse or social worker should be familiar with community agencies that can help.

● IMPLEMENTATION OF GOALS IN REHABILITATIVE AND RESTORATIVE CARE

Goal 1: Maintenance of Joint Function

The implementation of planned care for older people requires that a holistic approach be adopted. The major concern in implementing care is the prevention of deformities through passive exercises that keep joints movable, promote venous return and lymphatic flow, and help prevent excessive demineralization of bones. This goal and care depend on the physician's orders that identify the extent of the exercise program to be implemented. By means of a thorough assessment of the physical condition of the older adult and the specific illness and prognosis for recovery, nurses assume responsibility for the passive exercise program. Such a program may include ROM activities in which each joint is put through the normal activities of which it is capable—supine, prone, lateral, medial, anterior, and posterior positions. This approach maintains the wellness capability of the joints and reduces the complications of contractures, strictures, and limitation of activity. By implementing passive ROM, nurses assist the injured person to resume independence of function and perform at optimal levels.

Goal 2: Active Exercise

Active exercise is designed to improve function and performance. It entails transferring from bed to chair, ambulating with assistive devices, using crutches properly, knowing how to maneuver the wheelchair, using hand-eye coordination, and using assistive devices that promote independent living in a normal manner. In each of these activities, nurses, in the role of teachers, help motivate the person to be as active in personal care as possible. Always follow the physician's orders for active exercise. A physical therapist is an excellent resource for these activities as well.

Goal 3: Bladder Continence

In some situations, it is necessary for the LPN to initiate bladder-training programs. Achievement of continence avoids the use of indwelling catheters. Bladder training aids in reducing the chance for urinary tract infections and increases self-esteem. Retraining is based on the development of clear patterns of communication between staff, the older adult, and the family regarding the schedule for toileting (usually every 2 hours). It is necessary for the bladder to be emptied at set times throughout the day. Limiting fluids after 6:00 p.m. so that the bladder can retain urine throughout the night is another strategy. Periodic catheterization may be employed sometimes to develop reflex emptying when the sensation for voiding is diminished or absent.

Goal 4: Bowel Continence

In addition to bladder training, it is important to employ bowel-training techniques if they are needed. Bowel training requires the establishment

---

CRITICALLY EXAMINE THE FOLLOWING

You are working with the RN to do a holistic assessment on an 80-year-old victim of a motor vehicle accident. Sister Agnes, a Catholic nun, was walking to prayers when she was hit by a speeding car. She has multiple fractures that will keep her in bed for days. She is in pain, and the RN is working to resolve her discomfort. The RN asked you to do a spiritual assessment on Sister Agnes. How will you proceed?

Spirituality discussions make some people uncomfortable. If that is true for you, please work on your skills in this area to overcome such feelings. When considering this discussion with Sister Agnes, you already know two significant things about her that will influence your interview. First, because she is a nun, you can feel reassured that she is a spiritual person and will welcome the discussion. The second thing you know is counterproductive to the first. She is in pain and will not feel like having a lengthy discussion. What two questions could you ask her that would give you the basic information you need without causing her undue distress because of the pain?

I do not generally give the answers in this section, but I will share my thoughts with you in this situation. You may have different answers that are just as effective as mine. My responses are not the only ones that could be used. Thoughtfully write your questions and come to class prepared to share them.

1. Do you believe in a higher power or God? Note: For a Muslim, the higher power would be Allah; for an agnostic, it would simply be a higher power. For Sister Agnes, her response probably would be that she believes in God.
2. What can I do for you or with you, while you are here, to assist you in meeting your spiritual needs? Note: Some people may want you to pray with them, others may want religious artifacts in the room, and others may want a visit from their spiritual leader. Other people will want nothing.

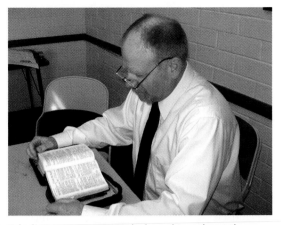

A holistic assessment includes asking about the older adult's spirituality. Religion has a significant role in the lives of most older people. You need to know about their spiritual needs and strive to meet them. This man takes great comfort in reading his scriptures. To do so, the scriptures need to be easily accessible, there should be good lighting, and he needs his glasses.

of a routine for emptying the bowel daily. This occurs most normally in the morning approximately 20 minutes after breakfast. The intake of breakfast stimulates the duodenocolic reflex, which assists in bowel elimination. A diet consisting of whole-grain breads, cereals, fresh fruits, whole bran, and increased fluid intake is helpful in providing the bulk and fluid needed for effective bowel training. This approach also reduces

the complication of constipation in the older adult. If constipation does occur, it may be necessary to provide medication to soften the stool and allow the bowel contents to move into the lower colon area for elimination. It also is helpful in bowel-training programs to request that the older adult use the toilet instead of the bedpan to facilitate bowel elimination. This is not always possible. Rectal suppositories are useful when initiating a bowel-training program. Enemas are rarely used as part of a bowel-training program.

Goal 5: Appropriate Sexual Expression

When implementing a holistic plan of care, the LPN must be aware of the older adult's sexual needs. This means building in time during the rehabilitation and restorative care process for partners to have privacy. It also can include offering the sense of touch by holding hands with the elderly adult in appropriate ways and, when given permission, for squeezing the shoulder or forearm with a firm but gentle touch.

Goal 6: Psychosocial and Spiritual Well-Being

It is crucial to include interventions that address the psychosocial and spiritual needs of older adults. Communicating, increasing self-concept and self-esteem, treating the person with dignity and respect, and meeting spiritual needs are essential to holistic nursing care. Examples could include uninterrupted time to pray, arrangements for visits from the local clergy, and allowing religious artifacts in the room.

In implementing rehabilitation and restorative care, nurses follow the plan of care outlined by the IDT. Such information comes from the database (MDS) of information collected during the admission assessment and periodically throughout the course of the care. The nurse must be alert to changes that need to be made in the plan of care as the older person improves, stays the same, or declines in physical abilities.

Final Thought About Implementing Goals

The implementation of care measures should focus on the older adult's previous coping skills. It is important that older adults become partners in the care regimen by sharing knowledge and adaptability. The goals are established by the

CRITICALLY EXAMINE THE FOLLOWING

You work in a long-term care rehabilitation facility. Recently, the adult children of a patient have come to the nurse manager to make a complaint. Every time one of the children comes to visit their mother, she is holding hands and talking in a quiet and intimate manner with a male resident. The children want the time together stopped. The nurse manager has asked you to look into the situation. What are you going to do?

Is there additional information you need to gather? If so, what is it? How important is sexual expression for older adults? Is it being expressed appropriately in this situation? Please carefully ponder your response and be prepared to share your thinking in class.

older person, the family, and the nurse as a member of the IDT based on the assessment data. When the goal is stated in specific, measurable terms, evaluation of the progress and outcome of care are easily measured. The terms of the goal are to be put in the framework of self-care and self-responsibility.

● ASSESSMENT OF GOALS

Goals are assessed at intervals—sometimes daily, sometimes weekly, sometimes monthly—depending on the goal to be accomplished. When the goals have been stated in observable, measurable terms, the assessment of their achievement is relatively easy. In the course of the disease or traumatic injury, in-depth documentation is extremely important for noting the progress of the person. A systematic approach to fulfill all the stated goals assures the patient, family, and health-care team that a holistic approach has been incorporated into the older adult's care. This approach reassures the older adult and the nurse that custodial care will be avoided and that rehabilitation and restorative nursing from a holistic perspective is in place.

Goals Specific to Elderly Adults

Restorative nursing goals specific to older adults include the following:

- Improvement of function
- Delay of deterioration
- Accommodation to dysfunction
- Comfort in the dying process

Improvement of Function

Functionality is defined as the ability to continue to live one's preferred lifestyle without disruption. In other words, each older adult can live independently, do activities of daily living (ADLs) and instrumental ADLs (IADLs), be mobile, and have self-care ability. To live independently suggests that there is no need for physical assistance or supervision from another person. Goal assessment on a daily or weekly basis is essential to good care.

To improve function, it is necessary to take into account the impact of the older person's social and environmental situation, the functional implications of acute or chronic disease processes, and the physical factors that may influence function. By combining these factors, a picture of the capability of older adults to live and function should emerge for the health-care team.

ROM exercises are exercises performed on a regular basis to preserve the function of the joints and muscles. It is crucial that this maintenance function be performed correctly and on a schedule so that no deterioration of the physical status of the person occurs. The nurse, under the direction of the physical therapist, does this activity or instructs another health-care team member to carry out the activity correctly.

Improving the strength of the muscles necessitates that some resistance be exerted so that the muscle works hard to maintain or improve its function. Resistance is often accomplished through the use of weights or by pushing against an object to provide resistance. The actual testing of the muscle strength and endurance is done by the physical therapist, and a plan of exercise is identified. This plan must be carried out meticulously so that every muscle and its function are duly exercised, and strength and endurance are improved.

Mobility is identified in various stages, depending on the type of injury or disease present in the older adult. The progression is usually from bed mobility, through transfer activities, to wheelchair or ambulatory locomotion. Transfer includes getting from bed to a chair and back to bed, on and off a toilet, and in and out of a bathtub or car. These activities involve standing, sitting, pivoting, turning, or side-slide movement (sliding from bed to chair using a transfer board). To promote function in mobility involves locomotion or moving from one point to another. Older adults may need to use a wheelchair, so the ability to propel and maneuver the wheelchair is important. Wheelchair use involves the development of arm strength with the use of weights or other forms of strength building. Other assistive devices such as crutches, braces, and splints may be needed to assist in locomotion. To help the individual reach optimal function, instruction needs to be given in the best approaches to maintaining balance and endurance and in the use of devices to prevent falls.

When the goal is to improve function, there is a positive outcome orientation. For example, if the nursing diagnosis is stated:

- Body Image Disturbance: functional—self-esteem disturbance related to function limitations, role and lifestyle change.

Then the goal should be written:

- The older adult will verbalize positive statements about self.
- The older adult will identify and demonstrate appropriate strategies to deal with functional limitations.

Some of these strategies could be the ability to manipulate buttons and zippers, to tie shoelaces, and to put on underwear. If the older adult is unable to perform these functions, devices such as long-handled reachers, button hooks, and elastic shoelaces may allow the person to perform more independently.

In helping older people retain functional ability and avoid deterioration, it is important to be aware of the disease processes that may interfere with their ability to achieve independent living. Such limiting problems most often involve cardiorespiratory, neurological, or musculoskeletal systems. Many of these conditions may impose significant functional limitations on the person. All of these factors must be kept in mind when implementing goals for rehabilitative and restorative care for the elderly person. Dedication to the restorative care plan helps older people keep motivated and engage in the purposeful and varied activities that promote function and performance.

Delay of Deterioration

A primary goal of rehabilitative and restorative nursing is the delay of deterioration in all functional aspects. If bouts of depression are noted on admission and during the course of treatment, the RN should be notified and a psychiatric consultation requested if it is determined to be appropriate for the individual. Depression signals initial deterioration of motivation. Helping the person maintain a spirit of hopefulness is one way to assist in the delay of deterioration.

Another approach to ensure delay of deterioration is to ensure that the nursing care plan calls for exercise of all mobile bodily parts—legs, arms, fingers, toes, neck, hips, and knees. Movement of all of these joints is essential in the maintenance of a healthy state. No nurse should ever allow a contracture to occur. Use of pillows, a footboard to prevent footdrop, and resting splints for wrists and fingers aids in proper alignment of the body to maintain function and delay deterioration. Properly aligned and supported body parts assume their natural posture and position. Passive ROM exercises for all joints can delay deterioration to a great extent. Caution

must be exercised, however. If care is not used in moving the joints, soft tissue injury can result from undue stretching of the muscles and joints; this could cause additional injury and slow the rate of recovery, or it could cause great pain when the person becomes active again.

Another priority concern is the prevention of pressure ulcers. Excellent skin care should be a daily part of nursing care for all persons. This is especially important for elderly people who have impaired nutritional status. Pressure ulcers may develop over any bony prominence and on the occiput, ear parts, sacrum, and greater trochanter. Special devices to cushion these parts need to be used as a preventive measure, such as special pillows, donuts, gauze dressings, and special mattresses (circulating water or air). Turning the person every 2 hours is the best preventive measure to ensure skin integrity. When turning the person, the support of limbs and back for good body alignment is essential to keep weakened muscles from further deterioration.

Cognitively impaired elderly persons are in need of individualized nursing care. These people need appropriate sensory stimulation to maintain their contact with the world. Putting the person in a position where others can be seen and the careful use of the radio and TV can help stimulate cognitive functions and lessen the possibility of further deterioration.

To delay deterioration, older adults should participate in out-of-bed activities as soon as they have achieved a medically stable condition. First, they should dangle their feet for several minutes to gain a sense of balance. When this activity is tolerated, the nurse should help the older adult to stand by the side of the bed with whatever assistive device is needed (e.g., a walker or cane). Finally, the person should be assisted to walk to a chair and sit with proper support for approximately 15 minutes at a time. You, as an LPN, are essential for providing the appropriate encouragement to the individual.

Accommodation to Dysfunction

The goal of helping elderly people accommodate to dysfunction requires a great deal of motivation on the part of the nurse. It is essential for the LPN to listen attentively and actively to the personal fears, hopes, thoughts, feelings, and values that are expressed by the person who is adjusting to the deficits left by an accident, injury, or stroke. Nurses should be aware that a rehabilitation program is primarily a learning and training process. Each person

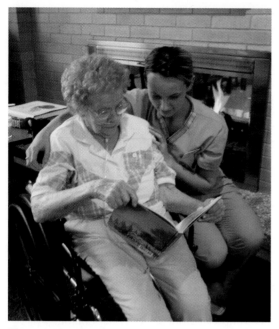

This woman was admitted to the nursing home in a weakened condition. Her family did not assist her out of bed because "she was too weak." After admission, it was determined that she did not have any acute conditions, but instead was deconditioned because of her prolonged time in bed. The first goal was to prevent her from deteriorating any further. As you can see, she now can be up in a wheelchair for short periods. This is the result of excellent nursing care.

must have the ability to absorb new information on how to use personal potential and how to practice new skills. If a person has sustained an injury that created a footdrop gait, the individual must learn to accommodate walking by lifting the foot intentionally so that it remains flat as weight is shifted from one side of the body to the next. This action requires major concentration until the old adage "practice makes perfect" becomes second nature to the walker. The nurse's role is to encourage the person to keep working for the highest outcome possible.

Holistic wellness occurs for the older adult receiving restorative care when:

- The psychological self-image of the person incorporates personal limitations into a healthy and acceptable image.
- Social activities and interactions with friends and family continue to be a major part of the person's life.
- The person exhibits gerotranscendence by accepting the new lifestyle with joy, peace,

and gratitude for the remaining strengths of his or her personhood.

These are the elements to be found when the goal of accommodation to dysfunction is achieved. As the grief and sense of loss diminish, older people adopt a healthier view so that life, once again, is worth living for them.

Comfort in the Dying Process

In older people experiencing trauma, 75% of deaths are caused by falls, thermal injury, and motor vehicle accidents. Falls are the leading cause of death in elderly men and women. Falls constitute approximately 50% of all fatalities. The most common injuries are associated with fractures of the hip, femur, and proximal humerus; Colles' fracture of the wrist; and head injuries. Death from thermal injury accounts for approximately 8% of all accidental deaths in people 65 years old and older. These injuries include burns and inhalation injuries, electrical injury, and contacts with sources of heat. The most commonly reported types of thermal injuries include scalds, flame burns, and contact with hot objects. In people 65 years old and older, 25% of deaths are due to motor vehicle accidents. As the population continues to age, this percentage of deaths and injuries will undoubtedly increase.

Restorative nursing may include providing comfort measures and palliative care to elderly people in the process of dying because of severe injury and trauma. Palliative care means providing the care requested by the older person in terms of advance directives and a living will. The individual's decisions must be honored by the nurse and family members. The older adult may have requested that no food or water be given after it has been determined that no benefits would be derived from such comfort measures. Life-sustaining technologies such as intravenous solutions or use of a respirator also may be terminated if no positive outcome is predicted. All of these wishes are to be followed using the Code of Ethics for Nurses.

Nurses are to be supportive of dying elderly persons and their family members. You must be accountable to the dying person for decisions that have been made and facilitate their implementation. All decisions are to be carried out in a humane and compassionate manner. Nurses need to approach death with reverence for the body, mind, and spirit of the older person who approaches the end of life. The nurse should attend to the dying person with dignity, respect, and appreciation for personal uniqueness. Chapter 10 contains more information on end-of-life issues.

CLINICAL IMPLICATIONS OF REHABILITATIVE AND RESTORATIVE CARE

Using the framework of the restorative care principles and guidelines that were cited earlier in this chapter, four clinical rehabilitative programs for older adults are outlined:

- Walking programs
- Bladder and bowel continence training
- Feeding and self-feeding programs
- Self-care—ADL programs

Walking Programs

Mobility is crucial to optimal functioning for older people. To be mobile means that the individual enjoys the satisfaction of independence in living. Nurses play a key role in providing motivation for a walking program. Depending on the type of assistive device needed by the older adult to aid in gait control, the nurse follows the directions given by the RN, physician, or physical therapist. Excellent foot care is critical to maintaining a walking program. Also, properly fitting shoes are important to establish proper posture while walking.

The older adult may need braces or crutches to walk. Leg and back braces are devices that are used to support body weight, limit involuntary movements, or prevent and correct deformities. Crutches are devices that may be necessary to help the person learn to walk again in a normal manner. Crutches may be used on a temporary or permanent basis, depending on the type of injury sustained during the trauma.

For successful crutch walking, it is important to strengthen the muscle groups used in this activity. This strengthening should begin as soon as the physician believes that the older adult has recovered sufficiently to consider walking. Strengthening exercises should be provided while the person is still confined to bed. These exercises include the muscles of the arms, shoulders, chest, and back. Before ambulation, the older adult should be taught how to move from the bed to the chair and should be capable of performing this movement without assistance. Older people who need assistance to learn to stand, balance themselves, and ambulate again sometimes experience difficulty. Patience on the part of the nurse is an important quality.

Important points in crutch walking include correct measurements for crutches so that they have a proper fit. Crutches need to have heavy rubber tips to prevent the crutch from sliding. The crutches need to be moved in a rhythmic way that propels the person forward. Finally, crutches should have padding on the underarm piece so that weight is not placed on the radial nerve. The handhold on the crutches may have padding to reduce irritation there as well. The nurse should emphasize good posture for a person who is crutch walking: The head should be held high, and the pelvis should be kept over the feet for excellent balance. Crutch walking is best taught in several short lessons to reduce fatigue in the older adult. When ambulation begins, it is important to have an attendant in front and in back of the person to provide stability and to reduce anxiety about possible falls.

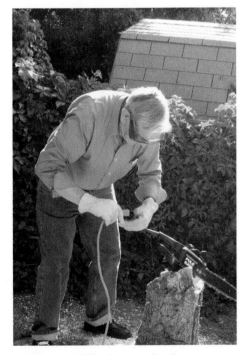

As people grow older, they need to keep moving. This 85-year-old man has spent most of his life working outdoors. He will never go to a gym because "they are for sissies!" He keeps busy with outdoor projects. They keep him moving, provide him with satisfaction, and a purpose in life.

Several types of gaits may be used in crutch walking, depending on the type of injury and the physician's orders, as follows:

- *Four-point gait*: The person bears weight on both feet and has four-point contact with the floor (both crutches and both feet).
- *Two-point gait*: There are two points of contact with the floor (crutches only).
- *Swing-to gait*: Crutches are placed ahead of the person, and, with weight on the crutches, the body swings through to the crutches.
- *Three-point gait*: Partial weight-bearing is permitted.

As the older adult practices the walking program outlined earlier, the person should master sufficient ADLs to be independent. This independence includes being able to get up and down steps and in and out of cars. It is important for nurses to be very familiar with all assistive devices used in walking programs.

Walking programs also are initiated for elderly adults without assistive devices. Walking for the older adult is an excellent physical fitness activity. It provides cardiovascular fitness and aerobic exercise. Walking for 20 to 30 minutes, three times a week, has been supported by research as a way to maintain good physical fitness and conditioning. Walking should be a lifelong program to promote wellness and joy in living.

Continence Training

A second major clinical challenge is maintenance of bladder and bowel continence in a traumatized, disabled older adult. An older adult who is the recipient of good nursing care should not experience urinary or bowel incontinence. The use of an indwelling catheter is ineffective bladder management. Urinary infection can result within 24 hours of catheter insertion. Catheter insertion also lowers the self-esteem and self-concept of the person trying to regain control of a traumatized life.

Bladder retraining is generally successful when a regular time schedule is established for emptying the bladder. Retraining of the bladder takes patience on the part of the older adult and the nurse. A similar program for bowel training should be initiated soon after admission. As noted earlier, increasing the patient's fiber and fluid intake and a regular toileting regimen promotes bowel elimination on a regular schedule. If constipation does occur, stool softeners are the treatment of choice to resolve this problem.

The use of enemas is not part of a retraining program. Enemas should be used only in an emergency.

Feeding and Self-Feeding Programs

The clinical challenge of maintaining nutrition adequate for tissue repair and health demands a high level of skill on the part of the LPN. In the early stages of rehabilitative and restorative nursing, the older adult may need to be fed through a nasogastric tube. A specially formulated feeding prepared to caloric specifications is administered through the tube on a regular basis. The tube should be patent, and sufficient fluid should be used to keep it clear and unclogged. After each feeding, the tube should be flushed according to the protocols in the facility.

As the older adult progresses in recovery, he or she may need to be placed on a feeding program in which manual assistance by the LPN or nursing assistant is needed until the person has sufficient strength for self-feeding. Older adults should be fed at regular mealtimes, and snacks should be provided. Promoting the older person to a self-feeding program is a definite sign of progress. Encouragement should be given by the nurse so that the older adult consumes sufficient calories to have adequate nutrition to meet the energy demands of rehabilitation.

Self-Promoting Behaviors and Activities of Daily Living

Independence in personal care is a challenge for older adults with disabilities that affect their ROM, mobility, strength, coordination, and dexterity. It is important that members of the nursing care team allow older adults to have time to perform aspects of their own care independently. Occupational therapists can provide assistive equipment that makes self-care easier. Built-up handles for toothbrushes and hairbrushes are easier for older adults to hold. A chair in the tub or shower may allow a weak individual to be able to bathe independently. Lowered sinks, counters, and mirrors might allow a wheelchair-bound person to sit up to the sink to wash and perform other personal care. Specially designed plastic devices with long handles to insert inside a person's socks and long-handled shoehorns allow older people who are unable to bend over to put on their own socks and shoes. Clothing with Velcro fasteners is easier to fasten and unfasten when dressing. Adjustments in the care environment and education of all of the personal care staff are essential to the success of self-care–ADL programs.

CONCLUSION

This chapter provides an overview of the principles that govern rehabilitation and restorative nursing practices for LPNs who care for older adults in various settings. Through appreciation of the uniqueness of older adults and their special needs, rehabilitative and restorative nursing care can help them achieve optimal functioning to live life to the fullest.

At age 60, Mr. A. suffered a severe, incapacitating stroke on the left side of his body. Mr. A. and his wife had planned to retire in 5 years and travel. The stroke created major difficulties regarding the couple's anticipated retirement.

While hospitalized, Mr. A. developed a footdrop condition that interfered with his rehabilitative program. He became despondent over his condition and refused to participate in the walking program.

Discussion

As the LPN responsible for Mr. A.'s care, you need to do an assessment of his holistic needs. What are the priorities of care?

Solution

1. Mr. A. needs assurance from the health professionals, nurses, and therapists that he will gain sufficient strength to walk with the aid of a walker and eventually to walk independently.
2. The LPN and Mr. A. contract to carry out the walking and exercise program on a daily basis to correct the footdrop problem.
3. By setting goals, Mr. A. perceives his condition in a more positive light and is encouraged by his progress.
4. The LPN also is concerned about Mr. A's despondency. She documents Mr. A.'s behavior and informs the RN about his psychological state. Together, the nurses talk with Mr. A. about his depression and seek his approval to obtain a psychiatric consultation. This problem is then referred to a mental health professional.
5. The LPN arranges for Mr. A. and his wife to become participants in a clinical conference in which the rehabilitative team reviews Mr. A.'s case and allows him to make informed decisions on how to proceed on discharge.

This may include referral to various social agencies that could assist him in obtaining medical equipment for home use, receiving nursing care in the home if his wife feels unable to take care of Mr. A., and seeking Social Security and pension payments if Mr. A. believes he can no longer work.
6. Mr. A. is encouraged to eat nutritious meals so that his tissue can make repairs. He needs sufficient energy from his nutritional intake to do his exercises and walking program properly.
7. Activities are scheduled for him so that he can regain his social skills and interact with people without embarrassment and hesitation. Mr. A. was discharged from the hospital within 2 weeks of the incident, feeling that he was in charge of his life and that life was worth living. He also could see that the goals he and his wife had established for retirement could be accomplished. Mr. A. learned to live with his disability, and because of good nursing care, the quality of his life was not diminished.

Select the best answer to each question.

1. The aim of rehabilitation for older adults is to:

   a. Engage in limited ADLs

   b. Deny function and performance that existed before the incident

   c. Keep food and fluids at a level so that energy and strength are minimized

   d. Restore an individual to his or her former or best possible function and environmental status

2. Which of the following directives most closely coincides with the desired goals of a successful rehabilitation program?

   a. Keep physical changes at a minimum and promote self-esteem.

   b. Promote independence and self-care, along with mobility and a holistic approach to living with the disability.

   c. Promote involvement in limited activities and ROM exercises.

   d. Promote the fulfillment of the patient's life goals despite mobility problems.

3. Principles of rehabilitation include the most important step in nursing care, which is:

   a. Doing passive ROM

   b. Understanding the patient's self-concept and encouraging feelings of dependency

   c. Beginning rehabilitation immediately on the patient's admission

   d. Giving selective information to the family

4. Rehabilitation goals specific to older adults include:

   a. ROM exercises, transfer skills from bed to chair, dependency on enema usage

   b. Improvement of function, delay of deterioration, development of codependent behavior

   c. Accommodation to dysfunction, comfort in the dying process, accommodation to an indwelling catheter

   d. Delay of deterioration, improvement of function, accommodation to dysfunction, comfort in the dying process

5. In continence training for bladder control, the nurse should:

   a. Increase fluids, especially during the evening hours, and toilet the patient every 4 hours

   b. Restrict fluids during the nighttime hours and toilet the patient at his or her request

   c. Increase fluids during the daytime hours and toilet the patient every 1000 mL

   d. Increase fluids during the daytime hours and toilet the patient every 2 hours

20 Pharmacology and Its Significance for Older Adults

Mary Ann Anderson

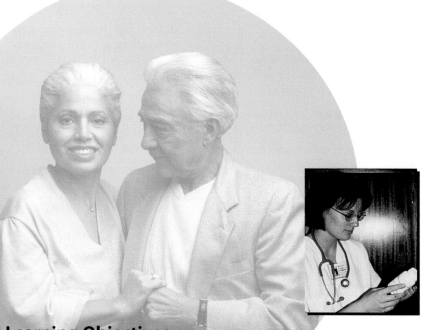

Learning Objectives

After completing this chapter, the student will be able to:

1. Identify physiological changes of aging that affect pharmacotherapeutics in older adults.
2. Identify sensory changes of aging that affect pharmacotherapeutics in older adults.
3. Identify psychological changes of aging that affect pharmacotherapeutics in older adults.
4. Identify polypharmacy problems in older adults and nursing interventions to compensate for them.
5. List four ways a licensed nurse can support the physician in implementing Beer's criteria.
6. Define the purpose of understanding chronopharmacology.
7. Develop a nursing care plan to synthesize interventions to assist older persons in maintaining proper pharmacotherapeutics.

INTRODUCTION

One of the biggest advances in medical care has been the discovery and rediscovery of plants and chemical compounds that formulate drugs. Drugs are prescribed to manage and sometimes cure physical and mental illnesses. Ancient civilizations used various herbs and other plant and mineral substances to prevent and treat physical and mental problems. Many modern drugs used in Western medical practice have a long history of effectiveness in healing. Some medicines that are prescribed today were originally discovered and used by medical practitioners and healers from other cultures. Quality medical care and medications are responsible for increasing the life expectancy of large populations of people. A dilemma of Western medicine is the heavy dependence on the use of medications for managing and treating diseases. Many people do not consider a medical treatment complete unless they receive a prescription for a drug. This can be a serious issue for older adults. This chapter examines issues related to drug use and older adults. Following are some basic terms related to drug use:

- *Pharmacology*—The study of medications.
- *Pharmacotherapeutics*—The use of medications to treat diseases. The benefit of a medication (desired effect) is weighed against the unwanted and dangerous effects (side effects) to measure the appropriate use of any medication.
- *Pharmacodynamics*—The effect of specific medications at the site of action. Pharmacokinetics, half-life, protein binding, disease processes, and aging affect pharmacodynamics.
- *Pharmacokinetics*—The study of how a medication moves into and through the body and how it is excreted from the body. The processes of absorption, distribution, metabolism, and excretion are affected by aging and diseases and influence the pharmacodynamics of any drug.
- *Half-life*—The time required for half the medication to be excreted or inactivated by the body.
- *Protein binding*—Binding properties of proteins. Proteins in the bloodstream are binding sites for many drugs. The portion of a drug that is bound to a protein is inactive (only a free drug is available to have a desired effect). Two drugs that are both highly protein-bound compete for protein binding sites. This competition significantly increases the level of free drug in the bloodstream (drug molecules that were bound to the protein and have been released). The significant increase has an impact on the effects and adverse effects of the drug.
- *Adverse drug reactions (ADRs)*—Unwanted effects or side effects of a medication. ADRs are related to changes in pharmacokinetics, dosage amounts, timing of doses, and interactions of medications with other medications or foods.

AGING CHANGES THAT AFFECT PHARMACOTHERAPEUTICS

Changes in Vision

Changes in vision can have a serious impact on the safe use of medications by older adults. As individuals age, they experience increased difficulty distinguishing colors, especially blue and green, because of the hardening and yellowing of the lens in their eyes. This yellowing often makes it difficult for older adults to differentiate shades of blue, purple, brown, and green, yet older people can see bright yellow, red, and black more clearly. Many older adults have difficulty distinguishing individual pills by color. When older adults are instructed to take the "pink pill in the morning and the blue one at night," they may make errors.

Reading small print is also a challenge for many older adults. Older people often have trouble reading the label on drug bottles because of the small print. Attaching a large-print tag to a bottle and having a magnifying glass by drug bottles can help an older person read the medication bottle label and avoid medication errors. Using a medication box or mediplanner is a good idea for many older individuals. Medication boxes are filled with the person's ordered medication. The box has a separate compartment for each time during the day that the older person has to take a medication. The box is usually filled for 1 week at a time, and the days of the week and times of medication doses are clearly marked in large, bold, raised initials and symbols. Family members and friends can be taught to assist the older person in preparing the medication box for a week at a time.

Sensitivity to glare is another visual challenge for aging eyes. Shiny surfaces such as plastic tape over medication labels can be difficult for older people to read. Portions of instructions written on paper that has been laminated may be missed or difficult to read because of reflecting glare. Labels for drug bottles should be printed on paper that is not shiny. Medication instructions should be in bold, large print on white or yellow paper to ensure they can be read.

Decreased Hearing Acuity

Hearing changes, such as presbycusis, increase the possibility that an older person may be unable to hear and understand instructions. Often, out of habit, older adults may nod their heads or state that they understand instructions even if they did not hear them all. Asking an older adult to repeat or demonstrate instructions is an excellent way to ensure that the instructions have been heard. Using large print instructions and following them when giving verbal instructions also helps older people. Many people with hearing difficulties develop lip-reading skills. Ensure that the older adult can see your mouth while you are giving instructions. Wearing lipstick if you are a woman and speaking slowly and intentionally, rather than louder, enhances an older person's ability to read lips. Throughout the time that you, the nurse, are giving verbal instructions, stop and ask older patients if they have any questions. Clarify information and have the older patient restate and demonstrate the teaching that is occurring.

Decreased Taste Acuity

With age, older adults experience changes in taste. It is most obvious in foods. A common complaint is that food is bland or has no taste. Changes in recognizing tastes and flavors result from changes in the taste buds and often in the sense of smell. The ability to differentiate medications by taste is inhibited, and the potential for unknowingly taking nonmedications or caustic poisons increases. Encourage older adults to throw away old prescription bottles and not to use them for storing household cleaning products and other poisons that may be mistaken for medications.

Changes in Touch and Dexterity

Older adults experience decreased touch sensitivity as they age. This decreased sensitivity can be worsened with decreased circulation and peripheral nerve deterioration in the hands and feet. Arthritic joint changes can combine with decreased touch to minimize strength, which can make it difficult to open modern packages. Childproof lids that require a person to push down and turn at the same time are very difficult for older people to open. Individual drug doses in plastic bubbles that require the plastic to be torn or the backing to be ripped off also are difficult to open. Pharmacists use alternative packaging for older adults if the older

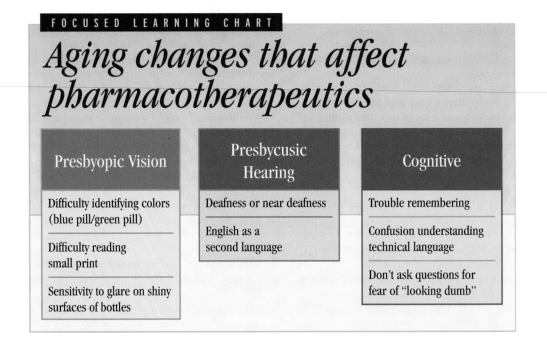

FOCUSED LEARNING CHART

Aging changes that affect pharmacotherapeutics

Presbyopic Vision	Presbycusic Hearing	Cognitive
Difficulty identifying colors (blue pill/green pill)	Deafness or near deafness	Trouble remembering
Difficulty reading small print	English as a second language	Confusion understanding technical language
Sensitivity to glare on shiny surfaces of bottles		Don't ask questions for fear of "looking dumb"

person requests it. Flip-top lids can replace the hard-to-twist childproof lids. Bubble-packed medications can be cut out of the packaging and placed in a pill bottle or a pill box.

Cognitive Changes

With increasing age and subsequent risk for disease, older adults may have changes in their thought patterns. It is important for the nurse to question what has caused the thought pattern changes. Are the causes pathological or drug-induced? Sometimes older adults have trouble remembering if they have taken their medications. Multiple drugs with varying dosages administered at different hours often create confusion.

The technical language that health-care professionals frequently use can be difficult for older people to understand, and they often are unwilling to ask questions. Many older adults do not want to seem uninformed and state that they trust the physician or nurse to do what is right.

Compliance Factors

Often individuals do not follow their drug regimen correctly. This can be intentional or the result of poor understanding. If older adults do not understand how a drug works or do not like the effect of a drug, they may make mistakes in administering their medications. Common problems are taking doses at the wrong time and altering the dosage amounts.

Forgetting to take medications is a routine compliance issue. When giving older people medication instructions, ask them to describe a typical day. Instructing older adults to take a medication everyday before breakfast rather than instructing them to take the drug at 8:00 a.m. may encourage compliance, especially if they sleep until noon or are up at 5:00 a.m. Studies have shown that more medication doses are forgotten when a drug is dosed frequently during the day rather than once a day. Simplified dosing schedules that consider the older person's daily routine and the use of medications that are dosed only once a day can help the person be compliant in taking medications.

Drugs are taken for the chemical effect that they have on the body. Unwanted effects or side effects are common for many medications. Individuals often choose to alter the dosages or quit taking an ordered medication because of the side effects. One of the most common side effects that older adults complain of is upset stomach; this often is caused by the medication dissolving in the stomach and irritating the stomach lining. Stomach irritation can be lessened if the older adult takes the medication with food, so instruct the older adult to do so as long as the medication does not need to be taken on an empty stomach. If the medication needs to be taken on an empty stomach, encourage the person to drink at least 8 oz (1 cup) of water with the medication. Drinking water washes the medication through the stomach faster and, it is hoped, lessens stomach irritation. Encourage people to talk about the uncomfortable side effects of their medications. Often by simply changing the timing of a medication dosage (from morning to bedtime dosing), unwanted or bothersome side effects may decrease significantly.

People commonly simply stop taking a medication. News in the media and advice from neighbors or friends may make older people uncomfortable with specific drugs or fearful of the drug's long-term effects on their bodies. Encourage older patients to discuss these concerns. Patients who are not accurately following

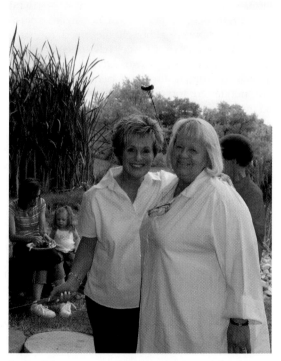

Both of these women take medications daily. Because they are compliant and follow their drug regimen correctly, they are able to attend, for example, this cookout. They also spend time with their families and give a great deal of service to their community. They both agree that their health is improved because of the medications they take.

prescribed drug regimens are reluctant to tell their physician. Not following orders could be interpreted as questioning the physician's skill and knowledge, and most older people do not want to be disrespectful. Many older adults manipulate drug routines to fit their beliefs about personal medication needs. Encourage an open dialogue about medications. Allow the expression of concerns or questions. Review magazines and newspapers that older people read to keep informed regarding potential questions and concerns they may have regarding their medications.

Polypharmacy and Chronic Health Changes

A good rule to follow for pharmacotherapeutics in older people is "the smallest number of drugs should be prescribed at the lowest possible dose." Two-thirds of physician office visits by older adults result in the prescription of one or more new drugs. Of these prescriptions, 50% do not have the desired therapeutic action for various reasons that range from too high or too low a dosage to not getting the prescription filled. Studies have shown that many physicians who prescribe for older people do not make adjustments in dosages, although the need for such adjustments related to age have been clearly established. Many physicians are not educated on dosage adjustment for older people. Most drugs are not tested for their effects on people age 65 and older. Studies on drug dosing, effects, and side effects are done most commonly with healthy middle-aged adults. The results of such studies are applied mistakenly to drug use for older adults. Such practices can lead to unanticipated drug effects and misdiagnosed drug side effects.

Older adults often have multiple chronic diseases. People with chronic health problems frequently have several drugs prescribed for each problem. The result for older patients often is complex and is called multiple drug medication regimen. This complexity is compounded when the older individual has multiple physicians prescribing medications. Pharmacists are skilled at identifying potential drug interactions, but their effectiveness depends on awareness of the total medication regimen. If an older person uses more than one pharmacy, a pharmacist cannot be aware of other drugs that the individual is taking. Increased numbers of medications and varied dosing schedules can lead to mistakes in taking medications and serious drug interactions. For example, an older adult with Alzheimer's disease may have periods of agitated behavior. A tranquilizer may be prescribed to decrease the agitation. The tranquilizer has a sedating effect that can increase drowsiness and cause the older adult to be at a higher risk for immobility and falls. This situation can lead to joint pain and pain associated with injuries that may require pain medications that can increase immobility further related to drowsiness and increased risk of falls. Using drugs to treat disease symptoms and using other drugs to treat the side effects of such drugs can lead to the severe adverse drug effects of polypharmacy. A thorough assessment of drug regimens in an effort to simplify them is an important step in avoiding adverse effects of polypharmacy.

Complex prescription routines are not the only cause of polypharmacy. Many older individuals take multiple nonprescription medications, such as laxatives, herbs, vitamins, and other home remedies. These widely available, over-the-counter (OTC) medications may interfere with prescribed medications, leading to adverse drug reactions (ADRs).

Older adults are significantly more prone than younger adults to having undesirable drug reactions. This potential increases in direct proportion to the number of medications being taken. Studies have shown that the potential for ADRs is 100% when an older adult is taking eight or more drugs a day. Common symptoms of ADRs or drug toxicity are changes in mood or behavior, restlessness, confusion, irritability, anxiety, insomnia, and hallucinations suggestive of mental deterioration. Many of these symptoms

---

POINT OF INTEREST

It is becoming common for older adults to purchase medications from Mexico or Canada either by traveling there or through the Internet. The medications in both countries are cheaper to buy and are a boon for the older adult's budget. Scientists suggest, however, that medications made in Mexico are not manufactured under the strict controls that drugs in the United States and Canada are manufactured. This is an important point for discussion with older persons.

can be confused with acute brain problems, and the ADR may go unrecognized. More medications may be prescribed to treat the symptoms of ADRs, and the cycle of problems continues.

Financial Concerns

Medications are expensive. Sometimes older adults self-prescribe rather than pay money for an office visit and a prescription. The end result of this behavior is the use of limited financial resources on OTC, self-prescribed medication that may or may not be beneficial. Older people spend three times more on nonprescription drugs than the general public.

Many older adults experience nutritional changes related to decreased financial resources; this may mean a decreased consumption of protein, resulting in decreased serum protein levels and decreased drug-binding ability. An increased use of alcohol, with resulting liver damage, may increase the metabolism time of the drug so that it circulates longer in the body.

The cost of physician office visits and getting prescriptions filled may be difficult for an older person to manage. Some people never get their prescriptions filled. Some save their prescriptions until they can get to the pharmacist with the right amount of money (this may result in not taking the medications for a month or more). Some people choose OTC medications for relief of the same symptoms as the prescribed drug and never get the prescription filled. Some older persons "save" their drugs by taking only one dose a day instead of two so that the medication lasts longer. For a home-bound individual, filling a prescription may necessitate the added expense of hiring someone to deliver the prescription or of being driven to the pharmacy and back home. Some people take the medications until the symptoms decrease and then put the rest away for "later." Other people share "over-the-fence" medications and health information with their friends and neighbors to save the money of an office visit or prescription filling. A scenario of use of an "over-the-fence" medication would be one in which an older woman has a pill that worked for her shoulder pain and a friend with shoulder pain then calls her to borrow some of the pills that helped the older woman. The friend may seem to benefit by not having to pay for and make a physician's office visit; the woman may feel good about helping another person; in actuality, however, the drug may not help or may be detrimental to the woman's friend.

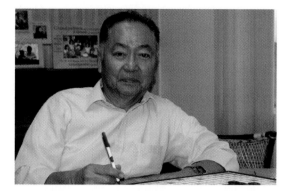

This is the man whose wife has rheumatoid arthritis. You met them playing Scrabble in a previous chapter. He feels concern over being able to pay for the medication necessary for her to move as little as she does. His commitment is to his wife, however, and the quality of her life. He says he always has made it work, and he will in the future as well.

PHARMACOKINETICS

Physiological changes related to normal aging and various disease processes affect the pharmacokinetics of many medications. When an individual takes a medication, there are certain expected events that assist the medication in getting to the intended site of action or effect. Medications in pill form are usually formulated to break down in the stomach acid or the small intestine. The dissolved medication is absorbed in the same place. If the individual has had a part of the stomach removed or has a low concentration of stomach acid, the pill may not be dissolved enough to be absorbed as expected. A good blood supply is necessary for the distribution of medication. Diminished blood supply to or from an area of the body alters the effective distribution of the medication. The liver metabolizes most medications. Liver disease or changes in the blood circulation to the liver change the expected metabolism of a medication. Excretion is the last step in pharmacokinetics. The kidneys have a major role in the excretion of most medications. Kidney disease or decreased blood flow to the kidneys can seriously change the intended excretion of medications. A discussion of the specific pharmacokinetic concerns for older adults follows.

Decreased Absorption

The overall effect of aging changes in older adults is decreased absorption. A major complaint by many older individuals is change in gastrointestinal (GI) motility, with resulting diarrhea or constipation. Drugs are absorbed poorly if they travel through the intestines at a rapid rate. Chronic diarrhea and overuse of laxatives move a medication through the intestines at a rapid rate and decrease the time that the drug is in contact with the intestinal wall to be absorbed. Drugs also are absorbed poorly if the intestine is impacted with stool, as in constipation.

Changes in the GI tract probably interfere with normal absorption of medications. Older adults often have changes in the quality and quantity of digestive enzymes that are important for dissolving and transforming medications into a form that can be absorbed through the intestine. Gastric pH becomes less acidic, and there is an overall decrease in the number of absorbing cells in the intestinal mucosa. The smooth muscle tone and motor activity of the GI tract decline with advancing age. These changes, along with slowed intestinal motility, decreased intestinal blood flow, and slowed gastric emptying time, serve to decrease potential drug absorption further. Atherosclerotic changes reduce the flow of blood to the major organs, resulting in slower disintegration of solid dosage forms such as tablets. Because of the changes in GI motility, drugs that are manufactured for normal adult GI motility are not suited to the slower geriatric bowel. Some drugs may be absorbed in lesser amounts. For example, acidic drugs are ionized to a greater extent, resulting in decreased absorption. Acetylsalicylic acid (aspirin) is more ionized in older people because their secretion of stomach acid is decreased. Absorption of aspirin may be decreased in older adults. Some drugs may be absorbed in greater amounts. Drugs that are absorbed from the intestines are more thoroughly absorbed if they remain in contact with the intestinal wall for a longer time.

Distribution

Drug distribution is greatly altered in older persons. As people age, the body mass becomes leaner with decreased parenchymal tissue and increased fat content. Increased fat results in increased absorption of fat-soluble drugs, resulting in decreased activity and prolonged effects for such drugs. Examples of drugs showing this effect are hypnotics, sedatives, fat-soluble vitamins, and heparin.

Changes in the cardiovascular system of older people may result in delayed arrival of the medication at the target receptors, slow release of the drug from the storage tissue, and slowed excretion of the drug. Decreased blood flow to the specific target tissue may result in decreased drug distribution.

Older people have decreased plasma protein concentrations. Plasma protein is an important factor in drug binding in the serum. Most drug dosages are set for people with normal plasma protein levels. If the older person has less plasma protein, more of the drug is free (i.e., unbound to the protein) and is free to act on the receptors and cause its effect. For example, warfarin (Coumadin) is 90% bound in the average adult. Its dosage is regulated because 90% of it is bound to protein and is unavailable to the person. If the person is elderly and has half the normal adult protein level, a normal dose of warfarin would be an overdose. Some researchers believe that the number and nature of drug receptors in the body change with aging. A decreased or increased response to a normal dosage of medication could result.

Another factor that influences drug distribution is the chronically dehydrated state that many older adults experience. Decreased fluid consumption frequently results in a lower blood volume; this factor decreases distribution in the blood.

Metabolism

Older adults experience a decrease in the rates of overall metabolism, microsomal metabolism, and hepatic biotransformation of the drug and a decline in the body's ability to transform active drugs into inactive drugs. The overall effect of these changes is that the drug remains for a longer time in an active form in older people. Some drugs may remain in the body twice as long as in younger adults.

Excretion

The altered filtration and decreased plasma volume that occur with dehydration commonly found in older people change the excretion of medications. Age-related renal changes result in slower excretion of the drug. Slowed excretion keeps drugs in the body longer and can lead to drug toxicity. Decreased respiratory and vital capacity, with increased carbon dioxide retention, results in decreased excretion of drugs normally excreted by respiration, such as anesthetics. Decreased and changed excretion results in an overall increased pharmacological effect of medications in older people.

The overall effect of aging changes in older adults is increased pharmacological effect. Although less medication is absorbed, it stays longer in the body and remains in the circulation for a longer time.

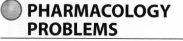

PHARMACOLOGY PROBLEMS

Pharmacology in older adults is frequently identified as a "can of worms." Problems include misuse, overuse, underuse, erratic use, and contraindicated use of drugs. Misuse phenomena include incorrect dosing, sharing of "over-the-fence" medications between neighbors and friends, and use of the same medications for a variety of purposes. Incorrect dosing involves physicians who prescribe dosages based on guidelines for middle-aged adults. As an individual ages, the dosage requirements for most medications decrease. Many medications given in normal adult doses to older adults result in an overdose. Another aspect of misuse occurs when a drug is taken for a variety of symptoms. An older adult may reason, "Well, this pill works for my upset stomach; it will probably work for my diarrhea."

Overuse may result from the theory that if one pill works well, then two pills will work better. People may believe that if they feel better with a vitamin supplement, then two vitamin supplements would definitely improve their health. This behavior may poison the older person's system.

In underuse problems, the person takes less medication than prescribed to "save" pills or money if finances are a problem. Many older adults are on fixed and limited incomes, the cost of medication is high, and medication is sometimes too expensive for the person to afford. Erratic use frequently occurs with short-term memory loss or forgetfulness; for example, a person may forget to take medications for 1 or 2 days.

Contraindicated use can apply in numerous situations. Sometimes older adults receive several drugs from several physicians. They also may have the prescriptions filled at several pharmacies. The end result is that the older population is at a much greater risk for drug interactions, allergic reactions, and problems with polypharmacy (taking multiple medications).

Specific Drug Problems for Older Adults

If all medications were carefully monitored and taken properly, and if the dosage were regulated and accompanied with instructions, the older adult would still be at greater risk than a younger adult for drug-specific problems because of aging changes in drug absorption, metabolism, and excretion. If an older person was prescribed the proper dosage of digoxin, understood the medication regimen, and was in full compliance, the older person would still be at a higher risk for complications to develop. Older people simply experience more side effects and difficulties.

Table 20.1 identifies categories of drugs that may precipitate side effects and adverse effects in older persons. It is important that you, as the licensed practical nurse (LPN), be aware of the possibility of potential problems and monitor for them. Another specific drug problem is the use of OTC medications. Antacids, laxatives, alcohol, and home remedies frequently interfere with the proper functioning of medication.

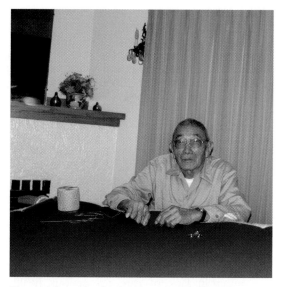

The problem of polypharmacy is a challenging one for older adults. This man quilts for a hobby and does not live a strenuous life. He still has multiple chronic diseases, however. The medication prescribed for him from his three physicians adds up to 22 pills each morning and 12 at night. It worries him, and he wants help in organizing the medications. Where would you refer him if he were your neighbor or family member?

TABLE 20.1 Specific Drug Problems of Elderly Patients

Effect	Drugs
Drugs that cause dry mouth	Analgesics, anticholinergics, antidiarrheals, antilipemics, antiemetics, antipsychotics, antiulcer medications, muscle relaxants, antihistamines, antiparkinsonian medications, antihypertensives
Drugs that promote gastroesophageal reflux	Anticholinergics, beta-blockers, diazepam, dopamine, theophylline
Drugs associated with ulcer formation	Adrenocorticotropic hormones, aspirin, indomethacin, iron, histamine, phenacetin, potassium
Drugs that alter absorption of nutrients	Colchicine, neomycin, cholestyramine, antacids, tricyclic antidepressants, sucralfate (Carafate)
Drugs that promote constipation	Aluminum-containing and calcium-containing antacids, narcotic analgesics, anticholinergics, diuretics, iron, tricyclic antidepressants
Drugs that may promote diarrhea	Analgesics, anti-inflammatory agents, antacids, antiulcer medications, antibiotics, antihypertensive medications, asthma drugs, cardiovascular drugs, diuretics, iron
Drugs that may promote hepatic damage	Acetaminophen (Tylenol), analgesics, anesthetics, antibiotics (especially penicillin and sulfa), antineoplastics, cardiovascular drugs, oral hypoglycemics, steroids
Drugs that may cause excessive depression	Antihistamines, antipsychotics, anxiolytics, cardiac glycosides, narcotics, sedatives/hypnotics
Drugs that may cause dysrhythmias	Antidepressants, cardiac glycosides, phenytoin
Drugs that may damage the kidneys	Aminoglycosides, antibiotics, colchicine
Drugs that may precipitate electrolyte imbalances	Corticosteroids, diuretics
Drugs that may precipitate blood dyscrasias	Antineoplastics, antipsychotics

Antacid Abuse

Some older people consume large amounts of antacids. Physically, a decreased amount of gastric acid has been documented with aging; paradoxically, antacid use usually increases with age. The antacids may be used by the elderly person for symptoms of chest pain. Early angina attacks may be considered heartburn and treated with antacids. Other pathological processes also may be perceived as heartburn. This behavior can result in lack of care for serious health problems. Many antacids are high in sodium content. Excessive use of antacids can increase the severity of cardiovascular and renal disease, exacerbate hypertension, and result in increased fluid load for the aged body. Antacids are notorious for altering the motility of the gut, with resulting diarrhea or constipation.

Use of home remedies frequently interferes with pharmacotherapeutics. Some home remedies have actual benefits, some have only psychological benefits, and some are detrimental. For example, the use of bicarbonate of soda for "acid stomach" is detrimental and may result in serious acid-base imbalance. The ingredients of the home remedy need to be evaluated. The LPN must evaluate the frequency of use and the possible interactions.

Laxative Abuse

Another class of drugs sometimes abused by older adults is laxatives. Laxatives may be taken once, twice, or more than three times a day. Some older people forget that they have had a bowel movement and take more laxatives to facilitate another bowel movement. Although there is no consistent alteration in frequency of bowel movements with advancing age, the ingestion of laxatives increases significantly.

Laxative abuse may result in damage to the intestinal mucosa. The ascending colon is often the site for this damage, and it may dilate and shorten, losing its typical muscular features, resulting in decreased absorption of other medications (and nutrients) that are administered orally. Laxatives also inhibit the absorption of medications from the intestine; this results in decreased levels of the available drug being absorbed, causing a decreased therapeutic effect. Laxatives also result in fluid and electrolyte imbalances that may exacerbate cardiovascular or renal problems. A person who is a frequent abuser of laxatives should be assisted in developing other bowel-training methods. Psychological intervention may be necessary.

Alcohol Abuse

Alcohol abuse is a social health problem in some older people. It is the primary drug of abuse worldwide. Alcohol abuse interferes with pharmacotherapeutics and frequently results in altered nutritional status. This may be seen in decreased serum protein levels (as discussed earlier in this chapter), decreased protein binding, and resultant overdosing of older people. Acid-base balance and fluid and electrolyte levels are adversely affected by alcohol abuse. Changes in these two homeostatic mechanisms result in changes in the pharmacotherapeutic effects of the medication regimen.

Alcohol impairs thinking, judgment, and psychomotor coordination, all of which may lead to decreased medication compliance. Alcohol increases or decreases the effects of several other drugs, and other drugs often increase or decrease the effects of alcohol. Alcohol is a central nervous system depressant that potentiates other central nervous system depressants, particularly barbiturates. When taken concurrently, these two drugs may result in central nervous system depression, coma, and death.

Alcohol has a vasodilating effect and consequently increases the hypotensive effects of most antihypertensive drugs. The effect of alcohol on oral anticoagulants varies. Alcohol intake decreases the effects of the anticoagulants until liver damage occurs, at which point the anticoagulant effects are increased.

Medication Administration Considerations

An evaluation of how older adults manage multiple medications and when they take their medications could reveal potential pharmacology problems. Beer's criteria and chronopharmacology

address these concerns and can help you to provide suggestions for more effective medication administration.

Beer's Criteria

Beer's criteria (Sandihya & Adithan, 2008) is a concept that has critical importance for elderly people who are taking multiple medications. Because aging is associated with a progressive decline in physiological function (which refers to the absorption, distribution, and elimination of medication) and multiple diseases, such as hypertension, arthritis, and diabetes, there is a strong need for oral medications to be given with attention to the personal needs of the older adult. Beer's criteria presents a standardized and collaborative approach for medication reduction and simplification.

The use of Beer's criteria is the responsibility of the physician because he or she is the person responsible for ordering the medication. There are several things you can do, however, to promote and support these criteria that would result in better medication administration for your elderly patients.

As the LPN, you need to be aware of Beer's criteria so that you can talk to older people and get the needed information, share that information with the registered nurse (RN), and ask about the possibility of a Beer's criteria review of the elderly person's medications. In general, a medication review is suggested for any older person who is taking eight or more oral medications.

Beer's criteria is "a medication simplification process," and it has seven steps, as follows:

1. *Remove or discard unnecessary or expired drugs to prevent confusion.* This can be done without a physician's order. If you are a home health nurse, go through all medications with the older person or family members. If you are in a hospital or nursing home and have someone with multiple medications, ask a family member to bring them all in to you. You or the pharmacist can go over the medication with the older person or a family member.
2. *Encourage the use of a single pharmacy to enhance regimen review and collaboration with the pharmacist.* This can be done without a physician's order. It is simply good common sense. When you review the medications at home or medications brought into the facility, you can note what

pharmacies are used and make suggestions to the family as to how to get them all transferred to one pharmacy.

3. *Consider nonpharmacological alternatives.* This can be done without a physician's order. You can suggest elevation of swollen feet, meditation and deep breathing for a headache, or mild heat for arthritis. Any alternative that can decrease the amount of medication being taken is considered a positive action.

4. *Coordinate administration times with established sleep and activity patterns.* This can be done without a physician's order. Ask for a list of times the medications are taken, and compare that with nap, sleep, and meal times. What can be changed to make compliance easier for the person who takes the medication? Associating medication administration with meal time or nap and sleep times encourages compliance in taking the drugs. Talk to the person about compliance and offer advice if you have it.

5. *Decrease administration frequency, using sustained-release or long-acting products.* This requires a physician's order. The fewer pills taken by the older adult, the less chance of a mistake being made by the elder or you.

6. *Reduce multiple medications to treat a single condition, unless combination therapy is intentional.* This requires a physician's order.

7. *Discontinue or substitute cautionary medications known to be problematic for older people (e.g., nonsteroidal anti-inflammatory drug for arthritis pain).* This requires a physician's order.

On the actual Beer's criteria list, you will find a list of 30 medications. With each medication, there is a list of what the side effects would be for an older person taking the drug, and an indication if drug is high or low risk for this age group. Here is one example:

Thioridazine (Mellaril): Greater potential for central nervous system and extrapyramidal adverse effects
Risk: High

This type of information is developed for the physician, but it should be of interest to you because of the amount of interaction that you have with your older patients. Your responsibility is to know about Beer's criteria and to work to complete the first four criteria on all people with more than eight oral medications.

Chronopharmacology

Do you know what a circadian rhythm is? You probably know about circadian rhythm if you have ever worked a night shift. Circadian rhythm is the normal, species-specific reaction to the rotation of the earth around its axis in 24 hours and around the sun in 365 days. We each have variations of our personal circadian rhythms, as do single cells, flowers, and animals. Owls stay up all night and sleep in the daytime. Some flowers bloom all day, others bloom all night, and others bloom for just a few hours in the evening; I also remember hearing about a flower that only blooms 1 day a year. There are people who stay up late, and others who get up early. Some nurses love to work the night shift, and others spend an entire career trying to avoid it. All of these things and many more behaviors are driven by our personal circadian rhythms.

The rhythms of the human body interact with medications. The study of circadian rhythms and medicine is called *chronopharmacology.* Research scientists have defined the major circadian rhythms in humans that impact the body's use of medications; they also recognize that diseases do not display characteristics that are consistent over a 24-hour period. For example, research indicates that most asthma attacks occur at night. What does that tell you about administering asthma medication? Other consistencies include allergic rhinitis symptoms, which are generally worse in the morning; gastric acid secretion, which peaks between 2:00 a.m. and 4:00 a.m.; and the incidence of gastric ulcers, which is greater in the winter (Touhy & Jett, 2010). Another example is cardiac disease: Angina, myocardial infarction, and thrombolytic stroke generally occur in the first 4 hours after waking. What does this indicate to you regarding compliance with administering morning medications?

Scientists have managed the most difficult aspect of chronopharmacology by inventing necessary timing elements for the medications that you deliver to the people in your care. These elements include enteric coatings, time-release capsules, and specific administration times. Your responsibility is to deliver medications on time and in the form they were ordered. Do not cut an enteric-coated pill in half or open a capsule and give just part of it. The science of developing medications for specific timed release is sophisticated and well established, and it is one that you need to honor.

Every persons' circadian rhythms are well established and are an important factor to consider when administering medications. Honoring circadian rhythms results in more effective use of medication by the body. It also can reduce the amount of medication needed by the older person because it is given at the time the body needs it. Both factors have the potential of decreasing toxic effects and improving therapeutic impact.

NURSING CARE OF OLDER ADULTS RECEIVING MEDICATIONS

When managing care of older adults receiving medications, the nurse should follow the nursing process as taught in Chapter 3. The five-stage nursing process consists of assessment, diagnosis, planning, implementation, and evaluation.

Assessment

Before administration of medication, a thorough assessment of the older adult should be completed. A thorough health history is extremely important. Ask the person about past diseases, illness, or symptoms and how they were handled. Inquire about the person's current health status. The history must include past use of drugs, present use of drugs, prescribed drugs, OTC drugs, "over-the-fence" drugs, and street drugs. Specifically ask about use of laxatives and antacids. Assess the person's allergies. Did the allergic reaction cause the person to have difficulty breathing? Hives? Nausea? Vomiting?

Assess the older person's social support network and home environment. Is the person able to get prescriptions filled? Are family members or friends available to help with medication compliance? Assess cognitive skills. Is the person confused or disoriented? Is this problem transitory? Is the person capable of understanding any teaching that occurs? Is depression present?

Assess the older adult's sensory status. Is vision impaired? Is hearing impaired? Is the person strong enough to open pill bottles? Assess the individual's current understanding of therapies and medication regimen. Does the person understand the drugs, dosage, side effects, or adverse effects of current medications?

Assess compliance. Does the person take medications at the proper time? For what reasons would the older adult miss a medication? Is there someone to provide transportation to the physician's office or the pharmacy?

A thorough physical examination must be performed. Watch the older adult for nutrition and fluid status. Is the person thin and emaciated? Is the person dehydrated? Is the person's serum protein level low? This finding may necessitate a reduction in some drug dosages. Is the person obese? If so, the person may require increased dosages of fat-soluble vitamins and medications.

Diagnosis

Many nursing diagnoses are applicable to the older adult receiving medication therapy. Applicable diagnoses include the following:

- Altered Health Maintenance related to insufficient teaching
- Ineffective Management of Therapeutic Regimen related to lack of motivation
- Noncompliance related to lack of financial resources
- Noncompliance related to inability to open bottles

Planning

To promote responsible medication habits in older adults, LPNs must help them become informed medication consumers. Because many

When setting priorities for teaching medication administration to older adults, you must think holistically. Before you begin any medication administration instructions, sit and talk with the older person you are teaching. Can the person hear what you are saying? Can the person read? Does the person have the visual ability to identify colors to differentiate pills? Does the person have arthritic hands that make it difficult or impossible to open medication wrappings and bottles? What are the person's financial resources; can the person afford the medication ordered? Who else should be invited to the teaching session (e.g., spouse, children, other caregivers)? Have a family member bring in the proverbial "brown bag" of medication that the older adult has been taking so that you can ensure there is nothing at home that is contraindicated.

After you have determined the answers to the previous questions, you can plan your teaching session. When you teach, sit close so that the older person can see and hear you. Be organized and have a plan ready that meets the needs you assessed previously. Those of you with more clinical experience may be thinking "no one has time for such a demanding teaching session." This is where you learn *the priority* for medication administration. You must take the time to assess, plan, and teach all older adults about their medications and how to take them!

What good is the power of modern medications—many of them actually miracle drugs—if the person taking them does not do it properly? It does no good. Many older persons take multiple medications with diverse administration schedules, such as diuretics every other day and potassium twice each day. If that person is admitted to the emergency department because of a fall from low potassium and dehydration, what could be the cause? Yes, you're right. The older adult mixed up the instructions and was taking the diuretic twice a day and potassium once every other day. The fall could easily result in a fracture and a prolonged hospital stay after surgery to repair the break.

The priority with medication administration is to assess, plan, and teach the person about all pertinent aspects of the medications given.

older people remain in acute-care settings for only a limited time, discharge planning and teaching must begin on admission.

Before beginning any teaching session, some preparations are important. Choose an environment with good lighting and minimal environmental distractions. Ensure that the older adult who has glasses and hearing aids is wearing them. Prepare visual aids and reading materials with strong colors and large print.

Plan the teaching session to be only 15 to 20 minutes long. Speak clearly and slowly. Use a low-pitched voice (some older people have difficulty hearing a higher pitch). Always face the person when speaking.

Whenever possible, relate the learning to prior life experiences. For example, when teaching about a thyroid drug, help the patient identify personal health problems that occurred before seeking medical treatment and relate those symptoms to how the patient will feel if the medication dose is too low. Tie administration times for medications to the person's daily schedule. If the older person eats oatmeal every morning without fail, the morning dose of digoxin can be associated with the oatmeal breakfast.

Treat older adults as the mature and capable people they are. Do not be patronizing in your teaching approach. Teach a family member, friend, or neighbor at the same time. Have the older person teach the other person and observe the integration of knowledge. Provide sufficient time for review, questions, and return demonstrations.

Consider the need for assistive devices. Medication boxes come in a multitude of styles with individual slots for different days and times. Consider the need for nonchildproof caps. Medication containers can be color-coded and accompanied by a wall chart with the color coding system shown. Teach the person to turn bottles upside down after the medication is taken. Allow the older person to be responsible for taking personal medication the last few days in the hospital. The nurse should monitor these actions and review any areas of knowledge deficit.

Encourage all older adults to carry a list of medications (including prescription and nonprescription drugs) at all times. Another family member should carry the same list. The older person should be encouraged to share the list with all physicians and pharmacists before receiving or filling any new prescriptions. Encourage all older adults to locate a pharmacy they like and fill all prescriptions there. On all admissions to the hospital, the nurse should review all medications and refer incompatibilities to the physician or pharmacist.

Implementation

In administering medications to older persons, several strategies are important. When administering medications by mouth, be aware of the medication form. Time-release capsules (e.g., many cold capsules) should not be opened or crushed and mixed with food. If the person is unable to swallow the capsule, contact the physician or pharmacist for a liquid form. Enteric-coated capsules should not be crushed or dissolved. Disruption of the enteric coating allows gastric acid to come into contact with the medication and inactivate it. Offer the most important medication first. Give the person enough fluid so that the medication reaches the stomach.

Parenteral injections should be given into the dorsogluteal or ventrogluteal sites. The deltoid muscle should be avoided because in most older people it has lost much of its mass. The vastus lateralis muscle should be avoided owing to its decreased muscle mass and decreased circulation. Avoid injections into edematous areas that have decreased circulation.

Intravenous therapy needs to be closely monitored in older people because many older adults are in a slightly dehydrated state. Fluid overload is especially critical in a person who may have underlying cardiac and renal disease that would be exacerbated by excess fluid.

Some older people experience visual changes with changes in a medication regimen. Recommend that the person not change prescription eyewear until the medication regimen is established.

Evaluation

Evaluation, the final step in the nursing process, is critical in administering medication for older adults. Evaluate the person's learning curve by doing a return demonstration teaching session. Ask questions about situations the older adult may encounter in the home setting. Allow the person to ask questions of you.

Evaluation of compliance is based primarily on personal and family report. Ask the older adult if medications are being taken, and then clarify how and when the medications are being consumed. Ask about the occurrence of side effects. If expected side effects do not occur, the nurse should question whether or not the medication is being taken. Blood levels (if available for a given medication) should be evaluated to determine whether the levels are commensurate with the person's report. Monitor the older adult's laboratory results to determine kidney and liver function. Ask for a personal evaluation of how the new medication is working. Does it help? What concerns does the person have?

POINT OF INTEREST

You are admitting an older person to the medical unit for chest pain, shortness of breath, and edema, and neither the older person nor the family member can recall the medications the older person is taking. A solution to this problem that is easy for the family is the "brown-bag" solution. Ask the family member to go home and put all medications the older person is taking into a brown bag and bring them to you. Be sure the family member brings prescription, OTC, and natural remedies. Assure the family member that all medications will be returned. This will give you the opportunity to make an accurate list of medications being taken by the older adult. It also gives you the opportunity to point out outdated medications that should be discarded.

The outcome of a successful medication plan can be evaluated by the following criteria:

- The older adult's ability to solve problems related to polypharmacy
- Communication of adverse reactions
- Adherence to regimen

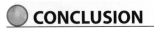

CONCLUSION

Pharmacology in older adults is a complex issue. The nursing care of the older adult must include attention to the details of the medication regimen. The LPN needs to be familiar with the aging changes that affect pharmacotherapeutics, including pharmacokinetic changes, sensory changes, psychological changes, problems of polypharmacy, chronic health changes, and financial changes. It is important that the nurse understand the drugs likely to be misused and be aware of specific drugs that are frequently misused by elderly patients: antacids, laxatives, alcohol, and home remedies.

The nurse needs to be able to implement the nursing process on behalf of older adults to assist them to develop into well-informed medication consumers. The ability to teach regarding medication administration and evaluate the impact of medications on the older person is a crucial skill for you to have.

Mr. W. is 74 years old and lives at home alone. He does fairly well on his own. He has difficulty seeing, but he can read soup can labels. He has arthritis in his hands and opens cans with an electric opener.

Mr. W.'s drug history includes heart, arthritis, diuretic, and potassium prescription medications. Mr. W. denies any use of street drugs and states that he "doesn't believe in that stuff." When asked about other medications, he states that he uses Mylanta "several times a day, just one tablespoon full," and Ex-Lax every day for a bowel movement. He also takes a small blue-and-white capsule that his brother gave him because it helps his brother's arthritis. He takes that capsule "once or twice, maybe three or four times a week."

Mr. W. is currently complaining of weakness, dizziness, and occasional chest pains that he treats with Mylanta. His feet and hands seem to be swelling lately.

Mr. W.'s neighbor called the home healthcare agency where you work and requested that a home visit be made because Mr. W. seems to be getting thinner and thinner. The agency assigns you to go visit. You find Mr. W. sitting on the porch with his feet propped up and half asleep.

Discussion

1. What is the first step in your home visit?
2. What nursing diagnoses may apply to Mr. W. at this time?
3. While looking at his brother's blue-and-white capsule, you discover the name of the drug on the side. What is your best course of action regarding this "over-the-fence" drug?
4. Mr. W. is wondering why his feet are swelling and he is feeling weak and dizzy. What drug interactions could be causing these symptoms?
5. What role does the Ex-Lax play in Mr. W.'s pharmacotherapeutics?
6. What referrals does the nurse need to make?
7. What should the nurse do to assist Mr. W. in becoming compliant?

Solution

1. Introduce yourself, explain why you have come, and begin a complete assessment. The history, drug history, and physical assessment need to be complete. View Mr. W.'s environment. Ask about support services, friends, family, and neighbors. Explore nutritional status and assess what food is available for Mr. W. Assess eyesight. Can he read drug labels? Assess compliance. Does he know when and how to take the medications?
2. Knowledge deficit related to medication regimen
   Noncompliance related to lack of understanding
   Ineffective management of therapeutic regimen
   Sensory deficit related to diminished visual acuity
3. Although the blue-and-white pill is a non-narcotic analgesic and nonsteroidal anti-inflammatory drug, it has not been prescribed for Mr. W. Identify his feelings about the medication. Does it seem to help his arthritis? Does he have side effects with the drug? Explain to the patient why it is important not to use this drug unless it is prescribed by the physician. Identify interactions of the drug with other prescribed medications (decreases the effectiveness of diuretics and antihypertensive therapy, increases gastric irritation, increases serum levels and risk of toxicity from digoxin). Stress the importance of not taking drugs unless his physician prescribes them. Offer to make an appointment for him to see his physician and ask for a prescription for a medication to relieve arthritis pain.
4. Increased sodium intake from use of Mylanta could result in peripheral edema. With increased body fluid volume, the heart could be working harder, increasing myocardial oxygen demand and causing angina.
5. Ex-Lax facilitates movement through the gut, decreasing absorption of all the other

Continued on page 362

medications; it probably contributes to fluid and electrolyte imbalance.

6. Refer to the physician for evaluation of chest pain (if this resembles cardiac angina, consider emergency referral) and to social services for necessary social support. Call on family members for assistance with medications and transportation, and suggest Meals-on-Wheels.

7. Set up a scheduling plan. Draw a calendar with medications depicted. Teach Mr. W. to take medications at specific times each day. Encourage discontinuance of Ex-Lax, Mylanta, and the blue-and-white pill. Build on the knowledge that he already has. Relate medications to events in Mr. W.'s lifestyle. If he seems unable to manage medications on his own, ask the physician for a referral for home-health nurses to administer medications as needed.

Select the best answer to each question.

1. Considering the pharmacokinetics in the older person, which of the following statements is true?

a. Overall absorption is decreased.

b. Overall distribution is enhanced.

c. There is an increase in receptors with aging.

d. Excretion is facilitated, resulting in a shorter duration of drug action.

2. Which of the following factors would be the strongest in influencing compliance in an older person on a fixed income?

a. Dietary habits

b. Cost of filling prescriptions

c. Body fat-to-lean muscle weight ratio

d. Family support

3. When working with Beer's criteria for medication simplification, the LPN should:

a. Discontinue all multiple medications.

b. Review all oral medications with the person who is ill and the family, and try to unify the prescriptions to one pharmacy.

c. Make a note to the physician with all of the high-risk medications the ill person is taking on it.

d. Ignore the oral medications except to give them as they are ordered.

4. Chronopharmacology relates to:

a. What time people wake up in the morning

b. The science of time-release and enteric-coated medications

c. The correlation between one's circadian rhythm and medication effectiveness

d. The correlation between one's circadian rhythm and injection effectiveness

5. Mrs. M., age 82, lives at home alone. Her daughter visits once a day and helps her bathe. Mrs. M. cooks her own meals and works in her home and yard. Which of the following factors could place Mrs. M. at risk of making a medication error?

a. Multiple medications

b. Visual changes

c. Different schedules for different drugs

d. All of the above

6. Mrs. M.'s daughter reports that she seems to take laxatives two or three times per day. What effect would laxative abuse have on the other medications Mrs. M. is taking?

a. Increased absorption owing to clearance of the GI tract

b. Increased absorption owing to facilitation of medication through the GI tract

c. Decreased absorption owing to increased gut motility

d. Decreased distribution owing to increased fluid consumption

7. Mrs. M. seems to have difficulty remembering whether or not she has taken her pills. Which of the following would be helpful to her?

a. Medication pill boxes with compartments

b. Turning the bottles upside down

c. Color coding the medications with a check-off list

d. All of the above

21 Laboratory Values and Older Adults

Mary Ann Anderson

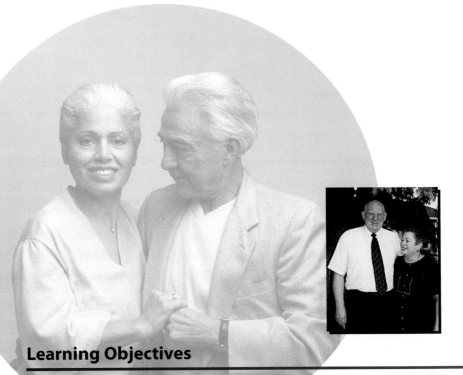

Learning Objectives

After completing this chapter, the student will be able to:

1. Identify laboratory tests that are important indicators of health and disease in elderly patients.
2. Apply an understanding of laboratory tests to the health of elderly persons.
3. Identify at least three reference resources for understanding laboratory values.
4. Identify medications that have an influence on laboratory tests for elderly patients.
5. Describe nursing actions appropriate for abnormal laboratory values.

INTRODUCTION

Laboratory tests are among the tools for health and illness measurement. Laboratory tests are done on admission to a hospital or nursing home, and they are often done for elderly persons when visiting the physician. As a licensed practical nurse (LPN), you have studied laboratory values and their meanings in your medical and surgical nursing classes. You also use laboratory resources at the facility where you work to interpret laboratory values of older adults correctly. The purpose of this chapter is not to repeat that information; instead, this chapter provides a ready reference of significant tests for elderly people along with specific and pertinent information that relates to elderly patients.

MEANING OF LABORATORY VALUES IN ELDERLY PATIENTS

Laboratory tests are a routine part of the health examination for all people. For many tests, the normal ranges are different for elderly people than for people younger than 65 years of age. For other tests, there is no change with age. Also, elderly people may have greater deviations from normal laboratory indicators when under stress, and return to normal levels is often slower in elderly people than in younger people. Conditions such as anemia, electrolyte imbalances, and infections are common in elderly people. They can be discovered and treatment can be monitored through the use of laboratory tests. The diagnosis and treatment of these conditions result in substantial improvement in health, even in elderly individuals with multiple health problems.

Relationship to Clinical Status

You, as the LPN, need to remember that all laboratory findings must be evaluated in relation to the individual's total clinical situation. The elderly person's gender, dietary pattern, activity level, use of tobacco and alcohol, current medications, and aggressive medical and nursing interventions can alter laboratory findings.

Laboratory values should never be considered in isolation, especially when dealing with often frail elderly persons seen in clinical settings. For example, abnormal laboratory values may indicate a physiological stressor such as

PRIORITY SETTING 21.1

Generally, laboratory employees are responsible for obtaining blood specimens from the people in your care. You, or a certified nursing assistant you supervise, will be responsible for obtaining any urine, stool, wound, or sputum specimens. The priority for you is to gather all specimens *perfectly*. That may seem a bit demanding, but there is no reason to send a specimen to the laboratory if it will not give you accurate results.

When an older person is asked to give you a midstream urine specimen, the individual may not understand what that means. Not wanting to look "dumb," the individual may not ask for clarification. You need to determine if the person understands the instructions by asking for feedback on what you want. When asked to cleanse the urinary meatus before voiding for a clean-catch specimen, an older person may think that is not "proper" and simply not do it. You are the person responsible to see that these things are done correctly so that the specimen gives accurate results.

When obtaining a sputum specimen, you are the person who must see that the specimen comes from a deep cough so that it is the best specimen possible. Most people do not like mucus, or perhaps it is painful for the older person to cough deeply. You need to plan ahead and be prepared with a strategy that will get the specimen needed for the proper treatment. As in all things you do, be patient and caring, as these are the hallmark behaviors of professionals in nursing.

dehydration or medication side effect rather than illness. It is essential that you consider all facets of the individual's health and habits when you review the laboratory results.

Routine Laboratory Evaluations

A routine laboratory evaluation generally consists of the following:

- Complete blood cell count
- Serum glucose
- Serum creatinine level

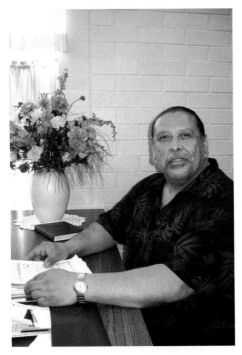

It is important to remember that behind every laboratory procedure there is a human being who is anxious about the procedure itself or the results of the procedure.

- Serum electrolytes
- Thyroid function tests
- Urinalysis
- Stool guaiac test

Other specific laboratory tests that are not part of the routine evaluation may be ordered to help diagnose illness and disease. These tests include the following

- Chest x-ray studies for individuals with symptoms or who are at risk of pulmonary disease
- Tuberculosis testing, which is recommended for individuals in group-living situations or for individuals who are at risk of exposure
- Baseline electrocardiograms, which should be done in all elderly persons and repeated when there is suspicion of heart rate or rhythm changes or myocardial infarction

This chapter discusses the most common laboratory tests ordered and their meanings for elderly people. The values shown under headings are normal reference values from *Harrison's Principles of Internal Medicine* (Fauci, 2008), unless otherwise indicated. As an LPN, you must refer to the reference intervals used by the clinical laboratory where you work for the most precise reference ranges.

COMMON SCREENING TESTS

There are three common screening tests that should be performed on elderly people. The physician may request additional tests, but these three are the most commonly used for general screening and are important for you to know.

Tuberculin Skin Test

Negative result   <10 mm of induration

General Information

The tuberculin skin test, using purified protein derivative (PPD), is the screening method of choice for the detection of tuberculosis. Up to 25% of older adults who are clinically ill with tuberculosis show no reaction (<10 mm of induration) to intradermal injections of 5 U of tuberculin. Some older adults who show no initial reaction to the test respond after the test is repeated 1 week later. Most people who react positively to the test have no clinical evidence of infection.

Nursing home residents, whose risk of infection is five times greater than that of nonresidents, should be screened with a tuberculin skin test on admission and annually thereafter. Although the incidence of infection is low, and treatment with isoniazid is known to be effective, congregate living poses the risk of epidemic infection.

Nursing Implications

Because anergy (lack of reaction to specific antigens) is common in elderly people, some clinicians recommend that all PPDs should be placed with appropriate intradermal technique and should be done annually.

Urinalysis

Appearance	Clear yellow/straw
Specific gravity	1.005–1.020
pH	4.5–8.0

General Information

Normal urine in an elderly person should test negative for glucose, ketones, blood, bilirubin, lupus erythematosus, protein nitrates, and calculi, although traces of protein may be present. There may be zero to three red blood cells (RBCs), zero to four white blood cells (WBCs), a few epithelial cells, and a few crystals per high-power field on microscopic examination. Elderly people commonly have the presence of zero to three hyaline casts on low-power field. In addition, 10% to 50% of older people have asymptomatic bacteriuria.

Nursing Implications

- Usually a midstream, clean-catch specimen is requested. For this sample, the urinary meatus is cleansed with soap and water or a mild cleaning solution, voiding is initiated, and then a sample is collected in midstream to allow clearing of contamination from outside the urinary meatus.
- First-morning and fasting urine specimens are collected when the individual awakes and can provide the most concentrated urine of the day. Analytic values for protein, nitrite, fasting urine glucose, and urinary sediment are highest at that time.
- A 24-hour urine specimen measures the average excretion for substances eliminated in variable amounts during the day.
- Urine specimens should be sent to the laboratory within 10 minutes or refrigerated to prevent growth of bacteria and to prevent the bacteria from using the glucose.

Urinary tract infection is a specific illness that is common in elderly people. The highest incidence of reported urinary tract infections is in long-term care facilities. This occurs because the urinary tract pathogens often become resistant to antibiotics in nursing homes.

1. Typical symptoms are:
   Frequency
   Burning
   Hematuria
2. In an older person, the only symptoms exhibited may be:
   Nocturia
   Incontinence
   Confusion
   Anorexia
   Lethargy

Stool for Occult Blood

Negative result   Absence of test color

General Information

Gastrointestinal (GI) bleeding is common in older people, especially in individuals taking aspirin-containing medications and nonsteroidal anti-inflammatory drugs (NSAIDs). Approximately 2.5 mL of blood per day normally appears in the stool. Hemorrhoids and colorectal cancer are the most common causes of minor bleeding in elderly people.

Abnormal bleeding from the GI tract may be either occult (hidden) or obvious by observation. Minor bleeding may be accompanied by a decrease in the hemoglobin and hematocrit and by symptoms of fatigue and weakness. The fecal occult blood test is useful in screening for colorectal cancer.

Nursing Implications

- There are various tests for fecal occult blood, all requiring the contact of a reagent with a stool specimen.
- A positive test result, indicated by color (usually blue), occurs when there is more than the normal amount of GI blood loss.
- Recommendations are to test at least three stool specimens and to sample from at least two areas of each stool.
- Instruct the person to avoid red meats, vitamin C intake, iron supplements, and aspirin for 2 to 3 days before and during stool testing to avoid invalidating the results. Check the manufacturer's directions for other restrictions.

● HEMATOLOGICAL INDICATORS

In addition to the three common screening tests, hematological tests are routinely done on all patients.

Complete Blood Count

The complete blood count (CBC) includes RBC count, hemoglobin, hematocrit, RBC indices, white blood cell (WBC) count, platelets, and frequently, but not always, a differential. Values for the CBC do not change with age.

Red Blood Cell Count

Men	$5.4 \pm 0.9 \times 10^{12}/L$
Women	$4.8 \pm 0.6 \times 10^{12}/L$

General Information

The RBC count is used to compute and support other hematological tests to diagnose anemia; polycythemia, and other bone marrow abnormalities.

1. Decreased RBC count may indicate:
   Anemia
   Fluid overload
   Kidney problems
   Bone marrow invasion of other cells or tumors
   Recent hemorrhage
   Chronic illness and autoimmune diseases
2. An increased RBC count may be caused by:
   Polycythemia
   Dehydration
   Hypoxia
   Congestive heart failure
   Impaired pulmonary ventilation
   Abnormal hemoglobin

Hemoglobin

Men	14–18 g/dL
Women	12–16 g/dL

General Information

Normal hemoglobin levels are maintained throughout life in healthy individuals. Hemoglobin concentration in whole blood correlates closely with the RBC count.

1. Increased hemoglobin levels may be caused by:
   Polycythemia
   Dehydration
2. Decreased hemoglobin levels may be caused by:
   Anemia
   Recent hemorrhage
   Fluid retention causing hemodilution
   Kidney disease

Hematocrit

Men	$47.0 \pm 5.0\%$
Women	$42.0 \pm 5.0\%$

General Information

Hematocrit measures the percentage by volume of packed RBCs in whole blood.

1. Decreased hematocrit levels may be caused by:
   Anemia
   Hemodilution
   Bone marrow disease
   Kidney disease
2. Increased hematocrit may be caused by:
   Polycythemia
3. Significant volume depletion occurs with associated increased blood urea nitrogen (BUN) and creatinine.

Red Blood Cell Indices

MCV	90 ± 7 fL
MCH	29 ± 2 pg
MCHC	$34 \pm 2\%$

General Information

RBC indices—mean corpuscular volume (MCV), mean corpuscular hemoglobin (MCH), and mean corpuscular hemoglobin concentration (MCHC)—aid in the diagnosis and classification of anemias by providing information about the size, hemoglobin concentration, and hemoglobin weight of an average RBC.

White Blood Cell Count

$4.5–11.0 \times 10^9/L$

General Information

The WBC count is also known as the leukocyte count. It is used to identify infectious or inflammatory processes, to evaluate the need for further tests, and to monitor the older person's response to chemotherapy or radiation therapy. There is a decrease in the WBC count with age because of a reduction in lymphocyte cells. This results in fewer lymphocytes to resist infection.

1. A decreased WBC count (leukopenia) may be caused by:
   Bone marrow depression, owing to primary disease (leukemia, myeloma, and other tumors)

Reactions to antineoplastics or other toxins
Viral infections (influenza, infectious hepatitis)
Sepsis
Radiation treatments
Drug use, including phenytoin, NSAIDs, and metronidazole

2. An increased WBC count (leukocytosis) may be caused by:
Infection
Inflammation
Tissue necrosis
Leukemia
Excessive exercise
Stress

In elderly persons, infection may not be accompanied by a normal increase in the number of WBCs (leukocytes). A WBC differential is required to detect and diagnose disease.

White Blood Cell Differential

Neutrophils $1.8-7.7 \times 10^9/L$ or 30%–60%
Eosinophils $0-0.45 \times 10^9/L$ or 1%–4%
Basophils $0-0.20 \times 10^9/L$ or 0%–0.5%
Lymphocytes $1.0-4.8 \times 10^9/L$ or 25%–35%
Monocytes $0-0.8 \times 10^9/L$ or 1%–4.0%

General Information

The WBC differential is used to determine the severity of an infection, detect allergic reactions and parasitic infections, identify various leukemias, and assess the individual's capacity to resist and overcome infection.

The following five types of WBCs are classified in the normal differential:

- Neutrophils
- Eosinophils
- Basophils
- Lymphocytes
- Monocytes

Platelet Count

130,000–400,000/mL

General Information

Platelets, also called thrombocytes, are necessary for the formation of the aggregate or plug necessary for clot formation and hemostasis. Platelets also supply phospholipids for the process of coagulation in the thromboplastin generation pathway. When the platelet count is less than $50,000/mm^3$, spontaneous bleeding may occur.

1. A decreased platelet count (thrombocytopenia) may be caused by:
Bone marrow disease
Folic acid or vitamin B_{12} deficiency
Disseminated intravascular coagulation
Drugs (antineoplastics, furosemide, indomethacin, penicillin, phenytoin, quinidine sulfate, salicylates, sulfonamides, thiazides, tricyclic antidepressants, and others)

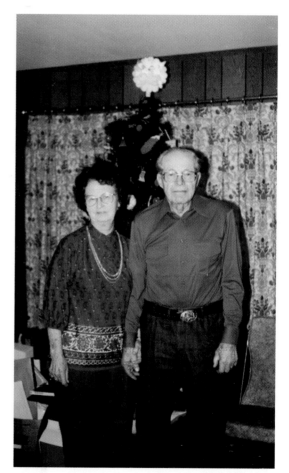

This older couple goes to the hospital outpatient department monthly to have blood drawn to assist in their medication management. The man has Alzheimer's disease and sometimes gets aggressive with his wife. The woman worries each time they have to go to the hospital, yet she perseveres because she knows how important the results are to their health.

Destruction resulting from immune disorders, radiation, or mechanical injury
Disseminated intravascular coagulation
2. An increased platelet count (thrombocytosis) may be caused by:
Iron-deficiency anemia
Hemorrhage
Splenectomy
Polycythemia vera
Malignancies
High altitudes
Persistent cold temperature
Strenuous exercise

Coagulation: Prothrombin Time (PT)

Normal   9.5–11.8 sec (control ± 1 sec)
Therapeutic   1.5–2.0 times normal control

General Information

Anticoagulation therapy is indicated in many conditions, such as pulmonary embolus, deep vein thrombosis, chronic atrial fibrillation, and heart valve prosthesis. Warfarin (Coumadin) is used in oral anticoagulation therapy. PT is an indirect measure of prothrombin and an overall evaluation of these extrinsic coagulation factors. PT is determined before initiation of warfarin therapy and then daily until maintenance dosage is established. Thereafter, PT determinations may be made at 1- to 4-week intervals, depending on the stability of the person's therapeutic level.

Nursing Implications

- Risk of serious hemorrhage is high in anticoagulated persons older than age 70, especially individuals at risk for falls.
- Many drugs have a potentiating or inhibiting effect on warfarin, so all medications being taken by an individual taking warfarin must be reviewed. Diets high in vitamin K should be encouraged.

Coagulation: Activated Partial Thromboplastin Time (APTT)

Normal   25–36 sec
Therapeutic   1.5–2.5 times normal control

General Information

APTT evaluates all of the clotting factors of the intrinsic pathway except for two by measuring the time required for formation of a fibrin clot. APTT is used to monitor heparin anticoagulation therapy aimed at increasing APTT to a therapeutic range. APTT is more sensitive and is often used in place of PT.

Nursing Implications

- If PT or APTT values are higher than the therapeutic range, or if bleeding or signs of bleeding such as hematuria, black tarry stools, hematemesis, bruising and petechiae, epistaxis, hemoptysis, continuous abdominal or head pain, faintness, or dizziness occur, withhold the anticoagulant dose, and notify the physician immediately.
- Periodic urinalyses and stool guaiac and liver function tests are carried out to detect hemorrhage or liver dysfunction.

BLOOD CHEMISTRY INDICATORS

Blood Glucose: Plasma

Fasting:

Normal   75–115 mg/dL
Diabetes mellitus   140 mg/dL on at least two occasions

Two hours after eating:

Normal   140 mg/dL
Impaired glucose   140–200 tolerance mg/dL
Diabetes mellitus   >200 mg/dL on at least two occasions

General Information

In elderly people, the exact definition of abnormal glucose tolerance is unclear. Using the National Diabetes Data Group and the World Health Organization diagnostic criteria, diabetes mellitus is present when the fasting (12- to 14-hour fast) plasma glucose is greater than 140 mg/dL on two separate occasions or greater than 200 mg/dL 2 hours after oral glucose administration.

Numerous drugs and conditions affect plasma glucose levels.

1. Decreased blood plasma glucose (hypoglycemia) is indicated by:
   Plasma blood glucose values less than 100 mg/dL
   Weakness
   Restlessness
   Hunger
   Nervousness
   Sweating
   Rapidly decreasing mental alertness in an elderly person without the above-listed common symptoms
2. Decreased plasma glucose levels may be caused by:
   Beta-blockers
   Ethanol
   Clofibrate
   Monoamine oxidase inhibitors
   Strenuous exercise
   Failure to refrigerate the blood sample and analyze it within a few hours of collection
3. Increased blood plasma glucose (hyperglycemia) is indicated by:
   Plasma glucose levels, which usually exceed 600 mg/dL. Plasma glucose greater than 160–180 mg/dL is the average renal threshold, resulting in glycosuria in older persons.
   Lack of symptoms
   Urinary frequency
   Dehydration
   Weakness
4. Elevation of plasma glucose levels may be caused by:
   Chlorthalidone
   Thiazide diuretics
   Furosemide
   Oral contraceptives
   Benzodiazepines
   Phenytoin
   Phenothiazines
   Lithium
   Epinephrine
   Nicotinic acid
   Corticosteroids
   Recent illness or infection

If undetected, worsening hyperglycemia results in alterations in mental status and hyperosmolar coma in an older person with non–insulin-dependent diabetes mellitus.

Electrolytes

Normal values for electrolytes are the same for young and old. Numerous conditions, medications, and dietary factors influence electrolyte values. Common electrolyte-related causes of weakness in elderly people are hypernatremia (high sodium), hyponatremia (low sodium), and hypokalemia (low potassium).

Sodium, Serum

136–145 mEq/L

General Information
Elderly people are at increased risk of serum sodium imbalance. Decreased sodium levels promote water excretion, and increased levels promote retention, primarily through stimulation or depression of aldosterone secretion. Loss of body water causes concentration of serum sodium (hypernatremia), whereas an increase in body water causes dilution of serum sodium (hyponatremia). Sodium also plays a role in acid-base balance, chloride and potassium levels, and neuromuscular function.

Hyponatremia
A sodium concentration of less than 136 mEq/L occurs when there is an excess of water in relation to total sodium.

1. Symptoms may be absent, or there may be:
   Fatigue
   Headache
   Restlessness
   Decreased skin turgor
   Nausea
   Muscle cramps and tremors
   Disorientation
   Confusion
   Coma
   Seizures
   Death
2. Conditions causing hyponatremia include:
   Vomiting
   Diarrhea
   Renal disorders
   Diuretics
   Congestive heart failure
   Cirrhosis
   Overhydration
   Adrenal insufficiency
   Use of nutritional support formulas without additional sodium

Syndrome of inappropriate antidiuretic hormone secretion associated with numerous drugs and diseases

Hypernatremia

A sodium concentration greater than 146 mEq/L is a result of a deficit of body water relative to total sodium content and is usually caused by dehydration.

1. Symptoms include:
   Weakness
   Thirst
   Restlessness
   Dry, sticky mucous membranes
   Flushed skin
   Oliguria
   Diminished reflexes
2. Conditions contributing to hypernatremia include:
   Inadequate fluid intake
   Diarrhea
   Polyuria associated with diabetes mellitus
   Diuretics
   Increased insensible water loss from fever and tachypnea
3. Conditions causing hypernatremia include:
   Hypertension
   Dyspnea
   Edema
   Kidney disease owing to a lack of response to antidiuretic hormone
4. Conditions causing excess sodium concentration are:
   Increased dietary intake
   Aldosteronism
   Intravenous infusion of normal saline for treatment of fluid loss or shock

Potassium, Serum

3.5–5.0 mEq/L

General Information

Potassium maintains cellular osmotic equilibrium and helps regulate muscle activity by maintaining electrical conduction within the cardiac and skeletal muscles. Potassium also helps regulate acid-base balance, enzyme activity, and kidney function. Potassium deficiency develops rapidly because the body has no effective way to conserve potassium.

1. Signs and symptoms commonly seen with hypokalemia (decreased serum potassium levels) include:
   Mental confusion
   Rapid, weak, irregular pulse
   Hypotension
   Anorexia
   Decreased reflexes
   Muscle weakness
   Paresthesia
2. Hypokalemia is caused by:
   Diuretics
   Diarrhea
   Vomiting
   Renal tubular acidosis
   Malnutrition
   Urinary potassium losses associated with glycosuria and ketonuria and with hyperaldosteronism
3. Signs and symptoms of hyperkalemia (increased serum potassium) are:
   Weakness
   Malaise
   Nausea
   Diarrhea
   Muscle irritability
   Oliguria
   Bradycardia
4. Hyperkalemia is caused by:
   Renal failure
   Cell damage from burns
   Injuries
   Chemotherapy
   Acidosis
   Addison's disease
   Diabetes mellitus
5. Several drugs may increase serum potassium levels, including:
   Spironolactone
   Triamterene
   NSAIDs
   Beta-blockers
   Angiotensin-converting enzyme inhibitors
   Penicillin G
   Amphotericin B
   Methicillin
   Tetracycline

Calcium, Plasma

9–10.5 mg/dL

General Information

Calcium absorption becomes less efficient with age in men and women. Inadequate dietary calcium is associated with the loss of bone that begins in the 40s. Calcium helps regulate and promote neuromuscular and enzyme activity, skeletal development, and blood coagulation. Parathyroid hormone, vitamin D, calcitonin, and adrenal steroids control calcium blood levels. Almost all of the body's calcium is stored in the bones and teeth. Serum calcium varies inversely with the body's phosphorus level. The body requires ingestion of about 1 g per day of dietary calcium because calcium is excreted in the urine and feces.

1. Signs and symptoms of hypocalcemia include:
   Circumoral and peripheral numbness and tingling
   Muscle twitching
   Facial muscle spasm
   Muscle cramping
   Seizures
   Dysrhythmias
2. Causes of hypocalcemia include:
   Insufficient activity of the parathyroid glands
   Hypomagnesemia
   Hyperphosphatemia owing to renal failure
   Laxatives
   Chemotherapy
   Corticosteroids
   Malabsorption
   Acute pancreatitis
   Alkalosis osteomalacia
   Diarrhea
   Rickets (vitamin D deficiency)
3. Signs and symptoms of hypercalcemia are:
   Hypertension
   Bone pain
   Muscle hypotonicity
   Nausea
   Vomiting
   Dehydration
   Mental confusion
   Coma
   Cardiac arrest
4. Causes of hypercalcemia are:
   Hyperparathyroidism
   Thiazide diuretics
   Cancer
   Addison's disease
   Hyperthyroidism
   Paget's disease
   Immobilization
   Excessive vitamin D intake
   Calcium-containing antacids
   Androgens
   Progestins or estrogens
   Lithium carbonate

Phosphate, Serum

3–4.5 mg/dL

General Information

Phosphate helps regulate calcium levels, carbohydrate and lipid metabolism, and acid-base balance. Adequate levels of vitamin D are necessary for absorption of phosphates from the intestine. About 85% of the body's phosphate is found in bone. Calcium and phosphate have a reciprocal relationship. The kidneys regulate phosphate excretion to maintain a balance with serum calcium.

Chloride, Serum

98–106 mEq/L

General Information

Chloride interacts with sodium to maintain the osmotic pressure of the blood. Chloride is important in maintaining the acid-base balance in the body and varies inversely with the bicarbonate level. Low chloride levels are usually seen with low sodium and potassium levels.

End Products of Metabolism

Blood Urea Nitrogen (BUN), Serum

10–20 mg/dL

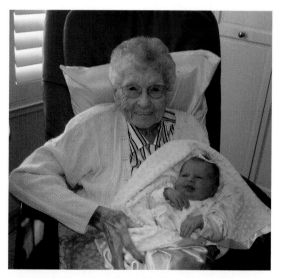

Family is this woman's greatest joy. She appreciates the monthly laboratory work that is done for her at the nursing home where she resides. She doesn't worry about the results because she knows the physician and nurses will manage the situation for her. That leaves her more time to be with her family.

General Information

BUN is the chief end product of protein metabolism. BUN level reflects protein intake, liver function, and kidney excretory capacity. The normal BUN value remains unchanged with age. Because protein intake is often low in elderly persons, BUN values may be normal even with impaired renal function. Elevation of BUN levels without serum creatinine elevation suggests dehydration.

There are usually no signs or symptoms of an increased BUN level other than the signs and symptoms associated with dehydration or other underlying renal disease. Likewise, with decreased BUN levels, the signs and symptoms are those of the underlying condition.

1. Increased BUN levels occur with:
   Renal disease
   Reduced renal blood flow
   Urinary tract obstruction
   Increased protein catabolism (starvation, burns)
   Drugs such as aminoglycosides, amphotericin B, and methicillin
2. Decreased BUN levels occur with:
   Severe liver failure
   Malnutrition
   Overhydration
   Chloramphenicol use

Creatinine, Serum

1.5 mg/dL

General Information

Creatinine values also are unchanged with age. Because lean body mass declines with age, however, the total daily production of creatinine also declines, remaining less than 1.2 mg/dL. This causes an overestimate of renal function in elderly persons based on static measurements of serum creatinine.

Creatinine clearance declines by almost 10% per decade after 40 years of age and is a more reliable indicator of kidney function than BUN and serum creatinine values. In elderly people, creatinine clearance is important for determining the dosage for drugs that are cleared by the kidney to avoid drug toxicity. Creatinine clearance (mL/min) is defined as a ratio. For men, the formula is:

$$[140 - age\ (yr)] \times body\ weight\ (kg) \div serum\ creatinine\ (mg/dL) \times 72$$

For women, multiply the result from the previous formula by 0.85.

An increase in serum creatinine may be caused by:

- Renal disease
- Diabetic acidosis
- Starvation
- Muscle disease
- Hyperthyroidism
- Use of ascorbic acid
- Barbiturates
- Diuretics

A high serum creatinine level indicating renal failure may be associated with nonspecific symptoms, such as weight loss and weakness. Because the kidneys easily excrete creatinine with minimal tubular reabsorption, serum creatinine levels are directly related to the glomerular filtration rate (GFR).

Bilirubin, Serum

Total	0.3–1.0 mg/dL
Direct	0.1–0.3 mg/dL
Indirect	0.2–0.7 mg/dL

General Information

Bilirubin is the major product of hemoglobin breakdown and is excreted as a pigment in bile. The excretion of bilirubin depends on the normal production and destruction of RBCs and a functional hepatobiliary system, where bilirubin is conjugated and excreted. The direct bilirubin value increases with the obstruction of the flow of bile through the biliary system because this causes uptake of direct bilirubin into the circulation. Levodopa may cause false increases in bilirubin.

Uric Acid, Serum

Men	2.5–8.0 mg/dL
Women	1.5–6.0 mg/dL

General Information

Uric acid, the major end metabolite of dietary and endogenous purines, is excreted through the kidneys. Cell breakdown and catabolism of nucleic acids, excessive production and destruction of cells, and inability to excrete uric acid are causes of hyperuricemia. An increase in serum uric acid is found in various conditions, including gout, impaired renal function, congestive heart failure, hemolytic anemia, polycythemia, neoplasms, and psoriasis.

Serum uric acid levels greater than 8 mg/dL in men and greater than 6 mg/dL in women are often associated with symptoms of gout. Gout is an acute inflammation of a joint, commonly the metatarsophalangeal joint of the great toe, caused by uric acid crystal accumulation.

Causes of increased serum uric acid levels include:

- Loop diuretics
- Thiazides
- Starvation
- High-purine diet
- Stress
- Alcohol abuse
- Chemotherapy

Levodopa, acetaminophen, ascorbic acid, and phenacetin may cause false elevations in uric acid levels.

Liver Function Tests

Most liver function tests remain unchanged in elderly people. The alkaline phosphatase level is frequently elevated in older adults. Total alkaline phosphatase may increase owing to Paget's disease, bone fracture, trauma, or osteoporosis. For people taking tacrine (Cognex) for Alzheimer's disease, liver function tests are very important.

Alanine Aminotransferase (ALT) or Serum Glutamic-Pyruvic Transaminase (SGPT)

0–35 U/L

General Information
ALT, an enzyme necessary for tissue energy production, is present predominantly in the liver. It also is present in the kidney, heart, and skeletal muscles and is a relatively specific indicator of acute liver cell damage.

Elevated ALT levels are caused by:

- Liver disease
- Different medications
- Cholecystitis
- Intrahepatic cholestasis
- Pancreatitis
- Hepatic congestion owing to heart failure
- Acute myocardial infarction
- Trauma
- Lead ingestion
- Carbon tetrachloride exposure

Falsely elevated ALT levels are caused by the use of barbiturates and narcotic analgesics.

Aspartate Aminotransferase (AST) or Serum Glutamic-Oxaloacetic Transaminase (SGOT)

0–35 U/L

General Information
AST is an enzyme found in cells of the liver, heart, muscles, kidneys, pancreas, and RBCs. Serum levels are highest during acute cellular damage and decrease during tissue repair. The AST level is useful in monitoring the progress of myocardial infarction and acute liver disease.

Elevations are found in:

- Myocardial infarction
- Liver disease
- Extensive surgery
- Hemolytic anemia
- Pulmonary emboli
- Delirium tremens
- Diseases of the brain, muscle, pancreas, spleen, and lungs

Alkaline Phosphatase Level

30–140 IU/L

General Information
Alkaline phosphatase is an enzyme that is active in bone calcification and in lipid and metabolite transport. Serum alkaline phosphatase levels are sensitive to biliary obstruction by space-occupying hepatic lesions, such as tumors or abscesses, and to metabolic bone disease. Alkaline phosphatase isoenzymes may be identified to differentiate hepatic and skeletal diseases.

Increases in alkaline phosphatase are found in:

- Gallbladder disease associated with obstruction
- Paget's disease
- Bone metastasis
- Hyperparathyroidism
- Liver disease
- Osteomalacia

Lactic Dehydrogenase (LDH), Serum

60–100 U/mL

General Information
LDH is most useful in diagnosing myocardial infarction, but it is also elevated in hepatic disease, pulmonary infarction, and anemias. It is present in almost all body tissues. Five tissue-specific isoenzymes may be measured; of these, LDH4 and LDH5 are found in the liver and the skeletal muscles. Elevated LDH values are

diagnostic in hepatitis, active cirrhosis, and hepatic congestion.

● NUTRITIONAL INDICATORS

Elderly persons require and consume fewer total calories per day than younger adults. Carbohydrate intake may increase slightly (40% of total calories), whereas fat and protein intakes generally decline in older people. Lean body mass and total body protein decrease, whereas the percentage of body fat increases with age.

It is crucial that you, as an LPN, recognize that elderly persons are often at risk for malnutrition. This risk is due to decreased mobility; cognitive and sensory deficits; chewing and swallowing difficulties; and loss of appetite because of medications, illness, or the environment. The increased occurrence of wounds, infection, and dehydration creates additional nutritional demands on elderly persons; however, the most significant causes of poor nutrition in older people are poverty and chronic illness.

Because of these physiological and societal factors, it is important to have baseline laboratory values for the following indices of nutritional status and to understand their significance:

- Total serum proteins measure visceral protein stores.
- Serum albumin is the most widely used indicator of protein status.
- Serum transferrin is an indicator of protein stores.
- Serum cholesterol indicates lipid mass.
- Serum creatinine indicates lean body mass.

The hemoglobin, hematocrit, and lymphocyte count included in the CBC reflect the body's ability to transport nutrients and resist disease. Other common nutritional indicators are iron and micronutrients such as vitamins and minerals.

Nutritional deficiencies are often identified only when an associated problem, such as weight loss, poor wound healing, or weakness, occurs. Treating an underlying cause such as medication use or an illness may correct the deficiency. Otherwise, an increased dietary intake of the nutrient or vitamin and mineral supplements may be indicated.

FOCUSED LEARNING CHART

Elderly persons often are at risk for malnutrition. Possible reasons are:

Physical	Psychological	Environmental
Chronic illness*	Depression	Poverty*
Decreased mobility	Cognitive deficits	Inability to travel to grocery store
Sensory deficits		
Loss of appetite due to medications		
Chewing and swallowing difficulties		

The most significant causes of malnutrition in the elderly.

Protein Indicators

Total Serum Protein

5.5–8.0 g/dL

General Information

The major blood proteins are serum albumin and the globulins, which together equal the total serum protein value. The measurement of total protein is performed by protein electrophoresis and aids in the diagnosis of protein deficiency; blood dyscrasias; and hepatic, GI, renal, and neoplastic diseases.

1. Symptoms commonly seen with low serum protein values are:
   Dermatitis
   Hair thinning
   Muscle wasting
   Weakness
   Poor wound healing
2. Total protein values are increased with:
   Dehydration
   Diabetic acidosis
   Infections
   Multiple myeloma
   Monocytic leukemia
   Chronic alcoholism
   Chronic inflammatory disease
3. Common causes are:
   Edema
   Tissue breakdown
   Poor wound healing
4. Total protein values decrease with:
   Malnutrition
   Hepatic disease
   Renal disease
   GI disease
   Hodgkin's disease
   Trauma, such as burns, hemorrhage, and shock
   Hyperthyroidism
   Congestive heart failure

Albumin, Serum

3.5–5.5 g/dL

General Information

Albumin values of less than 3.5 g/dL indicate protein malnutrition and are accompanied by an increased incidence of morbidity and mortality. Albumin maintains oncotic pressure and transports substances such as bilirubin, fatty acids, hormones, and drugs that are insoluble in water.

1. Albumin is increased only in: Multiple myeloma

2. Albumin is decreased in:
   Malnutrition
   Liver and renal disease
   Collagen diseases
   Rheumatoid arthritis
   Metastatic carcinoma
   Hyperthyroidism
   Essential hypertension
   Use of cytotoxic agents

Globulins, Serum

2.0–3.0 g/dL

General Information

The four types of globulins identified by protein electrophoresis are found in differing quantities in various conditions. Alpha$_1$ globulin, alpha$_2$ globulin, and beta globulin are carrier proteins that transport lipids, hormones, and metals through the blood. Gamma globulin is an important component of the immune system.

Globulins are increased in:

- Tuberculosis
- Chronic syphilis
- Subacute bacterial endocarditis
- Myocardial infarction
- Multiple myeloma
- Collagen diseases
- Rheumatoid arthritis
- Diabetes mellitus
- Hodgkin's disease

Nursing Implications

Because a consistent relationship between protein intake and serum albumin levels has not been established, a high-protein diet is not advised except for individuals with evidence of protein calorie malnutrition. Protein allowance is the same for older people as for younger people: 0.8 g/kg body weight. Protein should provide at least 12% of total calories for the healthy older person. The proteins from animal sources such as beef, poultry, fish, and dairy products are the most complete, whereas complementary vegetable proteins have less biological value. Some older people may need nutritional supplementation through oral, enteral, or parenteral routes if malnutrition is severe.

Iron Indicators

Iron, Serum

Men	80–180 mg/dL
Women	60–160 mg/dL

General Information

Iron appears in the plasma bound to the glyco-protein transferrin. Iron is essential in the production and function of hemoglobin and other compounds. Dietary iron is absorbed by the intestine and distributed in the body for synthesis, storage, and transport. The body has no mechanism for eliminating excessive iron; total body and bone marrow iron stores increase with advancing age, although serum iron may be depleted. Serum iron values should be interpreted together with the total iron-binding capacity (TIBC) and serum ferritin. Bone marrow and liver biopsy and iron absorption or excretion studies may be necessary to obtain a definitive diagnosis in iron-related disease. A decrease in serum iron with an increased TIBC occurs in iron-deficiency anemia, which is most commonly caused in elderly persons by GI blood loss or malabsorption.

Ferritin, Serum

15–200 ng/mL

General Information

Ferritin is an iron-storage protein. Serum ferritin level indicates the amount of available iron stored in the body. It is measured to distinguish between iron deficiency (decreased ferritin level) and chronic infection or inflammation (increased or normal ferritin level).

1. Serum ferritin is increased in:
   Hepatic disease
   Iron overload
   Leukemia
   Hodgkin's disease
   Chronic renal disease
   Hemolytic anemias
   Acute or chronic infection and inflammation
2. Ferritin is decreased only in: Chronic iron deficiency

Total Iron-Binding Capacity (Transferrin), Serum

250–460 mg/dL

General Information

TIBC decreases with age and reflects the transferrin content of the serum. Transferrin, a beta globulin protein, transports circulating iron that is stored in various forms in the bone marrow, liver, and spleen. In protein-energy malnutrition, TIBC is less than 250 mg/dL (see previous discussion under serum iron).

Lipoproteins

Total Plasma Cholesterol

Desired	<200 mg/dL
Borderline	200–239 mg/dL
High	≥240 mg/dL

High-Density Lipoprotein (HDL) Cholesterol

Desired	>35 mg/dL

Low-Density Lipoprotein (LDL) Cholesterol

Desired	130 mg/dL
Borderline	130–159 mg/dL
High	160 mg/dL
Triglycerides	160 mg/dL

General Information

Blood lipid and lipoprotein cholesterol levels, which are influenced by heredity, diet, and obesity, are directly related to atherosclerotic heart disease in elderly people. Higher HDL cholesterol, lower LDL cholesterol, and a decreased level of plasma triglycerides all are associated with decreased incidence of coronary heart disease.

In women, the increase in plasma total cholesterol with age is due primarily to an increase in LDL cholesterol. HDL cholesterol increases slightly in men older than 65 years but decreases in women of the same age. Without intervening therapy, the risk for coronary heart disease in elderly people gradually increases.

Total cholesterol and HDL cholesterol should be measured in screening tests for the elderly population. The findings of a high initial cholesterol value should be followed by two subsequent evaluations because there may be significant daily variations in values. Older persons may have a total cholesterol of less than 200 to 240 mg/dL but have elevated LDL cholesterol and decreased HDL cholesterol and so have an increased risk of coronary heart disease. Conversely, if HDL cholesterol is high, accounting for a total cholesterol level greater than 200 mg/dL, there is a reduced risk for coronary heart disease. Total cholesterol and HDL cholesterol may be obtained from nonfasting blood samples. Triglyceride levels are accurate only after a 12-hour fast. LDL cholesterol levels may be calculated after total cholesterol, HDL cholesterol, and triglycerides are known.

Lipid abnormalities are often familial, but secondary causes are common in elderly people and include the following:

- Diets high in saturated fat or cholesterol
- Excessive alcohol intake
- Estrogen supplements
- Thiazide diuretics
- Beta blockers
- Smoking
- Uncontrolled diabetes
- Hypothyroidism
- Uremia
- Corticosteroid use
- Sedentary lifestyle
- Morbid obesity

Cholesterol levels less than 120 to 156 mg/dL have been associated with increased mortality in nursing home residents. Cholesterol is decreased in:

- Malnutrition
- Hyperthyroidism
- Chronic obstructive pulmonary disease

Nursing Implications for Lipid Abnormalities

- Weight control
- Increased physical activity
- Restriction of alcohol
- Cessation of smoking
- Restriction of dietary fat

Dietary restriction must be made cautiously because maintaining adequate calorie and protein intake is a major concern among elderly people. Drug therapy to control lipid levels may be beneficial in older persons with known coronary heart disease or high risk of disease.

DRUG MONITORING AND TOXICOLOGY

Drug monitoring is important when the margin of safety between therapeutic and toxic blood levels is narrow. Drug blood levels are useful guides in maintaining therapeutic levels and in identifying toxic levels of drugs. Not all drugs have a known therapeutic blood level even though toxic levels have been identified. Some drugs, such as amphetamines, are monitored through urine testing. Elderly persons metabolize and eliminate drugs more slowly than middle-aged adults, which heightens the importance of drug monitoring.

Three commonly monitored drugs—digoxin, theophylline, and phenytoin—are discussed because they require close observation by the LPN. Numerous classes of drugs are commonly checked for therapeutic or toxic levels. Review the list in Box 21.1. Refer to a basic laboratory manual for specific drug therapeutic and toxic values.

Digoxin (Lanoxin) Level, Serum

Therapeutic	0.5–20 ng/mL
Toxic	2.5 ng/mL

General Information

Digoxin, used in the treatment of congestive heart failure and cardiac arrhythmias, has a prolonged half-life in elderly patients because of its reduced renal clearance. Serum digoxin level has a narrow therapeutic range, and digitalis toxicity is relatively common in elderly persons despite the availability of tests for serum drug levels.

The most common side effects of digitalis toxicity are:

- Visual changes
- Headache
- Nausea and vomiting
- Weakness and fatigue

Weakness and fatigue are sometimes the only indicators of digitalis toxicity in elderly people.

Quinidine significantly increases the serum level of digoxin. Consequently, the digoxin dose must be reduced when both of these drugs are prescribed. Also, a change from tablet to elixir preparation of digoxin increases the absorption and serum level, so that the digoxin dose again needs to be reduced. Low serum potassium levels and high serum calcium levels increase the risk of serious arrhythmias in persons receiving digoxin therapy.

Nursing Implications for Digoxin Blood Levels

- Draw blood samples for determining serum digoxin levels at least 5 to 6 hours after the

BOX 21.1 **Commonly Monitored Drugs**

Alcohol	Nortriptyline (Pamelor, Aventyl)
Ethanol	Desipramine (Norpramin)
Isopropanol (rubbing alcohol)	Doxepin (Sinequan and others)
Methanol (antifreeze)	Imipramine (Tofranil)
Amphetamines (Urine Testing)	Lithium (Lithobid)
Amphetamine	**Barbiturates and Hypnotics**
Dextroamphetamine	Amobarbital (Amytal)
Methamphetamine (Desoxyn)	Glutethimide (Doriden)
Phenmetrazine (Preludin)	Pentobarbital (Nembutal)
Antiarrhythmics	Phenobarbital (Luminal)
Disopyramide (Norpace)	Secobarbital (Seconal)
Lidocaine (Xylocaine)	**Bronchodilators**
Procainamide (Pronestyl)	Aminophylline
Propranolol (Inderal)	Theophylline (Theo-Dur and others)
Quinidine (Quinaglute and others)	**Cardiac Glycosides**
Verapamil (Calan, Isoptin)	Digitoxin (Crystodigin)
Antibiotics	Digoxin (Lanoxin)
Amikacin (Amikin)	**Hemoglobin Derivatives**
Gentamicin (Garamycin)	Carboxyhemoglobin (Hg = CO)
Kanamycin (Kantrex)	Methemoglobin
Netilmicin (Netromycin)	Sulfhemoglobin
Tobramycin (Nebcin)	**Non-narcotic Analgesics**
Anticonvulsants	Acetaminophen (Tylenol and others)
Carbamazepine (Tegretol)	Salicylates (aspirin)
Ethosuximide (Zarontin)	**Phenothiazines**
Phenobarbital (Luminal)	Chlorpromazine (Thorazine)
Phenytoin (Dilantin)	Prochlorperazine (Compazine)
Primidone (Mysoline)	Thioridazine (Mellaril)
Antidepressants	Trifluoperazine (Stelazine)
Amitriptyline	

daily dose and preferably just before the next scheduled daily dose.

- Check the apical pulse for 1 full minute.
- Suspect digitalis toxicity when there is a sudden change in heart rhythm or pulse (especially a decrease).
- Withhold the medication and report to the physician when there is a sudden change in pulse or rhythm.
- Monitor the serum potassium level, especially if the person is taking diuretics.

Theophylline, Serum

Therapeutic	10–20 µg/mL
Toxic	20 µg/mL

General Information

Theophylline, a bronchodilator, may or may not be associated with improved respiratory effort on spirometry testing. Nevertheless, theophylline improves mucociliary clearance of the lungs and may improve myocardial contractility, stimulate respirations, and act as a mild diuretic.

Wide variations in the rate and extent of absorption and rate of metabolism for theophylline result in peak-to-trough fluctuations in serum concentrations and subsequent subtherapeutic or toxic responses.

1. Indications of possible toxicity include:
   Anorexia
   Abdominal discomfort

Nausea
Vomiting
Dizziness
Shakiness
Restlessness
Irritability
Palpitations
Tachycardia
Hypotension
Heart arrhythmias and seizures
2. Dizziness is a common side effect at the initiation of theophylline use in elderly people.
3. Elimination of the drug is reduced in persons with:
Heart failure
Kidney or liver dysfunction
Alcoholism
Fever
4. Smoking and phenytoin use increase the elimination of theophylline so that an increase in dosage is required. Macrolide antibiotics (e.g., erythromycin) as well as others may increase serum theophylline levels and cause toxicity.

Nursing Implications

- Regular monitoring of serum concentrations of theophylline is necessary to determine therapeutic dosage.
- The serum level must be checked when signs or symptoms of toxicity develop or when medications affecting serum levels are added or discontinued.

Phenytoin (Dilantin), Serum

Therapeutic	10–20 µg/mL
Toxic	30 µg/mL

General Information

Phenytoin, an anticonvulsant that also has antiarrhythmic properties, is metabolized by the liver and excreted in the bile and partially by the kidneys. Phenytoin has many potentially serious adverse reactions and side effects that necessitate monitoring of several parameters, including liver, kidney, thyroid, and hematological functioning.

1. Potential adverse reactions and side effects are:
Drowsiness
Mental confusion

Tremors
Bradycardia
Hypotension
Photophobia
Blurred vision
Nausea
Vomiting
Epigastric pain
Abnormal blood counts
Fever
Skin eruptions
Pneumonitis
2. Acute kidney or liver dysfunction results in toxic drug levels.
3. Decreased phenytoin serum levels may result from:
Chronic alcohol abuse
Antacids
Antihistamines
Antineoplastics
Barbiturates
Excess of folic acid
Rifampin
4. Increased serum levels may result from:
Acute intake of alcohol
Anticoagulants
Aminosalicylic acid
Benzodiazepines
Cimetidine
Dexamethasone
Estrogens
Isoniazid
Methylphenidate
Phenothiazines
Salicylates
Sulfonamides
Phenylbutazone

Nursing Implications

- Liver and thyroid function tests, blood counts, and urinalysis are recommended before the initiation of therapy, at monthly intervals during early therapy, and at regular intervals thereafter.
- Lower doses are given to older adults and individuals with liver or kidney impairment.
- When phenytoin is given intravenously, vital signs and cardiac function must be monitored closely.
- Serum concentrations of magnesium, folic acid, vitamin D, and vitamin K may be decreased with phenytoin therapy and should be monitored.
- Symptoms of low serum magnesium may mimic symptoms of phenytoin toxicity.

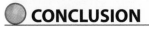

CONCLUSION

The use and interpretation of laboratory values are important in substantiating clinical judgment and providing comprehensive health assessment in elderly people. Physiological changes in older persons, presence of disease, use of medications, variance in diets, and exercise affect laboratory values. It is necessary to monitor changes in an individual's laboratory values and to compare an individual's values with values of other older adults in similar situations.

Understanding laboratory values in the elderly population is a continuing endeavor for all health-care practitioners. It is important to refer consistently to comprehensive laboratory manuals and individual laboratory reference intervals used in a particular locality and to specialized gerontological references. As new information becomes available, the interpretation of laboratory data will become more useful in determining care for older people.

Mr. K. is an 85-year-old resident of a small, independent group home where he has been caring for himself but sharing provided meals with the other residents. He underwent a transurethral resection of the prostate 4 years ago for benign prostatic hyperplasia. He has been treated for a heart irregularity and congestive heart failure in the past. Today he is being admitted to your intermediate care facility by his daughter because of several recent falls. Mr. K. reports that he has been nauseated and has not been eating well for the past few days. He also complains of wetting before reaching the restroom and blames this on his slow movement because of severe degenerative arthritis of his joints. Medications include the following:

- Furosemide (Lasix) 40 mg in the morning
- Digoxin 0.125 mg in the morning
- Ibuprofen (Motrin) 600 mg twice a day
- Acetaminophen (Tylenol) 500 mg every 4 hours as needed

On physical assessment, you find the following:
- Height 5 feet 10 inches
- Weight 135 lb
- Blood pressure sitting 120/70 mm Hg and pulse irregular at 80/min
- Blood pressure standing 90/60 mm Hg and pulse irregular at 90/min
- Respirations 20/min and unlabored
- Temperature 98.8°F (36°C)
- Lungs clear
- Skin warm and dry, with dry mucous membranes

Laboratory values available are:
- Potassium 3.2 mEq/L
- Sodium 132 mEq/L
- Chloride 106 mEq/L
- BUN 30 mg/dL
- Creatinine 1.4 mg/dL
- Glucose 130 mg/dL
- Urinalysis 3–5 WBCs, 0–3 RBCs, positive bacteria, specific gravity 1.022

Discussion

1. What problems have you identified based on the resident's history and physical assessment?
2. What other laboratory tests would be helpful?
3. What nursing actions should you take immediately?

Solutions

1. Underweight with risk of malnutrition
   Heart arrhythmia with possible orthostatic hypotension
   Probable urinary tract infection with urinary incontinence
   Anorexia and nausea possibly related to medications or urinary tract infection
   Recurrent falls with several possible causes, including weakness owing to decreased food and fluid intake, hypokalemia and hyponatremia, difficulty ambulating because of degenerative arthritis, orthostatic hypotension because of dehydration, and infection
2. CBC to assess for anemia and infection
   Digoxin level to check for toxicity as a cause of anorexia and nausea
   Urine culture and sensitivity to identify and quantify urine bacteria and determine antibiotic sensitivity
   Total protein to evaluate nutritional status
3. Safety measures to prevent falls, such as having Mr. K. call for assistance before getting up to go to the restroom. Advise him to change positions slowly from lying to sitting and then from sitting to standing. Consider a bedside commode because he has urinary incontinence and difficulty ambulating.
   Provide fluids and simple, easily digested foods in frequent small amounts.
   If nausea occurs, notify the physician.
   Withhold digoxin until the level value is obtained. Report to the physician.

Continued on page 384

Withhold the furosemide because Mr. K. is dehydrated and has hypokalemia and hyponatremia, probably as a result of the diuretic. Report to the physician.

Check any stools for occult blood because ibuprofen (an NSAID) is often the cause of GI bleeding. If the CBC indicates iron-deficiency anemia, the physician will probably discontinue this medication. Acetaminophen (Tylenol) may be used on a regular schedule to control arthritic pain.

Select the best answer to each question.

1. All laboratory test results for older adults should be:

    a. Evaluated against younger clients

    b. Evaluated against the other older adults on the unit

    c. Evaluated against the client's total clinical situation

    d. Evaluated against the person's CBC results

2. With the incidence of tuberculosis (TB) increasing among elderly people, it is critical for the LPN to know that:

    a. TB skin tests are inaccurate on people older than age 65

    b. When there is no initial reaction to the TB skin test in elderly people, it should be given again 1 week later

    c. It is unnecessary and expensive to do TB screening on nursing home residents

    d. Isoniazid is not an effective TB drug of choice for the elderly

3. The PT test is a measure of the overall coagulation factors. The risk of serious hemorrhage is high in the elderly person when:

    a. Warfarin is used

    b. Medication reviews on all medications are done

    c. PTs are drawn daily until the therapeutic dose is determined

    d. They are at risk for falls and subsequent bleeding

4. Potassium deficiency develops:

    a. Slowly in elderly persons

    b. In the kidneys

    c. Rapidly because there is no way to conserve potassium

    d. Only when using diuretics

5. Every elderly person with a low serum albumin level should be:

    a. Put on a high-protein diet

    b. Put on bedrest

    c. Put on a diet of 12% complete proteins

    d. Put on vitamin supplements

Unit Resources

The reader will note that some of the references in this section are older. They are used because they are "classic" references in that they are the original articles that defined the subjects discussed in them. I thought you would enjoy reading from the original work done on the topic.

UNIT ONE

AARP. (2007). *A profile of older americans.* Washington, DC: AARP.

American Heart Association. (2007). *American Heart association cook book* (7th ed.). New York, NY: American Heart Association.

American Hospital Association. (2008) http://www.aha.org/aha/issues/Communicating-With-Patients/py-care-partnership.html

Anderson, M. A. (2009). *Nursing leadership, management, and professional practice for the LVN/LPN* (5th ed.). Philadelphia, PA: F. A. Davis.

Behan, E. (2006). *Therapeutic nutrition: A guide to patient education.* New York, NY: Lippincott Williams & Wilkins.

Benner, P. (2001). *From novice to expert. Commemorative edition.* Upper Saddle River, NJ: Prentice Hall.

Bureau of National Health Statistics (2008). http://www.cdc.gov

Butler, R. M. (1969). Ageism: Another form of bigotry. *Gerontologist, 9,* 243–246.

Corrada, M. M., Kawas, C. H., Hillfisch, J., Muller, D., & Brookmeyer, R. (2005). Reduced risk of Alzheimer's disease with increased folate intake: The Baltimore longitudinal study. *Alzheimer & Dementia, 1,* 11–18.

Cruzan v. Director. Missouri Department of Health, 110 U.S. 2841 (1990).

Dossey, B. M., Keegan, L., & Guzzetta, C. E. (2005). *Holistic nursing* (4th ed.). Gaithersburg, MD: Aspen Publication.

Dudek, S. G. (2006). *Nutrition essentials for nursing practice.* New York, NY: Lippincott Williams & Wilkins.

Eliopolous, C. (2010). *Gerontological nursing* (7th ed.). Philadelphia, PA: J. B. Lippincott.

Engber, D. (2005). How does assisted suicide work? Slate.com/id/2/27629/#continue article

Erikson, E. H. (1963). *Childhood and society* (2nd ed.). New York, NY: Norton.

Goldsmith, T. (2008). http://www.azinet.com/aging

Hall, G., & Buckwalter, K. (1987). Progressively lowered stress threshold: A conceptual model for the care of adults with Alzheimer's disease. *Archives of Psychiatric Nursing, 1*(6), 399–406.

Health Care Financing Administration. (2005). Interpretative guidelines to OBRA. (No. 263-H). Washington, DC: U.S. Government Printing Office.

Insel, P., Turner, R. E., & Ross, D. (2006). *Discovering nutrition.* Sudbury, MA: Jones & Bartlett Publishers.

Kübler-Ross, E. (1969). *On death and dying.* New York, NY: McMillan.

Lichtenstein, A. H., Rasmussen, H., Yu, W. W., Epstein, S. R., & Russell, R. M. (2008). Modified MyPyramid for older adults. *Journal of Nutrition, 138,* 5–11.

Nightingale, F. (1946). *Notes on nursing, replica edition: What it is, and what it is not.* Philadelphia, PA: Lippincott-Raven Publishers.

Nix, S. (2005). *Williams' basic nutrition and diet therapy* (12th ed.). St. Louis, MO: Mosby.

O'Grady, T. (2001). The future of nursing. Presented at the National Gerontological Nursing Association Annual Convention, Washington, DC.

Ombudsman Reconciliation Act, '87. http://allhealth.org/BriefingMaterials/87summary.984.pdf

Random House College Dictionary (CD-ROM). (2008). http://www.randomhouse.com

St. Christopher's Hospice. (2001). http://www.stchristophers.org.uk/

Savage, C., & Money, K. (2005). The battle between caring and task oriented nursing. Paper presented at the Graduate Student Research Conference, University of Colorado, School of Nursing, Denver, CO.

Spector, R. E. (2004). *Cultural diversity in health and illness* (6th ed.). Upper Saddle River, NJ: Pearson/Prentice Hall.

Tabloski, P. A. (2006). *Principles of gerontological nursing.* (p. 13–21) Upper Saddle River, NJ: Prentice Hall.

Therrien, M., & Ramirez, R. R. (2001). The Hispanic population in the United States: March 2000. *Current Population Reports.* http://www.census.gov/prod/2001pubs/p20-535.pdf

Tornstam, L. (2005). *Gerotranscendence: A developmental theory of positive aging.* New York, NY: Springer Publishing.

U.S. Census Bureau. ACS Data Base (2008). http://factfinder.census.gov/home/saff/main.html?_lang=en

U.S. Department of Commerce. (2010). http://wwwanswers.com/topic/united-states-department-of-commerce

Watson, J. (1985). *Nursing: Human science and human care: A theory of nursing.* Norwalk, CT: Appleton-Century-Crofts.

Watson, J. (2000). Watson's Theory of Human Caring. http://www.nursing.ucdenver.edu/faculty/caring.htm

UNIT TWO

Bandler, R. (1985). Using your brain—for a CHANGE. In C. Andreas & S. Andreas (Eds.), *Neuro-linguistic programming*. Moab, UT: Real People Press.

CDC. (2006). Salmonella infection (salmonellosis) and animals. www.cdc.gov/healthypets/diseases/salmonellosis.htm

CDC. (2007). 2007 Guideline for isolation precautions: Preventing transmission of infectious agents in healthcare settings. http://www.cdc.gov/hicpac/2007IP/2007ip_part3.html

CDC. (2007). Infectious disease information: Cholera. http://www.cdc.gov/ncidod/diseases/submenus/sub_cholera.htm

CDC. (2007). Key facts about avian influenza (bird flu) and avian influenza A (H5N1) virus. http://www.cdc.gov/flu/avian/gen-info/facts.htm

CDC. (2008). Guidelines. www.cdc.gov

CDC. (2010). HIV/AIDS. http://www.cdc.gov/hiv/

CDC. (2010). Salmonella. http://www.cdc.gov/salmonella/

CDC. (2010). Tuberculosis. http://www.cdc.gov/tb/

CDC. (2010). West Nile Virus. http://www.cdc.gov/ncidod/dvbid/westnile/

Centers for Disease Control and Infection. (2010). *Recommended Adult Immunizations Schedule*. Washington, DC: U.S. Government Printing Office.

Fauci, A. S. (2008). *Harrison's Principles of Internal Medicine*. New York, NY: McGraw-Hill.

Feil, N. (1993). *Validation: The feil method*. Cleveland, OH: Edward Feil Productions.

Folstein, M. F., Folstein, S. E., & McHugh, P. R. (1975). Mini-mental status: A practice method for grading the cognitive state of patients for the clinician. *Journal of Psychiatric Research, 12*, 189.

Healthy People (2010). www.cdc.gov/ncdbbd/dh/hp2010.htm

Jacobs, J. W., Bernhard, M. R., Delgado, A., & Strain, J. J. (1977). Screening for organic mental syndromes in the medically ill. *Annals of Internal Medicine, 86*, 40.

Kahn, R., Goldfarb, A., Pollock, M., & Peck, A. (1960). Brief objective measures for the determination of mental status in the aged. *American Journal of Psychiatry, 117*, 326.

Kiernan, R. J., Mueller, J., Langston, J. W., & Vandyke, C. (1987). The neurocognitive status examination: A brief but differential approach to cognitive assessment. *Annals of Internal Medicine, 107*, 481.

Pfeiffer, E. (1975). A short portable mental status questionnaire for the assessment of organic brain deficit in elderly patients. *Journal of American Geriatrics Society, 23*, 433.

Sandhiya, S., & Adithan, C. (2008). Drug therapy in elderly. *Journal of the Association of Physicians of India, 56*, 525–531.

Touhy, T. A., & Jett, K. F. (2010). *Ebersole and Hess' gerontological nursing and healthy aging* (3rd ed.). St. Louis, MO: Mosby Elsevier.

U.S. Department of Agriculture and Human Services. (2006). My pyramid. www.mypyramid.gov

U.S. National Center for Health Statistics. (2004). Vital and health statistics. www.cdc.gov/chs/data/hus/tables/2004.

Venes, D. (Ed.). (2009). *Taber's Cyclopedic Medical Dictionary* (27th ed.). Philadelphia, PA: F. A. Davis Company.

Watson, J. (1988). *The science of human caring*. New York, NY: National Leagues of Nursing.

World Health Organization (WHO). (2010). Avian influenza. http://www.who.int/csr/disease/avian_influenza/en/

A Appendix

Sample Advance Directives: Living Will and Power of Attorney for Health Care

The following document is reproduced courtesy of Caring Connections, 1700 Diagonal Road, Suite 625, Alexandria, VA 22314. It is a sample for the state of California. To get a similar document for your state, please go to Caring Connection's Web site at www.caringinfo.org or call them at 800-658-8898.

Introduction to Your California Advance Directive

This packet contains a legal document, the California Advance Health Care Directive, that protects your right to refuse medical treatment you do not want, or to request treatment you do want, in the event you lose the ability to make decisions yourself.

1. Part 1, **Power of Attorney for Health Care,** lets you name someone to make decisions about your medical care—including decisions about life support—if you can no longer speak for yourself or immediately if you designate this on the document. The Power of Attorney for Health Care is especially useful because it appoints someone to speak for you any time you cannot or do not choose to make your own medical decisions, not only at the end of life.
2. Part 2, **Instruction for Health Care,** functions as your state's living will. It lets you state your wishes about medical care in the event that you can no longer speak for yourself.

   Although you have the option to complete only one part of this document, Caring Connections suggests that you complete Part 1 and Part 2 to best ensure that you receive the medical care you want when you can no longer speak for yourself.

3. Part 3, **Donation of Organs at Death,** is an optional section that allows you to record your wishes regarding organ donation.
4. Part 4, **Primary Physician,** is an optional section that allows you to designate your primary physician.

Note: This document will be legally binding only if the person completing it is a competent adult who is 18 years of age or older.

Introduction to Your California Advance Health Care Directive

How do I make my advance health care directive legal?

In order to make your Advance Health Care Directive legally binding you have two options:

1. Sign your document in the presence of two witnesses, who must also sign the document to show that they personally know you (or you provided convincing evidence of identity) and believe you to be of sound mind and under no duress, fraud, or undue influence.

Neither of your witnesses can be:

- the person you appointed as your agent,
- your health care provider, or an employee of your health care provider,
- the operator or employee of a community facility,
- the operator or employee of a residential care facility for the elderly.

In addition, only one of your witnesses may be:

- related to you by blood or marriage or adoption,
- entitled to any part of your estate either under your last will and testament or by operation of law.

OR

2. Sign your document in the presence of a notary public.

If you are a resident in a skilled nursing facility, one of the witnesses must be a patient advocate or ombudsman designated by the State Department of Aging.

Are there any important facts that I should know?

A copy of your California Advance Health Care Directive has the same effect as the original.

Completing Part 1: Power of Attorney for Health Care

Whom should I appoint as my agent?

A health care agent is the person you appoint to make decisions about your medical care if you become unable to make these decisions yourself. Your agent can be a family member or a close friend whom you trust to make serious decisions. The person you name as your agent should clearly understand your wishes and be willing to accept the responsibility of making medical decisions for you. The person you appoint as your agent **cannot be:**

1. your supervising health care provider or an employee of the health care institution where you are receiving care; or
2. an operator or employee of a community care facility or residential care facility at which you are receiving care.

Unless:

1. the employee is related to you by blood, marriage, adoption or is your registered domestic partner; or
2. the employee is your co-worker employed by the same health care institution, community care facility, or residential care facility for the elderly where you are a patient.

You can appoint a second and third person as your alternate agents. An alternate agent will step in if the person you name as agent is unable, unwilling, or unavailable to act for you.

Should I add personal instructions to my Power of Attorney?

You can use the space provided under paragraph (2) to limit your agent's authority. Unless the form you sign limits the authority of your agent, your agent may make almost all health care decisions for you, including:

a) consenting or refusing consent to any care, treatment, service, or procedure to maintain, diagnose, or otherwise affect a physical or mental condition;
b) selecting or discharging health care providers and institutions;
c) approving or disapproving diagnostic tests, surgical procedures, programs of medications, and orders not to resuscitate; and
d) directing the provision, withholding and withdrawal of artificial nutrition and hydration, and all other forms of health care.

Your agent is not authorized to consent to:

- commitment to or placement in a mental health treatment facility,
- convulsive treatment,
- psychosurgery,
- abortion,
- sterilization

One of the strongest reasons for naming a health care agent is to have someone who can respond flexibly as your medical condition changes and can deal with situations that you did not foresee.

We urge you to talk with your health care agent about your future medical care and describe what you consider to be an acceptable "quality of life." If you want to record your wishes about specific treatments or conditions, you can use Part 2 of this document, Instructions for Health Care.

What if I change my mind?

If you wish to cancel your Durable Power of Attorney for Health Care Decisions, you may do so by a signed writing or by personally notifying your supervising health care provider of your intent to revoke.

Are there any important facts I should know?

Paragraph (4) contains various statement about your agent's authority. Cross out and initial any portion of these statements that do not reflect your wishes. Paragraph (5) gives your the agent the authority to make anatomical gifts, authorize an autopsy, and direct the disposition of your remains after your death. Cross out and initial any portion of these statements that do not reflect your wishes. Paragraph (6) nominates your agent or alternate agents to be your court-appointed guardian should one become necessary. If this is not your intention, cross out and initial this section.

Completing Part 2: Instructions for Health Care

Can I add personal instructions to my Instructions for Health Care?

Yes. Paragraphs (7) and (8) allow you to include instructions about certain care and treatment. If there are any specific instructions that you would like to include that are not already listed on the document, you may list them in paragraph (9). For example, you may want to include a sentence such as, "I especially do not want cardiopulmonary resuscitation, a respirator, or antibiotics." If you have appointed an agent, it is a good idea to write a statement such as, "Any questions about how to interpret or when to apply my Instructions for Health Care are to be decided by my agent."

What if I change my mind?

You may cancel your Instructions for Health Care at any time and in any manner that communicates your intent to do so.

It is important to learn about the kinds of life-sustaining treatment you might receive. Consult your doctor or order the Caring Connections booklet, "Advance Directives and End-of-Life Decisions."

If you have questions about filling out your advance directive, please consult the list of state-based resources located in Appendix B.

You have filled out your Advance Directive, now what?

Your California Advance Health Care Directive is an important legal document. Keep the original signed document in a secure but accessible place. Do not put the original document in a safe deposit box or any other security box that would keep others from having access to it.

1. Give photocopies of the signed original to your agent and alternate agent(s), doctor(s), family, close friends, clergy, and anyone else who might become involved in your health care. If you enter a nursing home or hospital, have photocopies of your document placed in your medical records.
2. Be sure to talk to your agent and alternate agent(s), doctor(s), clergy, family, and friends about your wishes concerning medical treatment. Discuss your wishes with them often, particularly if your medical condition changes.
3. If you want to make changes to your document after it has been signed and witnessed, you should complete a new document.
4. Remember, you can always revoke one or both sections of your California Advance Health Care Directive.
5. Be aware that your California document will not be effective in the event of a medical emergency. Ambulance personnel are required to provide cardiopulmonary resuscitation (CPR) unless they are given a separate order that states otherwise. These orders, commonly called "non-hospital do-not-resuscitate orders," are designed for people whose poor health gives them little chance of benefiting from CPR. **Caring Connections does not distribute these forms.**

These orders must be signed by your physician and instruct ambulance personnel not to attempt CPR if your heart or breathing should stop. Currently not all states have laws authorizing non-hospital do-not-resuscitate orders. **Caring Connections does not distribute these forms.** We suggest you speak to your physician.

If you would like more information about this topic, contact Caring Connections or consult the Caring Connections booklet "Cardiopulmonary Resuscitation, Do-Not-Resuscitate Orders and End-Of-Life Decisions."

California Advance Health Care Directive—Page 1 of 8

Explanation

You have the right to give instructions about your own health care. You also have the right to name someone else to make health care decisions for you. This form lets you do either or both of these things. It also lets you express your wishes regarding donation of organs and the designation of your primary physician. If you use this form, you may complete or modify all or any part of it. You are free to use a different form.

Part 1 of this form is a power of attorney for health care. Part 1 lets you name another individual as agent to make health care decisions for you if you become incapable of making your own decisions or if you want someone else to make those decisions for you now even though you are still capable. You may name an alternate agent to act for you if your first choice is not willing, able, or reasonably available to make decisions for you. (Your agent may not be an operator or employee of a community care facility or a residential care facility where you are receiving care, or an employee of the health care institution where you are receiving care, unless your agent is related to you, is your registered domestic partner, or is a co-worker. Your supervising health care provider can never act as your agent.)

Unless the form you sign limits the authority of your agent, your agent may make all health care decisions for you. This form has a place for you to limit the authority of your agent. You need not limit the authority of your agent. if you wish to rely on your agent for all health care decisions that may have to be made. If you choose not to limit the authority of your agent, your agent will have the right to:

(a) Consent or refuse consent to any care, treatment, service, or procedure to maintain, diagnose, or otherwise affect a physical or mental condition;
(b) Select or discharge health care providers and institutions;
(c) Approve or disapprove diagnostic tests, surgical procedures, and programs of medication; and
(d) Direct the provision, withholding, or withdrawal of artificial nutrition and hydration and all other forms of health care, including cardiopulmonary resuscitation;
(e) Make anatomical gifts, authorize an autopsy, and direct the disposition of your remains.

Part 2 of this form lets you give specific instructions about any aspect of your health care, whether or not you appoint an agent. Choices are provided for you to express your wishes regarding the provision, withholding, or withdrawal of treatment to keep you alive, as well as the provision of pain relief. Space is provided for you to add to the choices you have made or for you to write out any additional wishes. If you are satisfied to allow your agent to determine what is best for you in making end-of-life decisions, you need not fill out part 2 of this form.

Part 3 of this form lets you express an intention to donate your bodily organs and tissues following your death.

Part 4 of this form lets you designate a physician to have primary responsibility for your health care. After completing this form, sign and date the form at the end. The form must be signed by two qualified witnesses or acknowledged before a notary public. Give a copy of the signed and completed form to your physician, to any other health care providers you may have, to any health care institution at which you are receiving care, and to any health care agents you have named. You should talk to the person you have named as agent to make sure that he or she understands your wishes and is willing to take the responsibility.

You have the right to revoke this advance health care directive or replace this form at any time.

Part 1: Power of Attorney for Health Care

<table>
<tr><td>

INSTRUCTIONS

PRINT THE NAME,
HOME ADDRESS,
AND HOME AND
WORK TELEPHONE
NUMBERS OF YOUR
PRIMARY AGENT

</td><td>

(1) DESIGNATION OF AGENT: I designate the following individual as my agent to make health care decisions for me:

(Name of individual you choose as agent)

(address) (city) (state) (zip code)

(home phone) (work phone)

</td></tr>
</table>

PRINT THE NAME, HOME ADDRESS, AND HOME AND WORK TELEPHONE NUMBERS OF YOUR FIRST ALTERNATE AGENT (OPTIONAL)

OPTIONAL: If I revoke my agent's authority or if my agent is not willing, able, or reasonably available to make a health care decision for me, I designate as my first alternate agent:

(Name of individual you choose as first alternate agent)

(address) (city) (state) (zip code)

(home phone) (work phone)

PRINT THE NAME, HOME ADDRESS, AND HOME AND WORK TELEPHONE NUMBERS OF YOUR SECOND ALTERNATE AGENT (OPTIONAL)

OPTIONAL: If I revoke the authority of my agent and first alternate agent or if neither is willing, able, or reasonably available to make a health care decision for me, I designate as my second alternate agent:

(Name of individual you choose as second alternate agent)

(address) (city) (state) (zip code)

(home phone) (work phone)

(2) AGENT'S AUTHORITY: My agent is authorized to make all health care decisions for me, including decisions to provide, withhold, or withdraw artificial nutrition and hydration, and all other forms of health care to keep me alive, except as I state here:

----

(3) WHEN AGENT'S AUTHORITY BECOMES EFFECTIVE: My agent's authority becomes effective when my primary physician determines that I am unable to make my own health care decisions unless I mark the following box. If I mark this box [ ], my agent's authority to make health care decisions for me takes effect immediately.

(4) AGENT'S OBLIGATION: My agent shall make health care decisions for me in accordance with this power of attorney for health care, any instructions I give in Part 2 of this form, and my other wishes to the extent known to my agent. To the extent my wishes are unknown, my agent shall make health care decisions for me in accordance with what my agent determines to be in my best interest. In determining my best interest, my agent shall consider my personal values to the extent known to my agent.

(5) AGENT'S POSTDEATH AUTHORITY: My agent is authorized to make anatomical gifts, authorize an autopsy, and direct disposition of my remains, except as I state here or in Part 3 of this form:

_____

_____

_____

(6) NOMINATION OF CONSERVATOR: If a conservator of my person needs to be appointed for me by a court, I nominate the agent designated in this form. If that agent is not willing, able, or reasonably available to act as conservator, I nominate the alternate agents whom I have named, in the order designated.

Part 2: Instructions for Health Care

INITIAL THE PARA-GRAPH THAT BEST REFLECTS YOUR WISHES REGARDING LIFE-SUPPORT MEASURES

If you fill out this part of the form, you may strike any wording you do not want.

(7) END-OF-LIFE DECISIONS: I direct that my health care providers and others involved in my care provide, withhold, or withdraw treatment in accordance with the choice I have marked below: **(Initial only one box)**

[ ] (a) **Choice NOT To Prolong Life**

I do not want my life to be prolonged if (1) I have an incurable and irreversible condition that will result in my death within a relatively short time, (2) I become unconscious and, to a reasonable degree of medical certainty, I will not regain consciousness, or (3) the likely risks and burdens of treatment would outweigh the expected benefits, OR

[ ] (b) **Choice To Prolong Life**

I want my life to be prolonged as long as possible within the limits of generally accepted health care standards.

ADDITIONAL INSTRUCTIONS (IF ANY)

(8) RELIEF FROM PAIN: Except as I state in the following space, I direct that treatment for alleviation of pain or discomfort should be provided at all times even if it hastens my death:

_____

_____

_____

(9) OTHER WISHES: (If you do not agree with any of the optional choices above and wish to write your own, or if you wish to add to the instructions you have given above, you may do so here.) I direct that:

Part 3: Donation of Organs at Death (Optional)

ORGAN DONATION
(OPTIONAL)

MARK THE BOX
THAT AGREES WITH
YOUR WISHES
ABOUT ORGAN
DONATION

(10) Upon my death: (mark applicable box)
[ ] (a) I give any needed organs, tissues, or parts,
OR
[ ] (b) I give the following organs, tissues, or parts only
[ ] (c) My gift is for the following purposes:
(strike any of the following you do not want)
(1) Transplant
(2) Therapy
(3) Research
(4) Education

Part 4: Primary Physician (Optional)

PRINT THE NAME,
ADDRESS, AND TELE-
PHONE NUMBER OF
YOUR PRIMARY
PHYSICIAN
(OPTIONAL)

(11) I designate the following physician as my primary physician:

(name of physician)

(address) (city) (state) (zip code)

(phone)

OPTIONAL: If the physician I have designated above is not willing, able, or reasonably available to act as my primary physician, I designate the following physician as my primary physician:

PRINT THE NAME,
ADDRESS, AND TELE-
PHONE NUMBER OF
YOUR ALTERNATE
PRIMARY PHYSICIAN
(OPTIONAL)

(name of physician)

(address) (city) (state) (zip code)

(phone)

© 2005 National
Hospice and Palliative
Care Organization
2006 Revised

SIGN AND DATE THE DOCUMENT AND THEN PRINT YOUR NAME AND ADDRESS

(12) EFFECT OF COPY: A copy of this form has the same effect as the original.

(13) SIGNATURE: Sign and date the form here:

_____   _____
(date)   (sign your name)

_____   _____
(address)   (print your name)

_____   _____
(city) (state)

WITNESSING PROCEDURE

(14) WITNESSES: This advance health care directive will not be valid for making health care decisions unless it is either:
  (1) signed by two (2) qualified adult witnesses who are personally known to you and who are present when you sign or acknowledge your signature; or
  (2) acknowledged before a notary public.

BOTH OF YOUR WITNESSES MUST AGREE WITH THIS STATEMENT

ALTERNATIVE NO. 1
STATEMENT OF WITNESSES
I declare under penalty of perjury under the laws of California (1) that the individual who signed or acknowledged this advance health care directive is personally known to me, or that the individual's identity was proven to me by convincing evidence, (2) that the individual signed or acknowledged this advance directive in my presence, (3) that the individual appears to be of sound mind and under no duress, fraud, or undue influence, (4) that I am not a person appointed as an agent by this advance directive, and (5) that I am not the individual's health care provider, an employee of the individual's health care provider, the operator of a community care facility, an employee of an operator of a community care facility, the operator of a residential care facility for the elderly, nor an employee of an operator of a residential care facility for the elderly, nor an employee of an operator of a residential care facility for the elderly.

HAVE YOUR WITNESSES SIGN AND DATE THE DOCUMENT AND THEN PRINT THEIR NAME AND ADDRESS

First Witness:

_____   _____
(date)   (signature of witness)

_____   _____
(address)   (printed name of witness)

_____   _____
(city) (state)

© 2005 National Hospice and Palliative Care Organization 2006 Revised

Second Witness:

_____   _____

(date)   (signature of witness)

_____   _____

(address)   (printed name of witness)

_____   _____

(city) (state)

ONE OF YOUR WITNESSES MUST ALSO AGREE WITH THIS STATEMENT

ADDITIONAL WITNESS STATEMENT

I further declare under penalty of perjury under the laws of California that I am not related to the individual executing this advance health care directive by blood, marriage, or adoption, and, to the best of my knowledge, I am not entitled to any part of the individual's estate upon his or her death under a will now existing or by operation of law.

_____   _____

(date)   (signature of witness)

_____   _____

(address)   (printed name of witness)

HAVE ONE OF YOUR WITNESSES ALSO SIGN AND DATE THIS SECTION AND PRINT THEIR NAME AND ADDRESS

_____   _____

(city) (state)

OR

A NOTARY PUBLIC SHOULD FILL OUT THIS SECTION OF YOUR DOCUMENT

ALTERNATIVE NO. 2: NOTARY PUBLIC

State of California   )
) SS.
County of _____   )

On _____ before me, _____

(insert name of notary public)

Personally appeared _____

(insert name of notary public)

personally known to me (or proved to me on the basis of satisfactory evidence) to be the person whose name is subscribed to the within instrument and acknowledged that he/she executed the same in his/her authorized capacity and that by his/her signature on the instrument the person upon behalf of which the person acted, executed the instrument. WITNESS my hand and official seal.

NOTARY SEAL _____

(signature of notary)

THIS SECTION IS TO BE COMPLETED ONLY IF YOU ARE A RESIDENT IN A SKILLED NURSING FACILITY

STATEMENT OF PATIENT ADVOCATE OR OMBUDSMAN

I declare under penalty of perjury under the laws of California that I am a patient advocate or ombudsman as designated by the State Department of Aging and that I am serving as witness as required by section 4675 of the Probate Code.

_____   _____

(date)   (signature)

_____   _____

(address)   (printed name)

_____   _____

(city) (state)

© 2005 National Hospice and Palliative Care Organization 2006 Revised

Courtesy of Caring Connections
1700 Diagonal Road, Suite 625, Alexandria, VA 22314
www.caringinfo.org, 800/658-8898

Index

Note: Page numbers followed by f refer to figures (illustrations); page numbers followed by t refer to tables.